Airway
Management
Paramedic

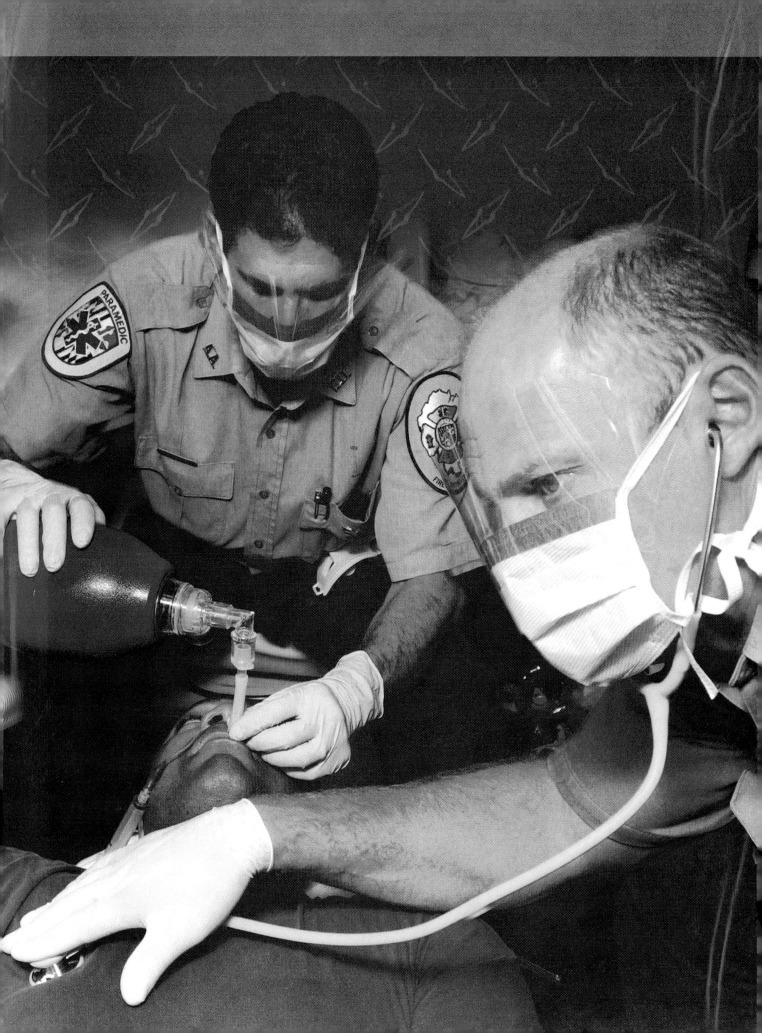

Airway Management
Paramedic

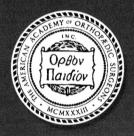

American Academy of Orthopaedic Surgeons

Gregg S. Margolis, MS, NREMT-P

Editor
Andrew N. Pollak, MD, EMT-P, FAAOS

JONES AND BARTLETT PUBLISHERS
Sudbury, Massachusetts
BOSTON   TORONTO   LONDON   SINGAPORE

Jones and Bartlett Publishers

World Headquarters
Jones and Bartlett Publishers
40 Tall Pine Drive
Sudbury, MA 01776
978-443-5000
info@jbpub.com
www.EMSzone.com

Jones and Bartlett Publishers Canada
2406 Nikanna Road
Mississauga, ON
Canada L5C 2W6

Jones and Bartlett Publishers International
Barb House, Barb Mews
London W6 7PA
United Kingdom

Production Credits
Chief Executive Officer: Clayton E. Jones
Chief Operating Officer: Donald W. Jones, Jr.
Executive V.P. and Publisher: Robert Holland
V.P., Sales and Marketing: William J. Kane
V.P., Production and Design: Anne Spencer
V.P., Manufacturing and Inventory Control: Therese Bräuer
Publisher, Public Safety: Kimberly Brophy
Associate Managing Editor: Jennifer Reed
Senior Production Editor: Linda S. DeBruyn
Production Editor: Scarlett L. Stoppa
Production Assistant: Carolyn Rogers
Director of Marketing: Alisha Weisman
Text and Cover Design: Studio Montage
Typesetting: Studio Montage
Printing and Binding: Courier Corporation
Cover Printer: Lehigh Press

American Academy of Orthopaedic Surgeons

Editorial Credits
Chief Education Officer: Mark W. Wieting
Director, Department of Publications: Marilyn L. Fox, PhD
Managing Editor: Lynne Roby Shindoll
Senior Editor: Barbara A. Scotese

Copyright © 2004 Jones and Bartlett Publishers, Inc.

Library of Congress Cataloging-in-Publication Data
Paramedic, airway management / American Academy of Orthopaedic Surgeons; editor, Gregg Margolis.-- 1st ed.
    p. ; cm.
Includes bibliographical references and index.
  ISBN 0-7637-1327-9
  1. Respiratory organs--Obstructions--Prevention. 2. Artificial respiration. 3. Trachea--Intubation. 4. Airway (Medicine)
  [DNLM: 1. Airway Obstruction--prevention & control--United States.
2. Emergency Medical Services--standards--United States. WF 140 P222 2004]
I. Margolis, Gregg S. II. American Academy of Orthopaedic Surgeons.
  RC87.9.P37 2004
  616.2'00425--dc22
                                                        2003015799
Additional Credits appear on page 331 which constitutes a continuation of the copyright page.

Printed in the United States of America
07 06 05 04 03   10 9 8 7 6 5 4 3 2 1

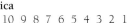

Brief Contents

Table of Contents

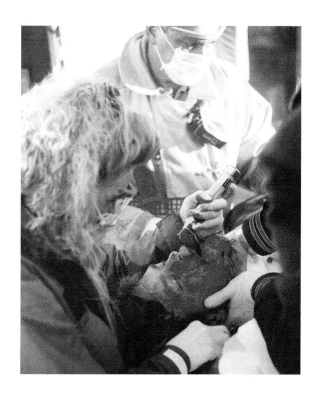

Chapter 4

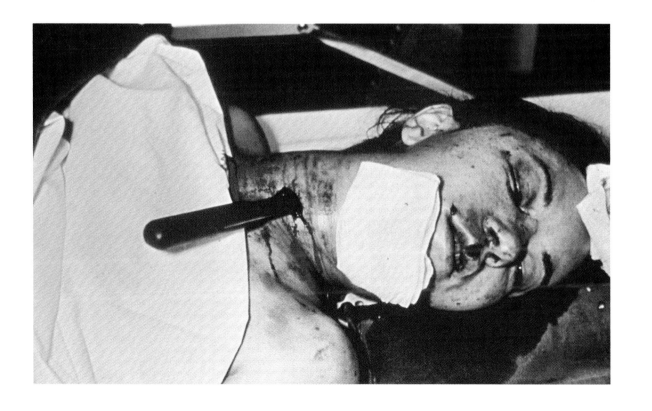

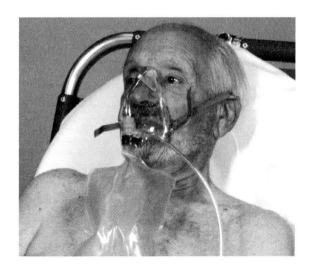

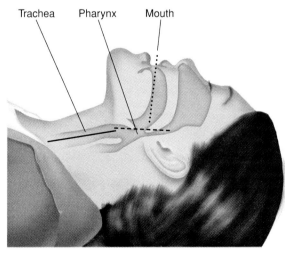

Trachea   Pharynx   Mouth

Table of Contents

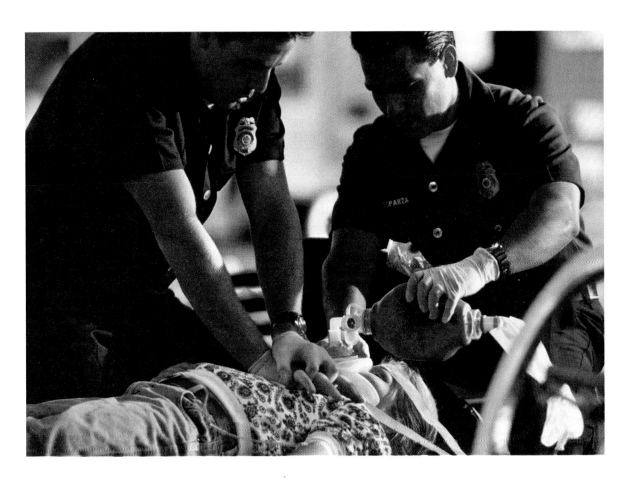

Chapter 7

Chapter 8

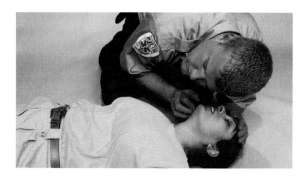

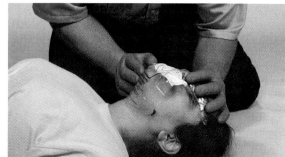

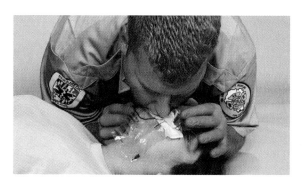

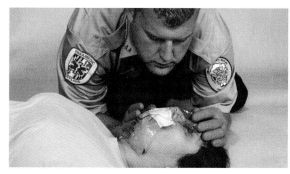

Chapter 9

Table of Contents

Chapter 10

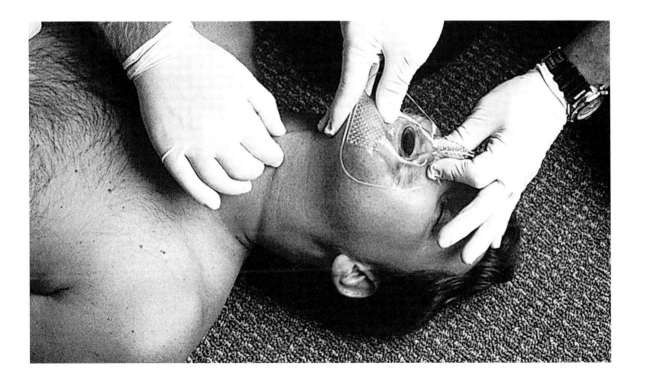

Chapter 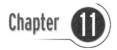 11

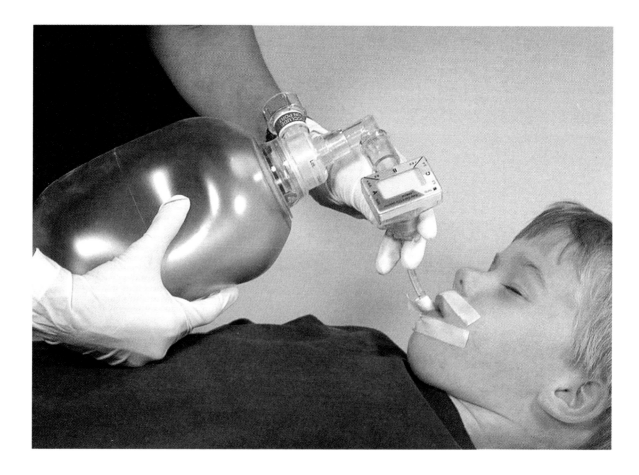

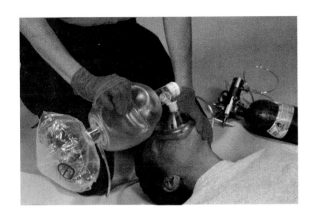

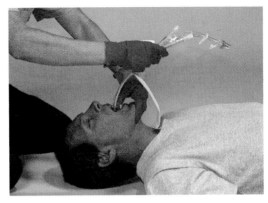

Chapter 12

Chapter 13

Table of Contents

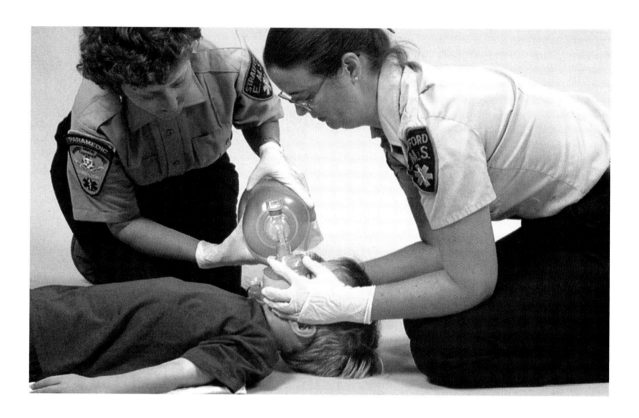

Chapter 14

Table of Contents

Chapter 15

Appendix

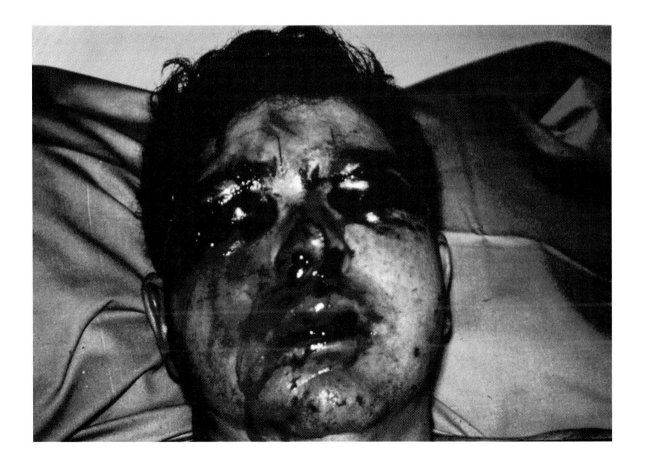

Chapter Resources

Paramedic: Airway Management is designed to give paramedic professionals the education and confidence they need to effectively treat patients in the field. Features that will reinforce and expand on essential information include:

Navigation Toolbar

Found at the beginning of each chapter, the navigation toolbar will guide students through the technology resources and text features available for that chapter.

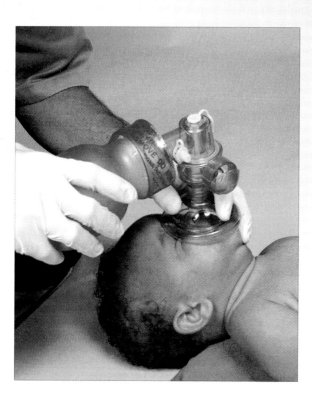

Evaluating Airway Patency and Ventilatory Efficiency 4

Objectives

Cognitive Objectives

2-1.6   Define gag reflex. (p 47)

2-1.9   Describe the measurement of oxygen in the blood. (p 65)

2-1.10   Describe the measurement of carbon dioxide in the blood. (p 66)

2-1.11   Describe peak expiratory flow (p 58)

2-1.12   List factors that cause decreased oxygen concentrations in the blood. (p 48)

2-1.13   List factors that increase and decrease carbon dioxide production in the body. (p 69)

2-1.20   List factors that affect respiratory rate and depth. (p 60)

2-1.22   Define pulsus paradoxus. (p 60)

2-1.23   Define and explain the implications of partial airway obstruction with good and poor air exchange (p 55)

2-1.24   Define complete airway obstruction. (p 51)

2-1.25   Describe causes of complete airway obstruction. (p 48)

2-1.26   Describe causes of respiratory distress. (p 60)

2-1.29   Describe complete airway obstruction maneuvers. (p 51)

Affective Objectives

2-1.77   Defend the need to oxygenate and ventilate a patient. (p 46)

2-1.78   Defend the necessity of establishing and/or maintaining patency of a patient's airway. (p 47)

Psychomotor Objectives

2-1.81   Perform pulse oximetry. (p 67) (Skill Drill 4-7)

2-1.83   Perform peak expiratory flow testing. (p 59) (Skill Drill 4-6)

2-1.87   Perform complete airway obstruction maneuvers, including:

- Heimlich maneuver (p 50) (Skill Drills 4-1, 4-2, and 4-4)
- Finger sweeps (p 50) (Skill Drills 4-1, 4-3, and 4-4)
- Chest thrusts (p 52) (Skill Drill 4-3)
- Removal with Magill forceps (p 56) (Skill Drill 4-5)

2-1.102   Perform retrieval of foreign bodies from the upper airway. (p 56) (Skill Drill 4-5)

www.Paramedic.EMSzone.com

Online Chapter Pretest

Vocabulary Explorer

Anatomy Review

Web Links

TECHNOLOGY

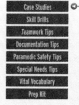

Case Studies

Skill Drills

Teamwork Tips

Documentation Tips

Paramedic Safety Tips

Special Needs Tips

Vital Vocabulary

Prep Kit

Chapter FEATURES

Skill Drills

Step-by-step explanations with a visual summary of key skills and procedures to enhance the student's comprehension.

Progressive Case Studies

Each chapter contains a progressive case study to make students start thinking about what they might do if they encountered a similar case in the field. The case study introduces patients and follows their progress from dispatch to delivery at the emergency department. The case becomes progressively more detailed as new material is presented. This feature, which includes additional diagnostic information, is a valuable learning tool that encourages critical thinking skills. Answers and rationales for the case study appear in the end of chapter Prep Kit.

Basic Airway Management Techniques   **Chapter 6**   105

Skill Drill
6-2 Head Tilt-Chin Lift Maneuver

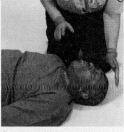
❶ Position yourself at the side of the patient.

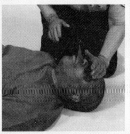
❷ Place your hand closest to the patient's head on the forehead.

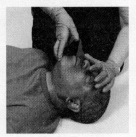
❸ With your other hand, place two fingers over the underside of the patient's chin.

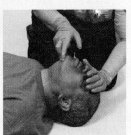
❹ Simultaneously apply backward and downward pressure to the patient's forehead and lift the jaw straight up. Be careful not to depress the submental triangle with your fingers, which causes the tongue to elevate, possibly pushing it against the roof of the mouth.

Positive Pressure Ventilation   **Chapter 7**   133

Case Study

Case Study Part 1

En route to a report of a "man down" you receive a report from the first responders on scene that "CPR is in progress." Your pulse quickens as you begin your mental checklist of equipment to bring onto the scene: paramedic bag, suction, medication kit, and monitor/defibrillator. You and your partner discuss role assignments; you jointly decide that you will manage the airway while she establishes an IV and operates the monitor.

Arriving at the scene, you can see the fire department first responders performing CPR on a middle-aged man lying on the sidewalk. The first responders report that a witness observed the patient stumble, sit down, and finally "pass out" as another bystander was dialing 9-1-1. Arriving on scene, the first responders found the patient pulseless and not breathing and began CPR. Using an AED, they delivered two shocks to the patient, with no return of spontaneous pulses, and continued CPR. It has been 3 minutes since they arrived on scene.

You quickly assess the patient's condition

Initial Assessment

Recording time:
0 minutes

Appearance
Cyanotic, with a pronounced distended abdomen

Level of consciousness
Unconscious, unresponsive to physical stimulus

Airway
Being managed by first responder

Breathing
Not breathing spontaneously

Circulation
No carotid pulse

As you set up your airway kit you observe something peculiar. It appears that the patient's stomach is growing larger with each ventilation!

Question 1: What is causing this to happen?

Question 2: How might this affect the patient?

Question 3: What can you do to change this situation?

the ventilation device. Small, disposable manometers are becoming common options on BVM devices. You should ventilate in a manner that keeps peak inspiratory pressure as low as possible, ideally below 15 cm of H_2O.

Unfortunately it is not always possible to keep the upper airway pressure below the esophageal opening pressure. In some conditions you must generate significant pressure to ventilate the patient. This is the case when the lungs are "stiff" (ie, have poor compliance), when there is high airway resistance (as occurs in bronchoconstriction), or when there is an airway obstruction. Large patients are another challenge. The larger the patient, the heavier the chest, and overcoming the weight of the chest with ventilation may require high pressures. All of these situations are true dilemmas. If you do not ventilate the patient with high enough pressure, you cannot effectively ventilate and hypoxemia will develop. As you ventilate the patient with sufficient pressure, the possibility of gastric distention increases.

Finally, the esophageal opening pressure is not a constant. Extensive research indicates that the esophageal opening pressure is generally between 15 to 25 cm H_2O in patients undergoing anesthesia. Unfortunately, the esophageal opening pressure has not been as extensively studied in emergency patients. While we do not know for certain, we must assume that alcohol, other drugs, food, and some diseases decrease the esophageal opening pressure. In cardiac arrest the esophageal opening pressure may fall as low as 0 to 5 cm H_2O. In such cases it is not possible to ventilate a patient who has not been intubated without exceeding the esophageal opening pressure.

Posterior Cricoid Pressure

Generally it is not possible to prevent all gastric distention, especially in cases of prolonged ventilation or cardiac arrest. An additional strategy is to apply posterior cricoid pressure to reduce the amount of

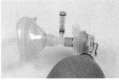
Manometer attached to a ventilation device.

air entering the stomach. The technique was first described by Sellick in 1961 and is often referred to as the **Sellick maneuver**.

The Sellick maneuver is based on the fact that the esophagus lies between the cricoid cartilage, which is a complete ring, and the cervical vertebrae (▶ **Skill Drill 7-1**). Pressure applied to the anterior portion of the ring is transmitted to the posterior portion of the ring without decreasing the internal diameter of the airway. Posterior cricoid pressure therefore partially occludes the esophagus by pinching it between two hard objects, the cricoid cartilage and the cervical vertebrae (▶ Figure 7-6).

Resource Preview

Documentation Tips

Provide advice on how to document patient care and highlight situations where documentation is crucial.

Special Needs Tips

Serve to highlight specific concerns for the elderly and/or pediatric patient.

Teamwork Tips

Provide voices of experience from masters of the trade (ie, experienced paramedics).

Supplemental Oxygen Therapy   **Chapter 5**   93

Special Needs Tip

Emergency situations can be frightening for all patients but especially for children. Most pediatric patients are uncomfortable with an oxygen delivery device on their face during times of high stress. If you believe the oxygen mask is significantly increasing the patient's anxiety, it may be better to remove the mask but continue to provide as much supplemental oxygen as possible through the use of an oxygen tent or hood.

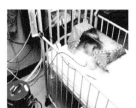

Figure 5-15 Oxygen tent or hood.

Patients with tracheostomies do not breathe through their mouth and nose. A face mask or nasal cannula therefore cannot be used to treat them. Masks designed specifically for these patients cover the tracheostomy hole and have a strap that goes around the neck. These masks are usually available in intensive care units, where many patients have tracheostomies, and may not be available in an emergency setting. If you do not have a tracheostomy mask, you can improvise by placing a face mask over the stoma. Even though the mask is shaped to fit the face, you can usually get an adequate fit over the patient's neck by adjusting the strap (Figure 5-14).

Delivery of Supplemental Oxygen to Pediatric Patients

The general principles of supplemental oxygen therapy apply to patients of all ages. To be effective, however, oxygen masks need to fit the patient. All of the

oxygen delivery devices discussed above are available in sizes for pediatric patients. It is important to have a variety of sizes immediately available.

Emergency situations can be frightening for all patients but especially for children. Most pediatric patients are uncomfortable with an oxygen delivery device on their face during times of high stress. If you believe the oxygen mask is significantly increasing the patient's anxiety, it may be better to remove the mask but continue to provide as much supplemental oxygen as possible. One possible alternative is an oxygen tent or hood (Figure 5-15). A hood covers the patient's entire head, and a tent is made of clear plastic to maintain an enriched oxygen atmosphere. The patient placed in a tent receives an increased FiO. Unfortunately, hoods and tents reduce access to the patient and often are not immediately available in emergency situations.

A quick alternative is to provide **blow-by oxygen**. Blow-by oxygen is administered by holding oxygen

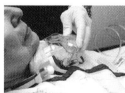

Figure 5-14 Using a face mask instead of a tracheostomy mask.

Teamwork Tip

Have you ever tried to administer oxygen to a critical patient only to find out that the tank was empty? This painful scenario is a reminder that someone needs to check the status of both the on-board and portable oxygen tanks at the beginning of each shift, as well as after the administration of oxygen.

Documentation Tip

There are two ways to express the amount of oxygen in the breathing gas. By a straight percentage or as a fraction of inspired oxygen (FiO.). FiO. is expressed as the decimal equivalent of the percentage of oxygen being delivered (ie, the FiO. of room air is 0.21; the FiO. of a nonrebreathing mask at 15 L/min is approximately 0.9)

Functional residual capacity is the amount of air left in your lungs after normal exhalation. Functional inspiratory capacity is the amount of air you inspire after normal exhalation. The vital capacity is the amount of air that you can forcefully exhale after a full inhalation—typically about 4,800 ml. The total lung capacity is the vital capacity plus the residual volume. Various respiratory and cardiac diseases affect the various lung volumes (Figure 3-5).

Oxygenation

Oxygenation is the process of assuring an adequate supply of oxygen molecules for delivery to the body's

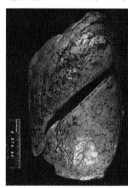

Figure 3-5 A diseased lung.

cells. Adequate oxygenation requires that the gas used for ventilation contains an adequate percentage of oxygen. The percentage and partial pressure of a given gas in a breathing mixture are important values. Understanding them requires an understanding of Dalton's law of partial pressure.

Dalton's law states that the total pressure of a gas is the sum of the partial pressure of the components of that gas. At sea level the total pressure of air is about 760 mm Hg. The major components of air are nitrogen (78.6%), oxygen (20.8%), carbon dioxide (0.3%), and water vapor (0.3%). The partial pressure of each of these gases is proportional to the relative percentage of each as shown in Table 3-4.

While you cannot oxygenate without ventilation, it is possible to ventilate without oxygenation. This occurs in places where oxygen levels in the breathing gas have been depleted, such as in mines and confined spaces. Ventilation without adequate oxygenation also occurs in climbers who ascend too quickly to an altitude of lower atmospheric pressure. At high altitude, the percentage of oxygen remains the same (20.8%), but the partial pressure decreases because the total pressure decreases. The low partial pressure of oxygen can make it difficult (or impossible) to adequately oxygenate tissues. Finally, oxygenation can be impeded when contaminants, in particular carbon monoxide, prevent oxygen from binding to hemoglobin.

Increasing the percentage of oxygen that the patient breathes is one strategy to increase the delivery of oxygen to the body's cells in times of respiratory or circulatory compromise.

Respiration

Respiration is the process of exchanging oxygen and carbon dioxide. This exchange occurs by a process of diffusion, in which a gas moves from an area of greater concentration to an area of lower concentration of the same gas. For example, diffusion occurs when you spray an air freshener in a room. The concentration of the air freshener vapor is very high near

Table 3-4
Partial Pressures of Gases in Air at Sea Level

Component	Percentage in Air	Partial Pressure
Nitrogen	78.6%	pN_2 = 597.36 mm Hg
Oxygen	20.8%	pO_2 = 158.08 mm Hg
Carbon dioxide	0.3%	pCO_2 = 22.8 mm Hg

Vital Vocabulary

Key terms are easily identified and defined. A comprehensive list follows each chapter.

Paramedic Safety Tips

Serve to reinforce safety concerns for both the paramedic and the patient.

Prep Kit

End of chapter resources reinforce important concepts with a chapter summary, comprehensive list of vital vocabulary, and case study answers and rationales.

The following are reduced-scale reproductions of textbook pages shown as examples:

Page 132 — Paramedic: Airway Management

or she can generally be adequately ventilated with 6 to 7 ml/kg because the endotracheal tube does not distend and there is less loss of gas volume than typically occurs with mask leakage.

Gastric Distention

Air drawn into the mouth and nose by negative pressure flows directly into the lungs. When air is forced under positive pressure into the mouth and nose, most of it goes into the lungs, but some of it may enter and become trapped in the stomach. The accumulation of air in the stomach leads to *gastric distention*. Gastric distention interferes with ventilation by pushing against the diaphragm and preventing complete lung expansion. Gastric distention causes a number of problems for airway management and ventilation and should be minimized as much as possible.

An understanding of how to prevent gastric distention is based on knowing why air accumulates in the stomach during artificial ventilation. The amount of air that goes into the stomach depends on the esophageal opening pressure and the pressure of the gas in the upper airway (▼ Figure 7-4).

The esophagus is a collapsible tube of tissue that is usually not open. The esophageal opening pressure is the amount of pressure required to force air though this flaccid tube. In unconscious patients, it takes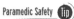

Paramedic Safety Tip

Recognize that gastric distention may lead to unexpected and often uncontrolled vomiting by the patient. If you are managing the airway be prepared for such incidents by wearing personal protective equipment such as protective eyewear and face shields.

overcome this difficulty, greater pressure is required, creating a vicious cycle of increased gastric distention. Although hypoventilation due to gastric distention is a potential problem in all patients, it is particularly problematic in pediatric patients.

In addition to decreasing the effectiveness of ventilation, gastric distention significantly increases the risk of vomiting. The stomach is a distensible organ but can hold only so much volume. As gastric distention increases, the intragastric pressure increases. Eventually this pressure will exceed the esophageal opening pressure, causing *passive regurgitation*. Any time a patient regurgitates stomach contents, the patient is at a serious risk for aspiration of vomitus into the lungs. Patients with a suppressed gag reflex are at an even greater risk. Aspiration of stomach contents into the

---

Pages 226–227 — Paramedic: Airway Management / Techniques of Endotracheal Intubation — Chapter 10

Prep Kit

Chapter Summary

Endotracheal tubes come in a variety of sizes and styles to accommodate varying airway presentations. Select a tube of the appropriate size to minimize chances of both mechanical trauma and barotrauma.

There are many techniques used to get a tube into the trachea. By far the most common in both emergency and elective situations is direct laryngoscopy. While this is the mainstay of advanced airway management by most paramedics, there are other techniques of intubation. Skilled paramedics are familiar with a number of alternative techniques that can provide advantages over direct laryngoscopy in some situations and with some patients.

The steps to oral intubation using direct laryngoscopy are as follows:

1. Check/prepare/assemble your equipment
2. Body substance isolation
3. Preoxygenate your patient
4. Position the patient
5. Insert the laryngoscope blade
6. Visualize the glottic opening
7. Pass the tube
8. Ventilate the patient
9. Confirm tube placement
10. Secure the tube

Each step is critical to the success of any intubation attempt.

The steps to a nasotracheal intubation attempt are similar to an oral intubation using direct laryngoscopy:

1. Check/prepare/assemble your equipment
2. Body substance isolation
3. Preoxygenate your patient
4. Position the patient in a supine, or semi-Fowler's position
5. Advance the tube to the glottic opening
6. Time insertion of the tube with the inspiratory effort of the patient
7. Ventilate the patient
8. Confirm tube placement
9. Secure the tube

Digital intubation can be used as an effective alternative to direct laryngoscopy. However, there is potential of being inadvertently bitten by the patient, so use this technique carefully!

As is the case with any alternative technique, transillumination of the upper airway during intubation can be effective under certain conditions. Practice with your equipment often in order to be comfortable with this (and any other) airway technique.

Vital Vocabulary

anode (armored) endotracheal tube A special type of endotracheal tube that has wire reinforcements built into the wall of the tube itself that prevents kinking of the tube. The tube is rarely used in the prehospital setting.

atlanto-occipital joint Joint formed at the articulation of the atlas of the vertebral column and the occipital bone of the skull.

BURP maneuver Acronym for **B**ackward, **U**pward, and **R**ightward **P**ressure.

digital intubation A blind technique of intubation in which you palpate and elevate the epiglottis with your middle finger while guiding the endotracheal tube into position by feel.

double-lumen endobronchial tube A specialty tube that is used when one lung must be isolated from the other. This tube is rarely used in the prehospital setting.

endotracheal intubation The technique of inserting an endotracheal tube through the vocal cords and into the trachea in order to maintain a patent airway.

endotracheal (ET) tube Tube that is placed into the trachea during intubation. The ET tube has a standard 15/22-mm fitting on its proximal end, which makes it compatible with any type of ventilatory device (such as a bag-valve-mask device or mechanical ventilator).

endotrol tube Tube made from a material that is more flexible than that of standard endotracheal tubes.

epiglottitis A bacterial infection of the epiglottis that results in laryngeal swelling and airway closure.

gastric insufflation Instillation of air into the stomach when the endotracheal tube is inadvertently placed into the esophagus instead of the trachea.

gum bougie A device that is placed in-between the vocal cords under direct laryngoscopy. The endotracheal tube is then advanced over the gum bougie and into the trachea. This device is useful when you are unable to obtain a full view of the glottic opening.

iatrogenic trauma Injury caused to the patient by the rescuer. In the case of intubation, this would include damaging the soft tissues of the mouth or breaking the patient's teeth.

laryngoscope An instrument used in conjunction with a straight or curved blade to give a direct view of the patient's vocal cords during endotracheal intubation.

malleable stylet Flexible wire that is placed into the endotracheal tube and makes the tube formfitting. This device facilitates maneuvering of the ET tube during intubation.

Murphy's eye The hole at the distal end of the endotracheal tube that enables ventilations to occur even if the tip becomes occluded by blood, mucus, or the tracheal wall.

nasotracheal intubation Intubation of the trachea via the nasopharynx.

pilot balloon Small pouch at the end of the inflation port on the endotracheal tube that indicates if the cuff is inflated or deflated once the distal end of the tube is inserted into the patient.

pulse oximeter Assessment tool that measures oxygen saturation of the blood through the capillary bed. The pulse oximeter reading is expressed as either the SpO₂ or SaO₂.

temporomandibular joint Joint that connects the mandible (lower jaw bone) to the temporal bone of the skull.

transilluminated intubation Technique in which a lighted stylet is used to illuminate the trachea and facilitate intubation.

Case Study Answers

Question 1: What are your main concerns about the patient's condition so far?

Answer: Managing this patient's airway quickly and decisively is critical. Besides the obvious signs of trauma and significant mechanism of injury, the blood coming out of the patient's mouth is of significant concern. Where is it coming from? Is the blood being aspirated by the patient? He clearly needs a definitive airway.

Question 2: What are your next immediate series of actions in the management of the patient's airway?

Answer: While maintaining manual cervical spine precautions, suctioning the airway is a critical first action step. If the airway can be cleared with suction, then basic ventilation procedures, followed by endotracheal intubation, can proceed. However, if the potential aspirate cannot be cleared adequately, intubation may have to occur much earlier, using techniques not involving direct laryngoscopy.

Question 3: What are some of your options in managing this patient's airway using endotracheal intubation? What are some of the drawbacks to each procedure?

Answer: Inserting an endotracheal tube in this particular patient with an unstable airway will require some quick decision making on your part.

Your options include:

A. Direct laryngoscopy–With the view of the glottic opening obscured by frank blood, it will be difficult to pass the tube through the vocal cords successfully. Additionally, as the patient exhales, blood may become aerosolized, splattering your face and eyes.

B. Nasal intubation–Although the patient is breathing, the presence of facial injuries and mechanism of injury may indicate the presence of a fractured cribriform plate, increasing the danger of brain injury if a nasal intubation procedure is selected.

C. Digital intubation–This may be a good option, although being bit by the patient is a potential drawback. However, in this case, the patient's level of consciousness appears to be appropriate for the use of the digital technique.

D. Transillumination–The potential drawback to this device is the level of ambient light that might obscure the view of the lighted stylet as it passes through the trachea.

www.Paramedic.EMSzone.com

CASE STUDY ANSWERS

Resource Preview

Instructor Resources

Instructor's ToolKit CD-ROM

ISBN: 0-7637-3126-9

Preparing for class is easy with the resources found on this CD-ROM, including:

- **PowerPoint Presentations** Providing you with a powerful way to make presentations that are educational and engaging to your students. The slides can be edited and modified to meet your needs.

- **Lecture Outlines** Providing you with complete ready-to-use lesson plans that outline all of the topics covered in the text. The lesson plans can be modified and customized to fit your needs.

- **Image Bank** Providing you with a selection of images found in the text. You can use them to incorporate more images into the PowerPoint presentation, make handouts, or enlarge a specific image for further discussion.

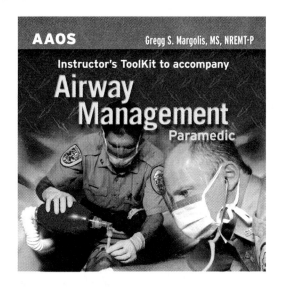

The resources on the Instructor's ToolKit CD-ROM that accompanies this text have been formatted so that instructors can seamlessly implement them into the most popular course administration tools. Please feel free to contact Jones and Bartlett technical support at any time with questions.

Technology Resources

- **Web Links** Present current information, including trends in paramedic care and new equipment.

- **Online Chapter Pretests** Prepare students for training with instant results and feedback on incorrect answers.

- **Vocabulary Explorer** Interactive online glossary to expand student's medical vocabulary.

- **Animated Flash Cards** Review vital vocabulary and key concepts.

- **Anatomy Review** Interactive anatomic figure labeling.

www.Paramedic.EMSzone.com

Acknowledgments

Contributors

Stephen J. Rahm, NREMT-P
Kendall County EMS Training Institute
Boerne, TX

Arthur B. Hsieh, BS, MA
Assistant Professor of Emergency Medicine
Emergency Health Services Program at
　George Washington University
Washington, DC

Reviewers

Vicki Bacidore, RN, MS
Loyola University Medical Center
Maywood, IL

Brenda Beasley
Calhoun Community College
Wedowee, AL

**Christopher Bell, BA, NREMT-P,
　CCEMT-P, FP-C**
Columbus State Community College
Columbus, OH

Gary Bonewald
Houston Community College
Houston, TX

Daniel Ellis, EMT-P
City of Chicago Fire Department
Chicago, IL

Chris Hobbs, AS, NREMT-P
Central Georgia Technical College
Macon, GA

Scott McConnell
Albert Einstein EMS Education Center
Philadelphia, PA

Frank Miller
Simply Critical Educators
Black River, NY

Bob Page, AAS, NREMT-P, CCEMT-P, I/C
St. John's Health System
Springfield, Missouri

Don Walsh, Ph.D., EMT-P
Emergency Medicine Researchers International
Chicago, IL

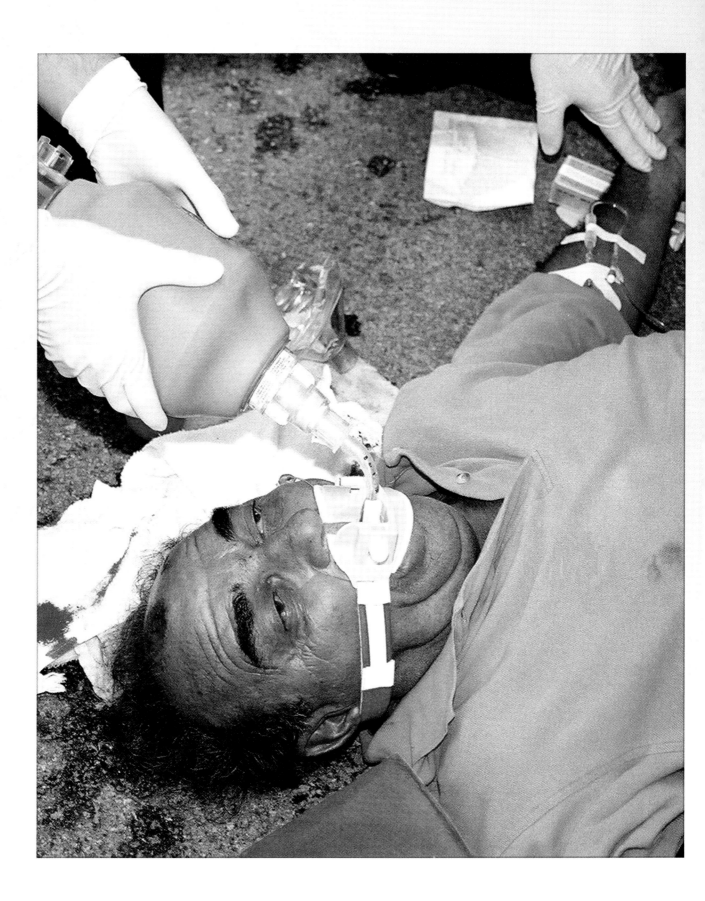

Introduction to Emergency Airway Management and Ventilation

Objectives

Cognitive Objectives

2-1.1 Explain the primary objective of airway maintenance. (p 4)

2-1.2 Identify commonly neglected prehospital skills related to airway. (p 4)

2-1.21 Explain the risk of infection to EMS providers associated with ventilation. (p 10)

Affective Objectives

2-1.77 Defend the need to oxygenate and ventilate a patient. (p 7)

2-1.78 Defend the necessity of establishing and/or maintaining patency of a patient's airway. (p 6)

2-1.79 Comply with standard precautions to defend against infectious and communicable diseases. (p 10)

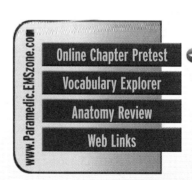

www.Paramedic.EMSzone.com

Online Chapter Pretest

Vocabulary Explorer

Anatomy Review

Web Links

TECHNOLOGY

Case Studies

Skill Drills

Teamwork Tips

Documentation Tips

Paramedic Safety Tips

Special Needs Tips

Vital Vocabulary

Prep Kit

Chapter FEATURES

You probably have heard that airway management and ventilation are the highest priorities in patient management. While this statement may seem like an oversimplification, few situations more rapidly cause disability and death than airway and breathing compromise. Maintaining the airway and ensuring breathing are almost always the very first considerations when treating emergency patients. The primary goal of airway management is to ensure a free and clear passageway for airflow. The primary goal of ventilation is to ensure a constant movement of air in and out of the lungs. These goals are not always easy to attain.

Despite the critical importance of airway management and ventilation, patients still die every day because of inadequate attention to or improper management of the airway and breathing. Many of these deaths are preventable. In some cases, EMTs become distracted and ignore these critical priorities. A more insidious situation arises when poor technique is misinterpreted as adequate, and the patient quietly deteriorates as cells die by the millions for every second of oxygen deprivation.

Airway management and ventilation involve time-sensitive interventions. Permanent brain damage begins when the brain is deprived of oxygen for more than 6 minutes. After 10 minutes, brain damage is often profound. Although research may find ways to increase this narrow time window, rapid and effective airway management and ventilation remain critical to patient survival and well-being.

To reduce the number of preventable deaths and disabilities resulting from airway and breathing difficulties, a number of different strategies are important. First, because many threats to the airway and breathing occur outside the hospital, even with rapid response, it is unlikely that EMS can get to the patient before some brain damage occurs. Therefore, the public must learn simple manual airway management and how to perform mouth-to-mouth ventilations. Second, all health care providers should understand the importance of early detection, rapid and effective intervention, and continual reassessment of airway and ventilatory threats.

Failure to correct airway or ventilation problems, resulting from either omission or poor technique, remains a major cause of morbidity and mortality in emergency medicine. This book addresses the management of the airway and breathing support in emergency situations and provides the knowledge and skills needed to prevent this problem.

Emergency Airway Management is Different

Every day, tens of thousands of people require airway management. The most common situation demanding diligent airway management occurs during surgery, when a patient is under general anesthesia. **Anesthesiologists** and **anesthetists** manage these patients. Most surgeries are planned and relatively predictable. Because anesthesiologists know the importance of airway management and ventilation, they take great care in making sure that as many variables as possible are controlled. Surgical patients have an extensive medical evaluation before undergoing anesthesia, do not eat or drink before surgery, are positioned on a table at an effective working height, and are in a well-lit and climatically controlled environment.

Although most of what we know about airway management comes from experience with anesthesia, airway management during surgery is fundamentally different from that in emergency situations. In an emergency, you rarely have the chance to assess or even question the patient before intervention is begun. All patients are assumed to have eaten recently. Often trauma is involved. Occasionally, patients are on the floor and not easily placed in an ideal position for treatment. Outside the hospital the environment is unpredictable, with variable lighting,

Teamwork Tip

The most important piece of "equipment" for airway management is your brain. The brain works best when it processes all of the information available to make a decision. So listen to your teammates! If you use your brain well, you and your team can solve almost any airway problem.

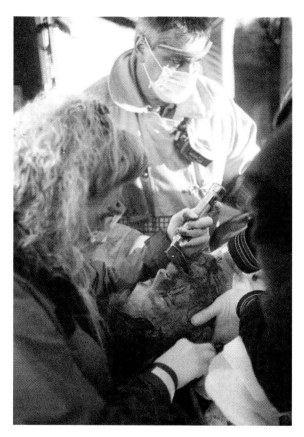

Figure 1-1 The paramedic must manage a patient's airway in less-than-ideal conditions.

Case Study

Case Study, Part 1

You have just told your partner that you have been accepted into paramedic school when your pagers go off. "BLS Seven, respond to a report of difficulty breathing, 676 Schoolhouse Road. ALS Three is responding from Middlesex Hospital." Your partner turns to you and says jokingly, "Well, Doctor, since it's your turn to attend, why don't you show me just how ALS is done!" He runs to the driver's seat while you get into the other side of the rig. You leave the ambulance bay with lights and siren on.

A few minutes later you arrive at a house set back from the road. Even from a distance you can see someone waving frantically from the front door. "Hurry!" she yells, as you pull the jump bag, oxygen kit, and AED out of the rig.

Question 1: As you begin walking toward the front door, what is your initial priority?

CASE STUDY

temperature, and noise levels. Finally, equipment and backup may not be present if a problem arises (▲ Figure 1-1).

In reality, EMT-Ps usually have less airway management and ventilation experience than do anesthesiologists and anesthetists, who manage airways every day. Most EMT-Ps encounter situations that require critical airway management and ventilation only a few times a month. In addition, local policy sometimes dictates that anesthesiologists perform all airway interventions, even in an emergency. This decreases the opportunity for those in other disciplines to maintain skill proficiency.

For all these reasons, airway management in emergency situations requires different techniques, approaches, and considerations than those used during surgery. Although EMT-Ps can learn from the expertise and experience of anesthesiologists, airway management and ventilation in emergencies present additional challenges (▼ Table 1-1).

Table 1-1
Differences Between Airway Management During Surgery and in the Field

Variable	During Surgery	In the Field
Frequency of managing airways	Many times a day	A few times a week or month
Patient assessment	Extensive medical assessment before anesthesia is given to identify potential problems	Rarely any history or physical available before intervention begins
Patient location	Waist height on an operating table	Can be anywhere
Stomach contents	Food and drink withheld for 12 hours	Assumed full
Planning and preparation	Planned	Unplanned

Technical Skills Versus Critical Thinking in Airway Management

Airway management and ventilation involve manipulative skills that require technical proficiency. However, airway management and ventilation also require a high degree of decision-making and thinking. Experienced EMT-Ps know that the decision *when* to intubate is much more difficult than *how* to intubate. The critical evaluation of the risks and benefits, and thoughtful decisions about the most appropriate technique to use, are much more difficult than simply being able to perform the skill.

Critical thinking

To develop the technical skills, you must practice, but that is only part of being a good EMT-P. Anyone can learn how to intubate a patient, but learning how to make the critical decisions about *why* to intubate, *when* to intubate, and *the best way* to intubate in a given situation, as well as evaluating whether the intubation is successful, are much more difficult. An EMT-P must have both good technical skill and clinical judgment to be effective. The combination of problem-solving skills with technical proficiency and experience will make your airway-management skills outstanding.

Definitions

The following sections define some of the terms that are used throughout this text.

Airway Management

The airway is the system of passageways through which air must travel to enable gas exchange. The airway includes all of the structures from the lips and the tip of the nose to the alveoli (▶ Figure 1-2).

Anything that interferes with the free passage of air in and out of the lungs is an immediate life threat because it affects the continual supply of oxygen to all body cells and the body's ability to get rid of carbon dioxide.

Airway management is the process of ensuring that the passageways remain open and free from obstruction, or **patent**. Obstructions can occur from either anatomic structures (such as the tongue or epiglottis), from objects or fluid in the airway (such as food, blood, vomit, saliva, broken teeth, or dentures), or from anatomic/pathologic abnormalities such as tumors or abscesses.

Managing an open airway includes ensuring that no anatomic structures occlude the airway and diligently assessing for and removing any foreign objects, fluids, or material. The airway is managed by a combination of patient positioning, manual techniques, removing foreign objects, and inserting

devices to minimize threats to the free and easy passage of air from the lips and nose all the way to the lungs. Effective airway management is necessary for ventilation to occur.

Ventilation

Ventilation is the process of moving air (or some other gas or combination of gases) in and out of the lungs. A patient who is not breathing is in **apnea**, or apneic. **Hypoventilation** indicates that not enough air is moving in and out of the lungs, possibly resulting from **bradypnea** (abnormally slow breathing), **hypopnea** (abnormally shallow breathing), or both. **Hyperventilation** indicates too much air is moving in and out of the lungs and can be the result of **tachypnea** (breathing too quickly), or **hyperpnea** (breathing too deeply), or both.

Normally ventilation is accomplished by the regular contraction and relaxation of the diaphragm and intercostal muscles in a process known as negative pressure ventilation. In this process air is pulled into the lungs. If a patient is apneic or hypoventilating, artificial ventilation is needed to increase the rate or depth of breathing, or both. All forms of artificial

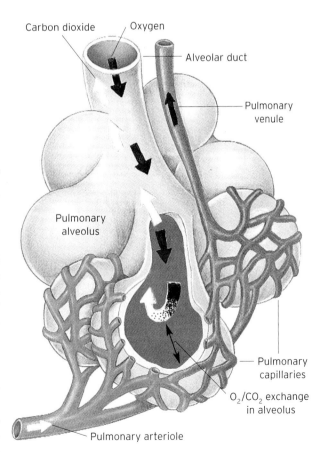

Figure 1-2 Illustration of the airway.

Special Needs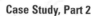

Today, older people are prescribed numerous medications to improve and prolong their lives. As with any other patient, you should inquire about any medications that the patient may be taking. Make certain that the patient is not having an allergic reaction.

Did You Know ?

Airway management and ventilation require a high degree of decision making and thinking. Experienced EMT-Ps know that the decision *when* to intubate is much more difficult than *how* to intubate.

Case Study

Case Study, Part 2

After establishing scene safety, you enter the dimly lit house. In the living room you see an elderly man sprawled out on the couch. Immediately you can see, even in poor lighting, that your patient is not doing well. Your initial assessment reveals the following findings:

Initial Assessment

Recording time
0 minutes

Appearance
His skin appears very pale, cyanotic (blue), and is diaphoretic (sweaty) to the touch.

Level of consciousness
You call out the patient's name. He moans slightly, but his eyes remain closed.

Airway
His chin is to his chest. You can hear loud, raspy noises as he breathes.

Breathing
His breathing is very slow, very irregular, almost gasping in nature.

Circulation
You can barely feel a radial pulse; the rate feels slow.

Question 2: How would you classify your patient's condition? What findings lead you to that conclusion?

Question 3: What is your treatment priority?

CASE STUDY

---

ventilation used in emergency situations use positive pressure ventilation. In this process, air is pushed into the lungs. Ventilation is necessary for oxygenation to occur.

Oxygenation

<u>Oxygenation</u> is the process of loading oxygen onto the hemoglobin and into the plasma for delivery to cells in the body. Every cell in the body requires a constant supply of oxygen for the effective conversion of glucose to energy. Any interruption in ventilation affects the influx of oxygen into the bloodstream and therefore threatens oxygenation. One of the strategies to increase oxygenation in cases of hypoventilation is to increase the percentage of inspired oxygen the patient is breathing. Oxygenation is required for respiration.

Respiration

<u>Respiration</u> is the process of exchanging oxygen and carbon dioxide. While oxygen is essential for the proper metabolism of glucose into energy, the removal of carbon dioxide is equally important.

Carbon dioxide is a waste product of the conversion of glucose into energy in the form of adenosine triphosphate. If carbon dioxide is not removed from the body through exhalation, it will accumulate and cause the blood to become acidic.

Respiration consists of external respiration and internal respiration. <u>External respiration</u> is the exchange of oxygen and carbon dioxide between the alveoli and the pulmonary circulatory system. <u>Internal respiration</u> is the exchange of oxygen and carbon dioxide between the systemic circulatory system and cells in the body. Internal respiration requires external respiration and movement through the circulatory system of blood from the lungs to the entire body. Internal respiration is the ultimate goal of airway management, ventilation, oxygenation, and external respiration.

It is important to remember that there must be a constant supply of oxygen and that carbon dioxide must be removed continually from each cell in the body. Unfortunately, many situations can threaten this chain of events. This text is primarily concerned with what EMT-Ps can do to ensure that external

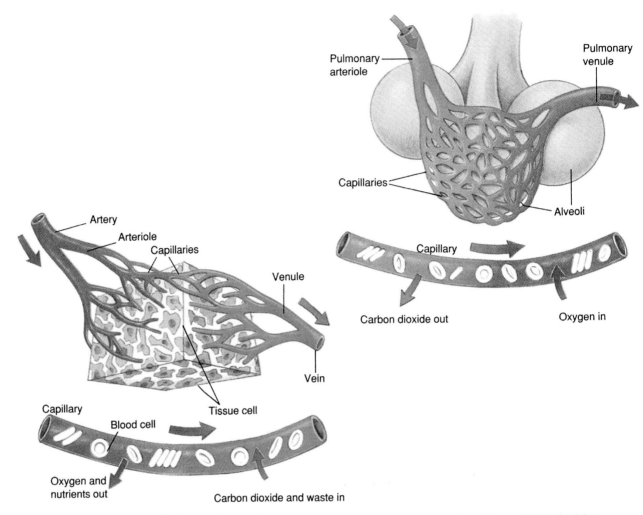

Figure 1-3 External respiration is the exchange of oxygen and carbon dioxide between the alveoli and the pulmonary circulatory system. Internal respiration is the exchange of oxygen and carbon dioxide between the systemic circulatory system and cells.

respiration occurs, with the hope that an intact circulatory system can deliver oxygen and remove carbon dioxide from the body. Remember that external respiration requires airway management, ventilation, and oxygenation (▲ Figure 1-3).

The Toolbox Concept

It may be useful to think of your airway management and ventilation skills as tools that make up a toolbox. You should carry and be proficient in the use of many tools so that you can perform different kinds of jobs. Having only one or two tools available would limit your ability to solve problems and consider alternatives when one technique does not work.

Often the most difficult decision is which tool to use. This text discusses the advantages, disadvantages, indications, contraindications, and complications of every technique. Your clinical judgment and problem-solving skills will be necessary to decide which tool is best suited for each situation. With experience you will find that it becomes easier to decide which tool to use. Even though you may use some tools more often than others, you need to carry and be able to use them all because you will never know which tool you will need and when you will need it.

Notes on Skill Practice

Most of the skills in this book are psychomotor skills, such as obtaining an airtight seal of the mask on the patient's face, ventilation, and intubation by a variety of techniques. Psychomotor skills require a cognitive knowledge base to be able to perform a series of discrete, coordinated, and precise actions. Driving, for example, requires you to learn rules, traffic laws, and basic physics. You studied this information and practiced the skills of driving. Although you probably could have learned to operate a vehicle without learning about traffic laws, you would not be a safe driver without that knowledge. The only way to fully develop and maintain psychomotor skills is through study *and* practice.

How Much Practice?

To become competent in your airway management skills, you need to practice them until you can do them easily and automatically without thinking about them—just as you drive a car. Studies have determined that it can take between 1,000 and 5,000 repetitions, depending on the skill complexity, to imprint the skill so that your muscles perform the tasks without thought. While this may seem repetitive, *the frequency matters.* You should plan on spending many hours practicing these skills until you can do them automatically.

Airway management and ventilation skills can degrade over time. The best EMT-Ps are not those who have the most years of experience or the highest education, but those who perform the skills the most frequently. If you do not perform these skills regularly, you must practice as often as is necessary to maintain your skill proficiency.

What Kind of Practice?

It is important to practice skills with perfection. Practice makes permanent, and the only way to develop perfect skills is to practice. It is tempting to take shortcuts and use sloppy technique during practice, perhaps telling yourself that you will correct your technique on a "real patient." Unfortunately, your muscles remember the way that you practice. You will likely take the same shortcuts and make the same mistakes when performing the skill on your patients. Therefore you need to commit yourself to *perfect practice.*

Excellent training manikins have been developed for practicing your skills. They are designed to simulate patients, with varying degrees of realism, and are a valuable training tool for learning airway skills.

The Advantages and Disadvantages of Practicing on Manikins

Training manikins are essential for learning airway management and ventilation skills, but there are drawbacks to their use. Although manikin designers and manufacturers have dramatically improved their product to improve realism, practicing on a manikin is still not like working on live tissue (▶ Figure 1-4). Table 1-2 summarizes the major advantages and disadvantages of practicing on manikins (▶ **Table 1-2**).

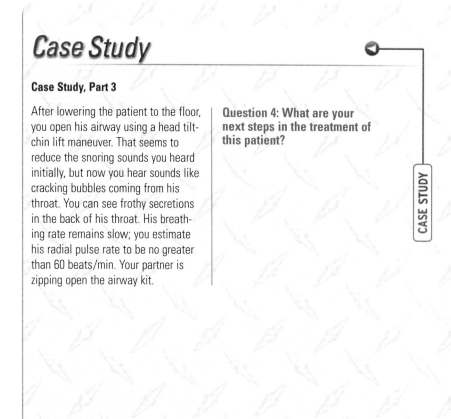

Case Study

Case Study, Part 3

After lowering the patient to the floor, you open his airway using a head tilt-chin lift maneuver. That seems to reduce the snoring sounds you heard initially, but now you hear sounds like cracking bubbles coming from his throat. You can see frothy secretions in the back of his throat. His breathing rate remains slow; you estimate his radial pulse rate to be no greater than 60 beats/min. Your partner is zipping open the airway kit.

Question 4: What are your next steps in the treatment of this patient?

CASE STUDY

The Advantages of Practice During Surgery

Manikins are effective for practice, but the only way you will become proficient in airway management and ventilation skills is by performing them on patients, such as patients under general anesthesia during surgery. Although managing airways and ventilating patients in emergency situations is different

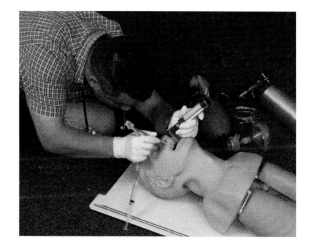

Figure 1-4 Practicing on manikins helps to prepare you to perform your airway skills on patients.

Table 1-2
The Advantages and Disadvantages of Practicing on Manikins

Advantages	Disadvantages
Skills can be perfected without jeopardizing patients	No anatomic variations; all manikins appear to be the same
No body secretions are encountered	Manikin tongues are plastic and easy to control, while patient tongues are not
Practice can be as frequent as necessary	Manikins are made of plastic and rubber for durability, which make them more forgiving of rough technique than a patient
Experimentation with other techniques is possible	Intubation of most manikins requires more strength than intubation of patients because the rubber is less resilient than human tissue

from surgery, you will learn a tremendous amount by practicing in a controlled environment under the supervision of anesthesia professionals. Keep the following in mind:

- Develop skills in a controlled setting with direct supervision and backup.

- Patients are much less likely to vomit because they have fasted before undergoing anesthesia.

- The hemodynamic and oxygenation status of the patient is known and closely monitored, allowing for longer periods to intubate.

- Secretions are typically reduced by medications.

- The patient is positioned at a good working level.

- The environment is climate-controlled and well lit.

The only disadvantage of practicing your airway skills during surgery is the possibility of developing habits that, although not detrimental in planned surgical cases, may present a problem in emergency situations, such as the time limits for intubation. During emergency treatment, ventilations are not interrupted for more than 30 seconds, but during surgery this is often done. Before patients undergo surgery, you know their medical history, laboratory values (specifically their hemoglobin and hematocrit), hemodynamic status, and oxygenation, or patients breathe 100% oxygen and have a significant oxygen reserve. These facts give you confidence that the information from patient monitoring devices is accurate. In emergency situations these variables are usually not known, and while many of the same

monitoring techniques are used, you should not have complete faith in their accuracy.

Paramedic Safety
Body Substance Isolation Precautions

In emergency situations it is impossible to have access to all of the information about a patient's medical history and the patient may have an infectious disease that could be passed on to you. For this reason, it is important to assume that all blood and body fluids are potentially infectious, and precautions should be consistently used for all patients. This approach, recommended by the Centers for Disease Control and Prevention, is referred to as "universal blood and body fluid precautions," or "universal precautions." This is also called body substance isolation.

Airway management and ventilation procedures often expose you to blood, vomit, and saliva. While blood is the most potentially infectious fluid, you should exercise great caution to avoid contact with all body fluids. You should wear gloves for all airway and ventilation procedures and when handling equipment that has been contaminated with body fluids. Because of the risk of splashing or droplets of body fluids coming in contact with your mouth, nose, and eyes, you should wear a mask and protective eyewear or face shields, especially when intubating. Masks with integrated face shields are fast and easy to put on and do not interfere with your performance. In cases with significant bleeding, such as in trauma, gowns or aprons also should be worn.

For cases with a lot of blood, consider wearing two pairs of gloves. Double gloving provides an extra layer of protection in the event that the outer glove rips, and also provides you with the ability to remove the outer glove to touch other equipment without contamination or exposing yourself.

You should thoroughly wash your hands immediately after you remove your gloves. Also be sure to wash any parts of your body that may have been exposed to body fluids. You also must thoroughly disinfect all equipment and surfaces exposed to mucous membranes or body fluids to prevent secondary transmission. Equipment can generally be cleaned with a chemical disinfectant that kills vegetative organisms, viruses, and bacteria.

The use of disposable equipment significantly decreases the need for cleaning supplies. Obviously, disposable equipment should be properly discarded after single patient use. Be sure to follow precautions when handling needles, scalpels, and other sharp instruments. Needles should never be recapped, purposely bent or broken by hand, removed from disposable syringes, or otherwise manipulated by hand. After they are used, disposable syringes and needles, scalpel blades, and other sharp items should be placed in the proper puncture-resistant receptacle. Plan ahead, and be sure to place a sharps container close to you before you begin the procedure.

Saliva has never been proven to transmit HIV. While the risk is low, saliva can transmit other diseases (including herpes simplex, meningitis, and tuberculosis). Most infectious diseases experts believe that the risk of contracting an infectious disease while performing mouth-to-mouth ventilations is low, but there should be no reason for you to take any such risk. You can virtually eliminate the need for emergency mouth-to-mouth ventilation by planning. Barrier devices and/or ventilation devices should be immediately available for use when the need for resuscitation is predictable.

Case Study

Case Study, Part 4

The wait for the paramedics to arrive seems to go on forever. However, your control of the patient's airway appears to be working, as you can see good chest rise and fall with each squeeze of your bag-valve-mask device. Your partner is able to establish the first set of vital signs:

Vital Signs

Recording time
4 minutes after patient contact

Skin signs
Remains pale

Pulse rate/quality
86 beats/min and regular

Blood pressure
170/96 mm Hg

Respiratory rate/depth
Assisted at 20 breaths/min

Pupils
Dilated, slow to react, equal

Soon you hear the siren of the hospital ALS unit as it arrives. Two paramedics come into the room, bringing their ALS equipment with them. You provide a concise, accurate report to one of them, describing how the patient presented and your interventions so far. They proceed to reassess his condition, paying particular attention to his airway and breathing status. In short order the patient is intubated, an IV of normal saline has been started, and a variety of medications administered.

As they load the patient into the ALS unit, one of the paramedics turns to you and says, "Great job! You really saved a life today." She shakes your hand and climbs into the ambulance. As the unit leaves, you silently thank yourself for having participated in the BLS airway drill at the station just a week ago. It certainly helped in this case!

CASE STUDY

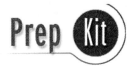

Chapter Summary

Airway management and ventilation skills are some of the most important and time-sensitive interventions in all of medicine.

By understanding how to maintain an airway and ventilate patients in emergency situations, you greatly increase your patient's chance of survival.

Airway management and ventilation skills take time and continual practice to perfect.

With practice, knowledge, and experience your airway management and ventilation skills will be excellent.

Time is critical to airway management and patient survival. Different strategies must be used to ensure a patient's airway is patent.

Ideal conditions for airway management do not exist in the field. This presents great challenges to the paramedic.

Technical expertise is not enough when it comes to managing a patient's airway. A paramedic must also have excellent critical thinking skills.

Anything that interferes with the free passage of air in and out of the lungs is an immediate life threat because it affects the continual supply of oxygen to all cells and the body's ability to release carbon dioxide. External respiration requires airway management, ventilation, and oxygenation.

Think of your airway management and ventilation skills as tools that make up a toolbox. You must be ready to use any or all of the tools in your toolbox at any time!

Practice makes perfect. You therefore must be certain that you practice your psychomotor skills with perfection. Practice the skills that you do not frequently use in the field—you never know when you will be called on to use them. When possible, practice your skills on patients in a controlled, supervised environment during surgery.

Vital Vocabulary

airway management The process of ensuring that airway passages remain open and free from obstruction of any kind.

anesthesiologist A physician who specializes in inducing, maintaining, and reversing anesthesia and the care of the anesthetized patient.

anesthetist A nurse who has received advanced specialty training in inducing, maintaining, and reversing anesthesia and in the care of the anesthetized patient.

apnea The absence of breathing. Apneic (adj).

bradypnea Abnormally slow breathing.

hyperpnea Excessive breathing.

hyperventilation A state in which too much air is moving in and out of the lungs.

hypopnea Abnormally shallow or insufficient breathing.

hypoventilation Breathing is too slow, shallow, or both.

oxygenation The process of loading oxygen onto the hemoglobin and into the plasma for delivery to body cells.

patent Open; the absence of obstruction.

respiration The process of exchanging oxygen and carbon dioxide.

respiration (external) The exchange of oxygen and carbon dioxide between the alveoli and the pulmonary circulatory system.

respiration (internal) The exchange of oxygen and carbon dioxide between the systemic circulatory system and body cells.

tachypnea Breathing too rapidly.

ventilation The process of moving air, or some other gas or combination of gases, in and out of the lungs.

Case Study Answers

Question 1: As you begin walking toward the front door, what is your initial priority?

Answer: Control of the scene and establishing scene safety for yourself, your partner, and your patient are your initial priorities in any situation!

Question 2: How would you classify your patient's condition? What findings lead you to that conclusion?

Answer: The patient's condition is classified as emergent. He is responsive only to verbal stimulus (V on the AVPU scale). His airway appears to be at least partially blocked, judging from the noises you hear, and his breathing rhythm and circulatory status are not within normal range.

Question 3: What is your treatment priority?

Answer: Establishing the patient's airway is your first priority. It will be difficult to perform any other treatments without ensuring a patent airway. In this case, you must try manually opening the airway using a head tilt-chin lift procedure with the patient in a supine position, probably on the floor.

Question 4: What are your next steps in the treatment of this patient?

Answer: You should attempt suctioning to try to clear the airway of the secretions. The patient, however, needs to be ventilated and oxygenated as soon as possible. This is a typical dilemma. Consistent, solid training coupled with accurate experiences will guide your treatment efforts with this patient and other patients in similar situations.

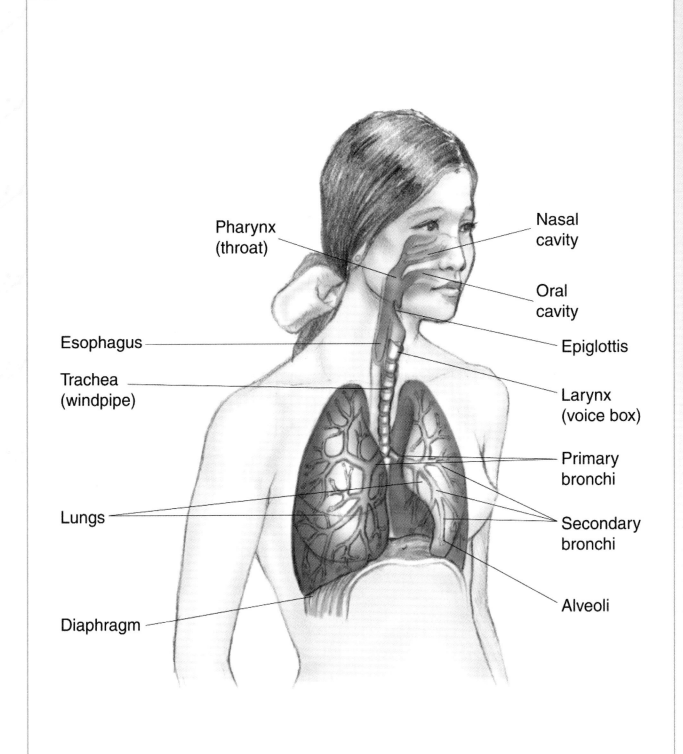

Pharynx
(throat)

Nasal
cavity

Oral
cavity

Epiglottis

Esophagus

Trachea
(windpipe)

Larynx
(voice box)

Primary
bronchi

Lungs

Secondary
bronchi

Diaphragm

Alveoli

Clinical Airway Anatomy

Chapter 2

Objectives

Cognitive Objectives

2-1.3 Identify the anatomy of the upper and lower airway. (p 16)

2-1.4 Describe the functions of the upper and lower airway. (p 16)

Chapter FEATURES / TECHNOLOGY

www.Paramedic.EMSzone.com

- Online Chapter Pretest
- Vocabulary Explorer
- Anatomy Review
- Web Links

- Case Studies
- Skill Drills
- Teamwork Tips
- Documentation Tips
- Paramedic Safety Tips
- Special Needs Tips
- Vital Vocabulary
- Prep Kit

A thorough knowledge of airway anatomy is critical for managing emergency patients. To perform airway interventions successfully, you must be able to identify and locate anatomic landmarks. You must also be able to locate all of the major anatomic landmarks in the upper airway when trauma has occurred, which may cause swelling, anatomic variations, and pathologic changes.

The <u>airway</u> is a conduit through which air flows between the external environment and the alveoli in the lungs, the functional level of gas exchange. These passageways must remain free from obstructions that could threaten the free and easy flow of air. These passageways vary in internal diameter and generally get smaller the further down the airway the air travels. In adults the trachea is about 2.5 cm in diameter, and the smallest bronchioles are less than 0.5 mm in diameter.

The airway is divided into the upper and lower airways. Although some disagreement exists about the dividing line between the upper and lower airways, this text will follow the convention that the <u>lower airway</u> includes the air passages below the vocal cords/glottis (▼ Figure 2-1).

The Upper Airway

The <u>upper airway</u> warms, humidifies, and filters air as it comes into the body. Air enters the body through the mouth and nose.

The Nose and Nasal Cavity

The nose and nasal cavity contain the major structures that provide the sense of smell, but they also serve the important function of warming, filtering, and humidifying the air that enters the body. The nose is composed of bone, cartilage, and fibrofatty tissue, with openings to the environment called nostrils, or <u>nares</u>. The nose, because of its position on the face, is often damaged by a direct blow to the face.

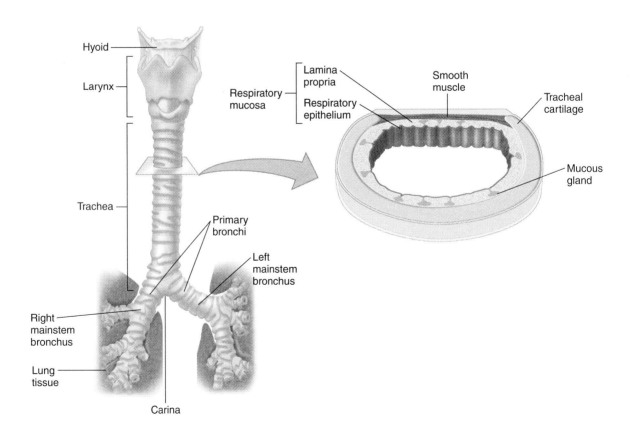

Figure 2-1 Illustration of the lower airway.

The entire nasal cavity is lined with a ciliated mucosal membrane. The mucosal membranes trap dust and small particles and prevent them from entering the respiratory system. Cilia help move contaminants out of the body. In illness, the body produces more mucus to trap potentially infectious agents. Mucus occasionally dries and encrusts the lining of the nasal passages. Some medications increase this drying effect. Dried mucus can interfere with airflow and must be removed if excessive.

Each side of the nose is divided into the floor, roof, lateral wall, and medial wall. The ethmoid and vomer bones form the medial wall, also known as the nasal septum. These bones are very thin and easily damaged. From the lateral walls, three bony shelves called turbinates extend into the nasal passageway. The turbinates serve to increase the surface area of the nasal mucosa, thereby improving warming and humidification. Along the lateral wall of the nasal passageway are numerous openings that extend into the frontal and maxillary sinuses. Because of their proximity to and direct communication with the nasal passage, the frontal and maxillary sinuses are referred to as the **paranasal sinuses** (▼ Figure 2-2).

The nasal passage and mouth are separated only by a thin piece of bone and soft tissue. The floor of the nasal cavity, which is the roof of the mouth, is oriented straight back from the nostrils. In sagittal section it can be seen that the nasal cavity is separated from the cranial vault by only thin plates of bone. In some cases of head injury, especially those involving fractures to the base of the skull, cerebrospinal fluid

Case Study

Case Study, Part 1

"Medic 14; please respond to 3586 Laurel Court for an elderly woman who is unconscious. Your time out is 12:15."

Four minutes later, you are at the scene of a home located in a well-to-do section of town. After you are led inside, you discover a woman who appears to be in her late 60s. She is sitting in a kitchen chair but slumped over the table with a partially eaten plate of food in front of her. She is unresponsive. A family member states that she passed out while eating lunch. Your initial assessment reveals the following findings:

Initial Assessment

Recording time
0 minutes

Appearance
She is slumped over in the kitchen chair, with a half-eaten plate of food in front of her.

Level of consciousness
She does not respond to verbal or physical stimulation.

Airway
You are able to bring her head into a neutral position.

Breathing
There is no air exchange, although she is making feeble attempts to breathe.

Circulation
Her skin is cyanotic. You can detect a weak, slow radial pulse.

Question 1: What is the first priority in her management?

CASE STUDY

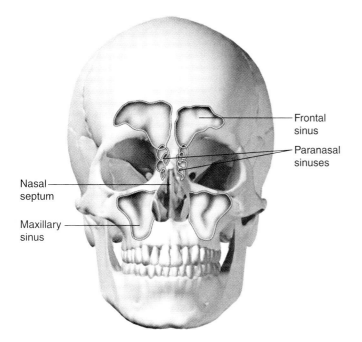

Figure 2-2 Illustration of the paranasal sinuses.

Frontal sinus
Paranasal sinuses
Nasal septum
Maxillary sinus

Did You Know

Keep the anatomy of the nasal passages in mind when you insert airway equipment into the nose. Insertion at an incorrect angle can damage the turbinates and cause extensive bleeding. Any insertion into the nose must be straight back, aiming for the ears (not the eyes), along the floor of the nasal cavity.

Be very careful when you insert airway devices into the nose of patients who have midface fractures or trauma. It is possible to enter the cranial vault from the nasal passages in cases of a cribriform plate fracture. The cribriform plate is essentially the floor of the cranium, which has jagged edges that can cause injury to the brain.

can leak into the nasal cavity. In addition, in such cases airway devices inserted into the nose could be passed directly into the brain.

The sinuses are pockets of tissue that are formed by the cranial bones and have a series of ducts that connect them to the airway. Bacteria tend to accumulate in the sinuses and cause infection. The bones forming the sinuses are very thin and fragile, and, if fractured, cerebrospinal fluid may leak through them and into the nasal passageways and ears.

The Oral Cavity

The mouth is divided into two parts, the vestibule and the <u>oral cavity</u> (▼ Figure 2-3). The vestibule consists of the space between the teeth and the lips and cheeks. The lips and cheeks are highly vascular structures lined with mucous membranes. Significant soft-tissue damage and bleeding therefore can result from a blow to the face or striking the face against an object or the ground. The patency of the airway may be seriously threatened in this situation, especially if the patient is unconscious or in a supine position.

The oral cavity is the anatomical space bordered by the teeth, gums, <u>palate</u>, tongue, and palatoglossal arch. The teeth, which are made of enamel, are the hardest structures in the body and are occasionally dislodged or broken by direct trauma. Dislodged or broken teeth can obstruct the airway.

The maxilla and palatine bones form the anterior three fourths of the roof of the mouth, which is

referred to as the <u>hard palate</u>. The posterior quarter of the palate is soft tissue. You may be able to feel the difference between your hard and <u>soft palate</u> by running your tongue across the roof of your mouth. Notice that towards the front of your mouth the roof is hard, but far in the back the roof becomes softer.

The tongue is a remarkably complex muscular structure. The tongue is covered by taste buds, which are the sense organs of taste. Very fine motor coordination is required for proper chewing and speech. The tongue is attached to the mandible and the <u>hyoid bone</u>—a small horseshoe-shaped bone to which the tongue, epiglottis, and thyroid cartilage are attached. Because the tongue lacks bony or cartilaginous structures to give it form, it is very floppy and can be a significant challenge to control in the patient with a decreased level of consciousness. When a patient with decreased sensorium is placed on his or her back, gravity causes the base of the tongue to come in contact with the back of the throat, potentially causing an obstruction to the airway.

The sensory nerves of the tongue carry taste and touch sensations to the brain through a number of major nerve bundles. The motor supply of the tongue comes from the hypoglossal nerve (cranial nerve XII), which lies superficially along the base of the tongue. This nerve can be permanently damaged by rough airway management.

The <u>palatoglossal arch</u>, the posterior border of the oral cavity, is an extension of the soft palate. The

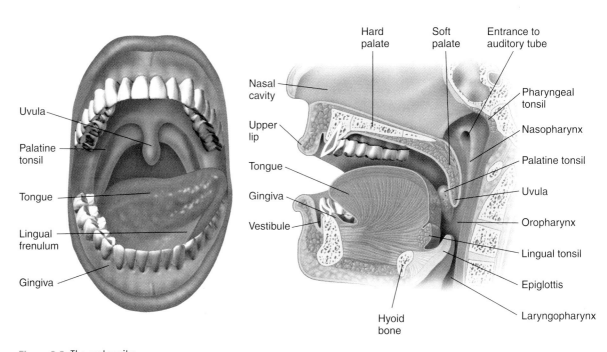

Figure 2-3 The oral cavity.

Documentation Tip

Completely assess and document the condition of the patient's mouth, lips, and teeth before and after all airway management procedures. Trauma to the teeth and soft tissues are common injuries caused by rough airway technique, but they may be present before you treat the patient. If a patient has damaged teeth or soft-tissue injuries before treatment begins, be sure it is documented.

uvula is the piece of soft tissue that looks like a punching bag extending into the archway. The **palatopharyngeal arch** is the entrance to the throat, or pharynx. The tonsils are masses of lymphatic tissue that help to fight infection. The **palatine tonsils** are paired structures that lie just behind the lateral walls of the palatoglossal arch, anterior to the palatopharyngeal arch. The palatine tonsils are often swollen in infections and are removed in a procedure called a tonsillectomy if they become chronically inflamed or problematic. The **pharyngeal tonsil**, also known as the **adenoid**, is located on the posterior nasopharyngeal wall. The **lingual tonsils** are at the base of the tongue (▶ Figure 2-4)

The Hyoid Bone

The hyoid bone is a small, horseshoe-shaped bone located between the chin and the mandibular angle. The jaw, tongue, epiglottis, and thyroid cartilage attach at this point. The muscles of the **submental triangle**, the block of tissue under the jaw, attach the hyoid bone to the jaw.

The Pharynx

The **pharynx** is the muscular tube that extends from the base of the skull to below the glottic opening (▶ Figure 2-5). It is divided into three regions. The most superior portion of the pharynx is the **nasopharynx**, the area directly behind the nasal cavity. The region directly behind the oral cavity is the **oropharynx**. Inferior to the oropharynx is the **laryngopharynx**, also called the **hypopharynx**. The posterior pharyngeal wall runs the entire length of the pharynx.

At the inferior portion of the pharynx are two potential passageways: the esophagus and the trachea. The esophagus is a muscular tube that is ordinarily collapsed. As food or liquid is swallowed, the tube expands and peristaltic contractions move the bolus into the gastrointestinal tract. The esophagus lies posterior to the airway, causing air and food to

Case Study

Case Study, Part 2

After moving the patient to the floor, your attempts to ventilate the patient with a BVM device and a good mask seal are unsuccessful, even with a satisfactory head tilt-chin lift procedure. Simultaneously your partner attempts to obtain a set of vital signs:

Vital Signs

Recording time
1 minute after patient contact

Skin signs
Cyanotic, diaphoretic

Pulse rate/quality
40 beats/min, faint at the radial aspect

Blood pressure
Not taken

Respiratory rate/depth
Agonal efforts at 4 breaths/min

Pupils
Dilated

SpO2
Does not register

Electrocardiogram
Not taken

Question 2: Considering the circumstances surrounding the incident, why have you been unsuccessful in establishing an airway?

Question 3: From an anatomic perspective, what can be done to relieve the problem?

CASE STUDY

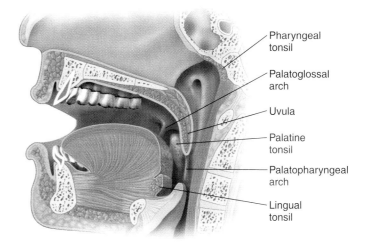

Figure 2-4 The tonsils.

- Pharyngeal tonsil
- Palatoglossal arch
- Uvula
- Palatine tonsil
- Palatopharyngeal arch
- Lingual tonsil

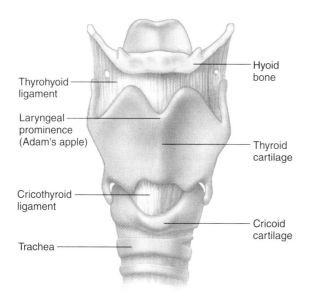

Figure 2-7 The larynx.

few nerves. It is bordered laterally and inferiorly by the very vascular thyroid gland.

The location and characteristics of the cricoid membrane make it useful for surgical and nonsurgical access to the airway, but because of its close proximity to the thyroid gland, carotid arteries, and jugular veins, it is very important that you locate the landmarks carefully.

The Trachea

The trachea begins immediately below the cricoid cartilage. The trachea is 10 to 12 cm long, composed of a series of C-shaped cartilaginous rings, and is the conduit for all the air that passes into the lungs. The shape of the tracheal rings enables food to pass down the esophagus easily during swallowing. The trachea is lined with ciliated mucous cells that secrete a sticky lining that traps small particles and other potential contaminants. A transected or crushed trachea is usually a lethal injury.

As the trachea extends into the chest, it splits into two major branches at the **carina**, the right and left mainstem **bronchi**. The carina is located approximately at the level of the sternal angle of Louis. Each of the mainstem bronchi is a conduit for all the airflow to its respective lung. Because the angle of the branch leading to the left lung is more acute than that for the right, airways or foreign objects are more commonly lodged in the right mainstem.

Lungs

The lungs consist of the entire mass of tissue that includes the smaller bronchi, bronchioles, and alveoli (▼ Figure 2-8). All of the blood vessels and the mainstem bronchi enter each lung at the hilum. The right lung has three lobes, and the left lung two lobes, each made of parenchymal tissue. The lungs are covered with a thin, slippery outer lining, known as visceral pleura, which enables the delicate tissue to move along the inside of the chest without damage. In total, the lungs

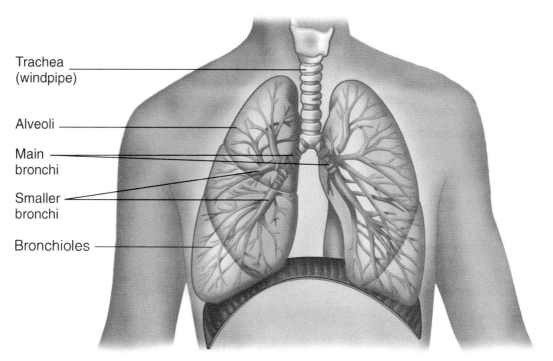

Figure 2-8 The trachea and the lungs.

Special Needs Tip

Patients who receive ventilation for a long time usually have a tracheotomy (surgical hole through the front of the neck into the trachea). A tracheotomy tube is generally placed through the surgical opening (stoma), providing the patient with an airway. Occlusion, obstruction, or accidental dislodgement of the tracheotomy tube is a serious emergency. You must be as vigilant in assessing the patency of a tracheotomy as you are in maintaining any other airway.

hold about 6 L of air. The parietal pleura lines the inside of the chest wall. There is a small amount of fluid between the two slippery tissue layers, which decreases friction during the respiratory cycle.

Bronchioles

After the trachea splits into the mainstem bronchi, it continues to branch into the secondary and tertiary bronchi, leading to the lobes of the lungs. The airway continues to divide into smaller and smaller branches. Initially these branches, like the trachea and bronchi, are made of cartilage. As they get smaller, the airways become softer and more pliable and are made of muscle rather than rigid cartilaginous tissue. These smaller branches of the airway are known as **bronchioles**. The bronchi branch as many as 22 to 26 times before they reach the terminal bronchioles.

The bronchioles, which are made of smooth muscle, can constrict to decrease their internal diameter. **Bronchoconstriction** is a defense mechanism to prevent the absorption of potentially harmful substances. Widespread bronchoconstriction, however, such as in asthma, can decrease airflow and become a life-threatening emergency.

Alveoli

Technically, the **alveoli** are not part of the airway itself, but rather, they are the termination of the airway. The alveoli are single-layered air sacs that are the functional site for the exchange of oxygen and carbon dioxide. This gas exchange occurs by simple diffusion between the alveoli and the capillaries of the pulmonary circulatory system. Alveoli function to increase the surface area of the lungs. As the alveoli are expanded during deep inhalation, they become even thinner, making diffusion easier.

The alveoli are lined with a proteinaceous substance known as **surfactant**, which decreases surface tension and helps keep the alveoli expanded. If the amount of surfactant is decreased, the alveoli collapse, which results in a condition known as **atelectasis**.

Case Study

Case Study, Part 4

Adjustments to your ventilation technique result in minimal abdomen rise. The chest appears to be rising fairly normally over the left side, and less so on the right. A rapid reassessment of the patient reveals that she is beginning to breathe spontaneously, although she remains unresponsive to physical stimulus. Her vital signs are noted as follows:

Vital Signs

Recording time
5 minutes after patient contact

Skin signs
Dusky extremities and face, returning color to trunk

Pulse rate/quality
80 beats/min, stronger than before

Blood pressure
80/50 mm Hg

Respiratory rate/depth
8 breaths/min, shallow

Pupils
Dilated, reactive

SpO$_2$
87%

Electrocardiogram
Sinus rhythm

Question 5: What are some of your concerns about both her short- and long-term recovery?

Case Study

Case Study, Part 5

Extrication and transport of the patient are uneventful. En route to the hospital the patient becomes conscious, although she remains confused. A physical exam reveals right-sided body weakness and reduced grip strength in the right hand. Slurred speech is also noted. At the time of patient transfer at the emergency department her vital signs are as follows:

Vital Signs

Recording time
10 minutes after patient contact

Skin signs
Pale, dry

Pulse rate/quality
100 beats/min, regular and strong

Blood pressure
156/86 mm Hg

Respiratory rate/depth
Assisted at 12 breaths/minute; spontaneous respirations at 8 breaths/min

Pupils
Equal, reactive

SpO$_2$
95% on 100% oxygen

Electrocardiogram
Sinus rhythm

Follow up at the hospital revealed the patient had probably experienced an acute stroke while she was eating lunch.

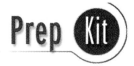

Chapter Summary

As in the rest of the human body, airway anatomic structures are complex, with each piece seemingly "designed" for a specific purpose.

The overall interaction of these structures results in a highly effective and efficient process of conducting airflow from the outside atmosphere to the internal sites within the body where gas exchange occurs.

On occasion this airflow is interrupted by disease, sudden illness, or injury.

Due to the potentially catastrophic outcomes, these problems will require the EMT-P to evaluate, analyze, and manage them quickly and accurately.

Air from the atmosphere flows through a series of airway structures in order to reach the lower portions of the respiratory tract for gas exchange.

Your solid comprehension of the different anatomic structures of the upper airway and their relationships to each other will lead to better management of emergencies that occur in this crucial region of the body.

The lower airway consists of structures that continue airflow from the upper airway. Airflow terminates in the alveoli where gas exchange within the body occurs.

Vital Vocabulary

adenoid The pharyngeal tonsil.

airway The conduit through which all air flows between the external environment and the functional level of gas exchange in the lungs.

airway, lower The portion of the airway below the glottic opening.

airway, upper The portion of the airway above the glottic opening.

alveoli Single-layered air sacs that are the functional site of the exchange of oxygen and carbon dioxide.

arytenoids Cartilaginous structures that articulate with the corniculate and cuneiform and make up the posterior attachment of the vocal cords.

atelectasis A condition of airless or collapsed alveoli that causes pulmonary shunting, ventilation-perfusion mismatching, and possibly hypoxemia.

bronchi The main branches of the airway that conduct air to and from each lung.

bronchioles Small airways made of smooth muscle that lead to the alveoli.

bronchoconstriction Constriction of the smooth muscle in the bronchioles, resulting in decreased airway diameter.

carina The point where the trachea bifurcates into the right and left mainstem bronchi.

cricoid cartilage The signet ring-shaped cartilaginous structure between the thyroid cartilage and the trachea.

cricothyroid membrane The thin membrane between the cricoid cartilage and the thyroid cartilage.

epiglottis The leaf-shaped flap located between the base of the tongue and the glottic opening, which prevents food and liquid from entering the lower airway.

glossoepiglottic ligament The ligament between the tongue and the epiglottis.

glottis The opening into the airway between the vocal cords, also known as the glottic opening.

hyoid bone The small horseshoe-shaped bone to which major upper airway structures are attached.

hypoepiglottic ligament The ligament between the hyoid bone and the epiglottis.

hypopharynx The inferior-most region of the pharynx located behind the larynx, also known as the laryngopharynx.

laryngeal prominence The Adam's apple, formed by the thyroid cartilage.

laryngopharynx The inferior-most region of the pharynx located behind the larynx, also known as the hypopharynx.

laryngospasm Spasmodic closure of the vocal cords.

larynx A complex structure formed by the epiglottis, thyroid cartilage, the cricoid cartilage, the arytenoid cartilage, the corniculate cartilage, and the cuneiform cartilage.

lingual tonsils Paired tonsils located at the base of the tongue.

nares/nostrils/nasopharynx The superior-most portion of the pharynx, located behind the nasal passages.

oral cavity The mouth.

oropharynx The region of the pharynx located behind the oral cavity.

palate The roof of the mouth.

palate, hard The anterior three-fourths of the roof of the mouth, formed by the maxilla and palatine bones.

palate, soft The posterior one-quarter of the palate that is composed of soft tissue.

palatine tonsils Paired lymphatic tissues that lie on the lateral walls of the palatoglossal arch, and anterior to the palatopharyngeal arch.

palatoglossal arch The posterior border of the oral cavity.

palatopharyngeal arch The entrance from the oral cavity into the pharynx.

paranasal sinuses The frontal and maxillary sinuses.

pharyngeal tonsil Single tonsil located on the posterior nasopharyngeal wall, which is also known as the adenoid.

pharynx The throat.

pyriform fossae Hollow pockets on the lateral sides of the glottic opening.

submental triangle The block of tissue under the jaw.

surfactant The proteinaceous substance that lines the inside of the alveoli and allows for easy expansion and recoil of the alveoli.

thyroepiglottic ligament The attachment of the thyroid cartilage to the epiglottis.

thyroid cartilage The shield-shaped cartilaginous structure that forms the laryngeal border.

uvula The piece of soft tissue that extends into the palatoglossal arch.

vallecula The anatomic space between the base of the tongue and the epiglottis.

Valsalva maneuver Straining against a closed glottis.

vocal cords The fibrous bands of tissue that vibrate to create speech.

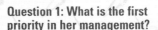

Case Study Answers

Question 1: What is the first priority in her management?

Answer: The first priority in managing this patient is to establish an airway and provide ventilation.

Question 2: Considering the circumstances surrounding the incident, why have you been unsuccessful in establishing an airway?

Answer: Because the patient lost consciousness while eating, some partially chewed food is likely to be lodged in the airway, usually at the level of the hypopharynx.

Foreign body airway obstructions in unconscious patients are relieved by abdominal thrusts, or removal under direct visualization with a laryngoscope and Magill forceps.

Statistically, the most likely cause of any airway obstruction is the tongue making contact with the posterior pharyngeal wall and the epiglottis partially occluding the glottis.

Question 3: From an anatomic perspective, what can be done to relieve the problem?

Answer: The ideal initial way to open the airway is to control the hyoid bone. In most cases this is accomplished by performing the head tilt-chin lift maneuver. When the jaw is lifted, the muscles of the submental triangle, which are attached to the jaw and hyoid bone, indirectly affect the position of the epiglottis and the base of the tongue. In this situation the head tilt-chin lift maneuver will likely be unsuccessful in providing a patent airway. Foreign body airway obstructions may be relieved by providing abdominal thrusts (Heimlich maneuver).

Question 4: What is the most likely cause of an airway obstruction now?

Answer: Considering the fact that there was initially a foreign body airway obstruction, the most likely explanation of a unilaterally decreased breath sound is a lower airway obstruction. In this case, it is most likely that a smaller object became lodged in the major bronchiole that aerates the right lower lobe.

Question 5: What are some of your concerns about both her short- and long-term recovery?

Answer: In the near term, aspiration of food particles causing a potentially fatal lung infection is of significant concern. The question of hypoxia-induced brain damage poses a greater, long-term issue for her ultimate outcome.

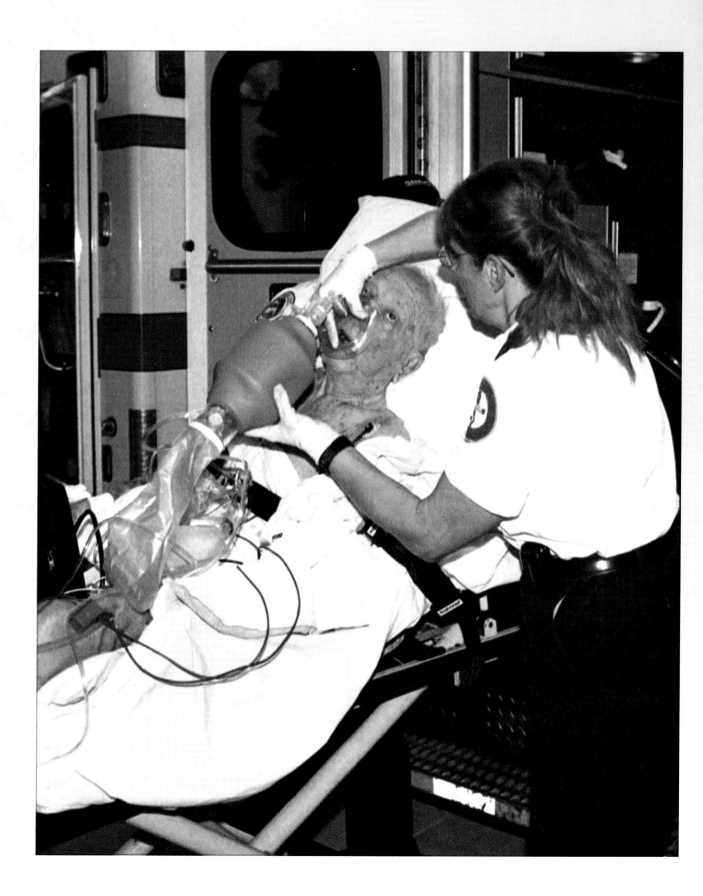

Physiology 3

Objectives

Cognitive Objectives

2-1.7 Explain the relationship between pulmonary circulation and respiration. (p 28)

2-1.8 List the concentration of gases that comprise atmospheric air. (p 36)

2-1.10 Describe the measurement of carbon dioxide in the blood. (p 30)

2-1.12 List factors that cause decreased oxygen concentrations in the blood. (p 30)

2-1.13 List the factors that increase and decrease carbon dioxide production in the body. (p 30)

2-1.15 Define FiO_2. (p 36)

2-1.16 Define and differentiate between hypoxia and hypoxemia. (p 40)

2-1.17 Describe the voluntary and involuntary regulation of respiration. (p 36)

2-1.18 Describe the modified forms of respiration. (p 38)

2-1.19 Define normal respiratory rates and tidal volumes for the adult, child, and infant. (p 34)

2-1.20 List the factors that affect respiratory rate and depth. (p 28)

www.Paramedic.EMSzone.com

Online Chapter Pretest
Vocabulary Explorer
Anatomy Review
Web Links

TECHNOLOGY

Case Studies
Skill Drills
Teamwork Tips
Documentation Tips
Paramedic Safety Tips
Special Needs Tips
Vital Vocabulary
Prep Kit

Chapter FEATURES

P hysiology is the study of function. A thorough understanding of the underlying physiology of respiration helps you appreciate the importance of airway management and respiratory care. A solid foundation in physiology is necessary in order to develop your problem-solving skills.

The respiratory and cardiovascular systems work together to ensure a constant supply of oxygen and nutrients to every cell in the body and the removal of carbon dioxide and waste products from every cell. The following three separate but mutually dependent processes must occur to achieve this: ventilation, oxygenation, and respiration.

Ventilation

Ventilation is the process of moving air into and out of the lungs. Normally, ventilation is necessary for oxygenation and respiration to occur. Adequate, continuous ventilation is essential for life and therefore is one of the highest priorities in treating any patient. If a patient is not breathing, or is breathing inadequately, you must immediately intervene to ensure adequate ventilation.

Apnea is the absence of ventilation. Brain damage begins after 4 to 6 minutes of apnea and can become permanent and profound after 10 minutes. Ventilation has two phases: inspiration and expiration. Inspiration is the process of air moving into the lungs. Expiration is the process of moving air out of the lungs. One ventilation cycle consists of one inspiration and one expiration.

The two major variables of ventilation are rate and depth. The ventilation rate (also called the respiratory rate) is the number of ventilatory cycles in a unit of time, usually 1 minute. The ventilatory depth, also known as the tidal volume, is the volume of air, usually measured in milliliters, that is exchanged in one ventilatory cycle.

Normal Ventilation

A person's need for oxygen varies depending on his or her level of activity and physiologic demands. The body can alter the amount of oxygen reaching the cells by changing the respiratory rate and depth. This complex process involves a number of interrelated feedback mechanisms, some of which can be consciously overridden. Fortunately, most of the time we do not need to think about breathing and the body automatically adjusts its respiratory rate to maintain the delicate balance of oxygen delivery to the blood and carbon dioxide removal from the blood.

The Control of Ventilation

The body's need for oxygen is constantly changing. The respiratory system responds to the demand for oxygen by altering the rate and depth of ventilation. Changes in the rate and depth of ventilation are primarily controlled by the acidity of the cerebrospinal fluid, which is directly related to the amount of carbon dioxide dissolved in the plasma portion of the blood ($PaCO_2$). The control of ventilation involves a complex series of receptors and feedback loops. Three basic types of control mechanism influence ventilation: neural, chemical, and mechanical. At any given time, a person's ventilatory rate and depth are influenced by these three control mechanisms.

Neural Control

The neural control of breathing originates in the brain and brainstem. The voluntary control of the respiratory pattern and rate is based in the cerebral cortex, which sends impulses through the corticospinal nerve tracts to the muscles of respiration. Voluntary control of respiration is important when a person is talking, laughing, singing, or playing a musical instrument.

The involuntary control of breathing originates in the brainstem, specifically in the pons and medulla. The impulses for automatic breathing descend through the spinal cord, not the corticospinal nerve tracts, and can be overridden (to a point) by voluntary control. The motor nerves of respiration are the phrenic nerve, which innervates the diaphragm, and the intercostal nerves, which innervate the external intercostal muscles.

The respiratory center, located in the medulla, is divided into three regions: the respiratory rhythmicity center, the apneustic center, and the pneumotaxic center. The respiratory rhythmicity center sets the pace of breathing and maintains that pace even in the absence of input. During normal, quiet respiration, the respiratory rhythmicity center gradually increases the stimulation for inhalation over 2 seconds and then relaxes over 3 seconds, allowing passive exhalation, and then repeats the cycle. This results in a resting breathing rate of 12 to 15 times a minute.

The respiratory rhythmicity center contains inspiratory neurons and expiratory neurons. In one respiratory cycle, the inspiratory neurons fire while the

Did You Know ?

Respiratory Patterns in Brain Lesions and Head Trauma

Understanding the control of breathing allows you to predict what types of respiratory patterns may be expected if a brain lesion or trauma occurs at different levels of the spinal cord or brain stem. A lesion in the brain stem below the level of the pneumotaxic center results in an increase in the rate and depth of ventilation, known as central neurogenic hyperventilation.

Central neurogenic hyperventilation results from the loss of inhibition of the apneustic center by the pneumotaxic center. Injuries or lesions between the apneustic center and the pons result in Cheyne-Stokes respiration, which is an irregular form of crescendo-decrescendo breathing, followed by periods of apnea. When there is a loss of neural control of breathing, the respiratory pattern is entirely controlled by chemoreceptors. Blood chemistry changes lag slightly behind respiratory changes. Cheyne-Stokes respiration therefore is a continuous attempt to catch up. Transections of the spinal cord between the brain stem and the third cervical spinal nerve root result in apnea because motor impulses through the phrenic nerve are interrupted, leaving a person unable to contract the diaphragm and inhale. Spinal cord injuries below this point usually do not directly affect respiration except when lesions are above the thoracic levels, causing paralysis of the intercostal muscles. The respiratory rate, although not immediately affected, becomes affected over time because of decreased tidal volume.

expiratory neurons relax. As the chest expands, mechanical receptors in the chest wall and bronchioles send a signal to the apneustic center via the vagus nerve to inhibit the inspiratory center, and expiration occurs. This feedback loop, a combination of mechanical and neural control known as the **Hering-Breuer reflex**, terminates inhalation and prevents lung overexpansion.

The apneustic center influences the respiratory rate by increasing the number of inspirations per minute. This is balanced by the pneumotaxic center, which has an inhibitory influence on inspiration. Respiratory rate, therefore, results from the interaction between these two centers. In times of increased demand, the pneumotaxic center decreases its influence, therefore increasing the rate.

Case Study

Case Study, Part 1

Your third attempt to eat your now late afternoon meal is interrupted once again by the Communications Center. "ALS 7, respond to 327 Albion Street, 2nd-floor apartment, report of sudden shortness of breath. Respond code 3." Your partner drops the transmission into gear, and several minutes later you arrive on the scene. Family members lead you upstairs to a 28-year-old woman in acute respiratory distress.

After you establish scene safety, you make your way into the kitchen, where the patient is sitting upright at the kitchen table. Several metered-dose inhalers (MDIs) are lying on the tabletop. She appears awake, but is focused on her breathing efforts. Your rapid initial assessment reveals the following:

Initial Assessment

Recording time
0 minutes

Appearance
Pale, diaphoretic skin; struggling to breathe

Level of consciousness
Alert

Airway
Appears patent

Breathing
Her respiratory rate is rapid, with obvious accessory muscle use. She is unable to speak more than one or two-word sentences.

Circulation
She appears pale with diaphoresis. A rapid, strong radial pulse is detected.

Question 1: What is involved in the initial management of this respiratory emergency?

CASE STUDY

Chemical Control

The goal of the respiratory system is to keep the blood's concentrations of oxygen and carbon dioxide, and its acid-base balance within a very narrow normal range. This is challenging because many factors influence these variables (▶ **Tables 3-1 and 3-2**). The body has a number of receptors that monitor these variables and provide feedback to the respiratory centers to modify the respiratory rate and pattern based on the body's needs. These **chemoreceptors** have important effects on respiratory rates.

Chemoreceptors that constantly monitor the chemical composition of body fluids are located

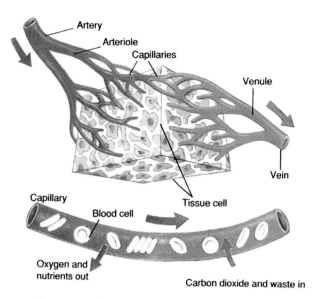
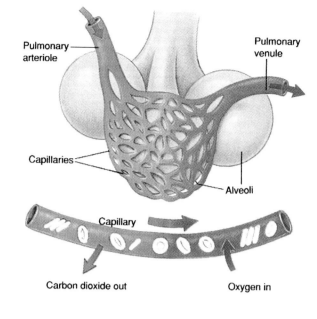

Figure 3-6 Internal and external respiration.

External respiration occurs in the lungs between the alveoli and the capillaries of the pulmonary circulatory system. Internal respiration is the exchange of oxygen and carbon dioxide between the blood and each cell in the body to provide oxygen to the cells and remove carbon dioxide and waste products. Internal respiration occurs between the capillaries of the systemic circulatory system and the body's tissues.

The Exchange and Transport of Gases in the Body

External Respiration

Fresh air that is inspired into the lungs contains about 21% oxygen, 78% nitrogen, and 0.3% carbon dioxide. As this air reaches the alveoli, it comes into contact with surfactant, which is a combination of phospholipids in a near-saline solution that lines the inside of the alveoli. The phospholipids reduce the surface tension of the saline, making it easier for the lungs to expand and decreasing the work of breathing.

Surfactant is also an important component of gas exchange. Components of inspired air dissolve in the surfactant. Once dissolved, oxygen molecules are transported in the blood in two forms. Approximately 97% of the oxygen transported throughout the body is bound to hemoglobin, which is an iron-containing molecule that has a great affinity for oxygen molecules. Hemoglobin is located in the red blood cells.

The hemoglobin in blood that is pumped to the lungs from the right side of the heart is low in oxygen. As this blood passes through the capillaries of

the pulmonary circulatory system it is in close proximity to the fresh alveolar air, rich in oxygen. The hemoglobin molecules pick up the oxygen molecules that are dissolved in surfactant. Under normal conditions, 96% to 100% of the hemoglobin receptor sites contain oxygen as the blood returns to the left side of the heart from the lungs. The percentage of hemoglobin that contains oxygen molecules is referred to as the arterial saturation of oxygen (SaO_2).

Dissolved oxygen is also transported through the body in the blood plasma. Although this involves only about 3% of the total amount of oxygen transported to the cells, it plays an important component in physiology. The amount of oxygen that can be dissolved in plasma is a function of the partial pressure of oxygen in the inspired air; this is expressed as the lab value PaO_2. While breathing room air, a person's normal PaO_2 is about 100 mm Hg. In cases of acute respiratory crisis, patients often receive higher percentages of inspired oxygen even if their SaO_2 is normal. This is done to increase the amount of oxygen available to the cells by increasing the oxygen dissolved in the plasma. While breathing 100% oxygen, a patient's PaO_2 can increase to 300 to 400 mm Hg. This additional oxygen available for metabolism can improve a patient's ability to supply oxygen to meet body demands.

After the blood plasma and hemoglobin are oxygenated in the pulmonary circulation, they are returned to the left side of the heart to be pumped to the rest of the body.

Internal Respiration

Internal respiration is the goal of the entire respiratory and cardiovascular system. Internal respiration is the exchange of oxygen and carbon dioxide between the systemic circulatory system and the cells of the body. Every cell in the body needs a constant supply of oxygen to survive. While some tissues are more resilient than others, eventually all cells will die if deprived of oxygen. Oxygen is used by the mitochondria of the cells to convert glucose into energy. In the presence of oxygen, **aerobic** metabolism is very efficient and produces energy (in the form of adenosine triphosphate), carbon dioxide, and water.

Most cells can survive for short periods of time under **anaerobic** conditions. Without adequate oxygen, the cell does not completely convert glucose into energy, and lactic acid and other toxins accumulate in the cell. Eventually, without an adequate supply of oxygen, the cell cannot meet its metabolic demands and will die.

When arterial blood that is high in oxygen reaches the capillary level, it comes in contact with interstitial fluid, which is relatively low in oxygen. Oxygen follows the diffusion gradient from high concentration (in the capillaries) to lower concentration (in the interstitial fluid). Because cells never stop using oxygen, the concentration of oxygen is lower in the cell than in the interstitial fluid, and oxygen constantly diffuses into the cell.

When the mitochondria within each cell use the oxygen to convert glucose to energy, carbon dioxide, the main waste product, accumulates in the cell. Carbon dioxide is transported from the cell to the lungs for exhalation in three ways: dissolved in plasma, as carbaminohemoglobin, and as bicarbonate.

Like other gases, carbon dioxide is soluble in liquid. As carbon dioxide levels rise in the cell, the diffusion gradient drives carbon dioxide from the area of high concentration (within the cell) to the area of low concentration (the interstitial fluid). Because blood in the capillaries has a lower concentration of carbon dioxide than the interstitial fluid, diffusion continues, and about 9% of the carbon dioxide is transported back to the lungs as molecules dissolved in the plasma.

While the main purpose of hemoglobin is to transport oxygen, the amino groups on the polypeptide portions of hemoglobin are capable of binding reversibly with carbon dioxide. This molecule, called carbaminohemoglobin, accounts for approximately 24% of the carbon dioxide transported from the cells to the lungs for elimination from the body.

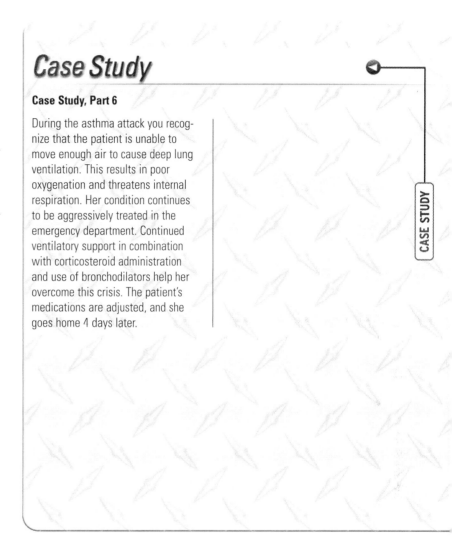

Case Study

Case Study, Part 6

During the asthma attack you recognize that the patient is unable to move enough air to cause deep lung ventilation. This results in poor oxygenation and threatens internal respiration. Her condition continues to be aggressively treated in the emergency department. Continued ventilatory support in combination with corticosteroid administration and use of bronchodilators help her overcome this crisis. The patient's medications are adjusted, and she goes home 4 days later.

CASE STUDY

Most of the carbon dioxide is removed from the body as the bicarbonate ion. Carbon dioxide reacts with water molecules in the body to form carbonic acid (H_2CO_3), which dissociates into hydrogen ions (H^+) and bicarbonate ions (HCO_3). These ions are important components in the acid-base balance of blood and body fluids and serve as a sponge that resists changes in pH. Approximately 67% of the carbon dioxide generated by the cells is transported to the lungs for exhalation as bicarbonate ions.

The Oxyhemoglobin Dissociation Curve

Hemoglobin is necessary for life. Approximately 95% of the protein in a red blood cell is hemoglobin. A common laboratory test to ensure that a patient has enough hemoglobin is the hemoglobin and hematocrit test. Hemoglobin levels are reported in grams per 100 milliliters; normal values are 14 to 16 g/100 mL for men and 12 to 14 g/100 mL for women. Hematocrit values indicate the percentage of red blood cells in whole blood when the sample is spun in a centrifuge. A normal hematocrit value is 45% to 52% for men and 37% to 48% for women.

One molecule of hemoglobin reversibly binds with four molecules of oxygen. Remember that the percentage of the receptor sites occupied with oxygen, expressed as SaO_2, under normal conditions is 98% to 100%. The SaO_2 is proportional to the amount of oxygen dissolved in the plasma component of the blood, denoted as PaO_2. The relationship of PaO_2 and SaO_2 is represented by the oxyhemoglobin dissociation curve (▶ Figure 3-7). Notice that under normal conditions ($PaO_2 = 105$ mm Hg), the corresponding SO_2 is approximately 98%.

While *deoxygenated* is often the term used to describe the venous blood returning to the heart during circulation, the blood is not completely devoid of oxygen. Some oxygen is still bound to the hemoglobin, because the ability of the respiratory system to supply oxygen to the rest of the body exceeds the demand in normal resting conditions. When metabolism increases, the demand for oxygen increases, and venous blood contains less oxygen. As blood is circulated to the tissue level, the PaO_2 begins to drop. At this point, the hemoglobin releases its oxygen molecules to make them available for cellular respiration. The lower the PaO_2 of a tissue drops, the more oxygen is unloaded into the interstitial fluid around it.

Hemoglobin has the ability to change how tightly it holds on to oxygen in response to changes in metabolic conditions. More oxygen molecules are released as acidity increases. This results in a shift in position of the oxyhemoglobin dissociation curve. Various other conditions can also shift the entire curve to the right or left. A shift to the right causes the hemoglobin to give up its oxygen faster and earlier. A shift to the left has the opposite effect. Acidosis and increased carbon dioxide levels cause the curve

to shift to the right. Alkalosis and a decrease in carbon dioxide levels cause the curve to shift to the left, causing the hemoglobin to hold on to more oxygen.

Fetal blood lacks a phosphorus-containing metabolite called 2,3 DPG. A decrease in 2,3 DPG causes the oxyhemoglobin curve to shift to the left, increasing the affinity of hemoglobin for oxygen. This enables the blood of the fetus to draw oxygen from the mother's circulatory system.

Causes of Hypoxia

If cells are deprived of oxygen, they will die. When too many cells die, survival of tissues or organs is threatened. Death is the ultimate result. Regardless of the underlying cause, when a critical number of cells in the body die, the individual dies. Brain and neural tissue are particularly sensitive to interruptions in oxygen delivery. Clearly, the first goal of all emergency care is to ensure an adequate supply of oxygen to the body's cells.

<u>Hypoxia</u> is the condition that occurs when the supply of oxygen to the tissues is inadequate. The four main causes of tissue hypoxia are hypoxemic hypoxia, anemic hypoxia, stagnant (or ischemic) hypoxia, and histotoxic hypoxia.

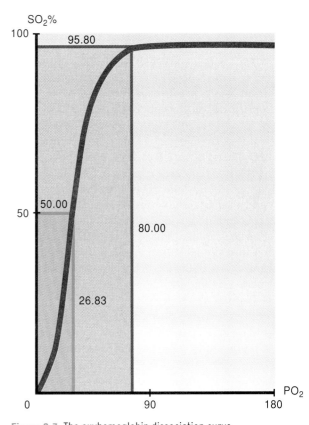

Figure 3-7 The oxyhemoglobin dissociation curve.

Did You Know ?

Some types of poisons cause histotoxic hypoxia because they affect the ability of hemoglobin to release oxygen or the ability of cells to use oxygen. Fortunately, this is a relatively uncommon situation, but it can be life threatening.

<u>Hypoxemia</u> is a decrease in the amount of oxygen in the bloodstream. Hypoxemia leads to hypoxia because inadequate oxygen is supplied to the body's tissues. Hypoxemia can be caused by a number of conditions such as respiratory arrest, hypoventilation, airway obstruction, breathing air containing inadequate oxygen (such as in confined spaces), breathing air that is too low in atmospheric pressure (such as at high altitude), lung trauma, pulmonary edema, and obstructive diseases. All of these conditions result in decreased oxygen content in the blood. Hypoxemia leads to tissue hypoxia. In hypoxemic hypoxia the hemoglobin saturation is below 96%.

<u>Anemia</u> is an inadequate supply of red blood cells in the blood. Because red blood cells are comprised predominantly of hemoglobin, a decrease in the hematocrit value (ratio of red blood cells to plasma) significantly alters the oxygen-carrying capacity of the blood. In anemic hypoxia, the oxygen saturation may be normal, but the blood does not contain enough oxygen-carrying capacity to support the metabolic demands of the tissues, and hypoxia results. The most common causes of anemia are iron deficiency, blood loss, and genetic disorders such as sickle cell anemia.

Stagnant hypoxia results from a local or systemic interruption in blood flow. If the heart stops completely, all tissues rapidly deplete the oxygen from the stagnant blood. Without a continual supply of oxygenated blood, hypoxia will result. Stagnant hypoxia can also occur if the heart is not beating with enough force. In this case, the blood moves through the circulatory system too slowly. While the arterial oxygen saturation may be high, the blood moves too slowly to meet the body's need for oxygen.

Stagnant hypoxia can also occur locally from a blockage in blood flow. In this case, a specific area of the body is affected, such as heart muscle tissue during a myocardial infarction or the brain during a stroke.

Some types of poisons cause histotoxic hypoxia because they affect the ability of hemoglobin to release oxygen or the ability of cells to use oxygen. Fortunately, this is a relatively uncommon situation, but it can be life threatening.

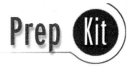

Chapter Summary

A strong background in respiratory physiology provides the paramedic with the foundation necessary to make thoughtful decisions regarding airway management and respiratory care.

When faced with a situation that requires immediate action, you must act quickly and decisively.

Certain circumstances demand a more contemplative approach that requires your decision-making skills.

Understanding the basic physiologic concepts of ventilation will lead to accurate assessment and treatment of patients experiencing ventilatory-related disorders. Under normal conditions, a person will adequately adjust both ventilatory rate and volume in response to the amount of carbon dioxide dissolved in plasma using a series of chemoreceptors and feedback loops.

Control over ventilation is largely involuntary via respiratory nerve centers found in the pons and medulla regions of the brain stem. The physical movement of gases through ventilation depends on mechanical and diffusion processes. Under abnormal conditions, failure of one or more ventilatory processes may cause significant hypoventilation, resulting in the use of artificial ventilations by the health care provider to support a patient's condition. Maintenance of a patient's tidal volume and minute volume is essential for adequate gas exchange in the lungs.

Ensuring and maintaining adequate amounts of oxygen to be delivered to the body's tissues is an essential skill. Remember that oxygenation does not equal ventilation, and vice versa!

Vital Vocabulary

aerobic Occurring in the presence of oxygen.

alveolar air The amount of gas that reaches the alveoli with each breath.

alveolar ventilation Exchanging the gas in the alveoli with fresh air.

anaerobic Occurring in the absence of, or without, oxygen.

anemia A decreased number of red blood cells in the blood.

apnea The absence of ventilation.

chemoreceptors Peripheral and central receptors that monitor the levels of chemicals in the blood.

dead space The amount of inhaled air that does not participate in respiration.

expiration The process of moving air out of the lungs.

expiratory reserve volume The amount of air that can be exhaled following normal exhalation.

Hering-Breuer reflex The nervous system mechanism that terminates inhalation and prevents lung overexpansion.

hypercapnia Elevated levels of carbon dioxide in the blood.

hypoxemia A decrease in the amount of oxygen in the bloodstream.

hypoxia Inadequate supply of oxygen to the tissues.

hypoxic drive Condition in which patients with chronic hypercapnia increase their respiratory rate exclusively in response to decreased oxygen levels in the blood.

inspiration The process of air moving into the lungs.

inspiratory reserve volume The maximum amount of air that can be forcefully inhaled following a full inhalation.

mechanoreceptors Peripheral receptors that detect stretch or pressure.

minute volume The amount of air moved in and out of the respiratory tract per minute, which is determined by the tidal volume multiplied by the respiratory rate.

negative pressure ventilation The process of pulling air into the lungs by decreasing intrathoracic pressure.

oxygenation The process of assuring an adequate supply of oxygen molecules for delivery to the body's cells.

positive pressure ventilation The process of pushing air into the lungs by increasing the pressure of the gas outside of the body.

residual volume The air that remains in the lungs after a maximal expiration.

respiration The process of exchanging oxygen and carbon dioxide.

respiratory center The area of the brainstem located in the pons and medulla that is responsible for involuntary control of breathing.

respiratory rate The number of ventilatory cycles in a unit of time, usually 1 minute, also known as the ventilation rate.

tidal volume The volume of air, usually measured in milliliters, which is exchanged in one ventilatory cycle, also known as the ventilatory volume.

ventilation The process of moving air into and out of the lungs.

ventilation cycle One inspiration and one expiration.

ventilation rate The number of ventilatory cycles in a unit of time, usually 1 minute, also known as the respiratory rate.

ventilatory depth The volume of air, usually measured in milliliters, which is exchanged in one ventilatory cycle, also known as the tidal volume.

Case Study Answers

Question 1: What is involved in the initial management of this patient's respiratory emergency?

Answer: Any patient with signs of respiratory distress must receive oxygen as soon as possible. Since her airway appears patent, 100% high-flow oxygen via a nonrebreathing mask would be a minimum approach to this patient. Assisted ventilations with a BVM device may be necessary; careful monitoring of the patient's condition is critical.

Question 2: Explain the mechanism causing the patient's respirations of 40 breaths/min.

Answer: The predominant mechanism for tachypnea is the chemical control of respiration. The bronchoconstriction of the asthma attack is decreasing deep lung aeration, and the patient is unable to get an adequate amount of oxygen and rid her body of carbon dioxide. The result is hypoxemia and hypercapnia. The increased carbon dioxide in the blood decreases pH (increases acidity of the blood). Central and peripheral chemoreceptors detect this change quickly and increase the respiratory rate in an attempt to blow off carbon dioxide. Unfortunately, the underlying bronchoconstriction makes this impossible, and the process continues as a vicious cycle.

Question 3: Given her respiratory status, is the nonrebreathing mask adequate to correct her condition? What other interventions would you consider?

Answer: She is breathing fairly rapidly (40 breaths/min), limiting her ability to achieve adequate tidal volume and subsequent gas exchange. Nonrebreathing masks can only provide supplemental oxygen; they do not affect the release of carbon dioxide buildup. The consideration of the use of a BVM device becomes much stronger now in order to increase ventilatory volumes.

Question 4: The patient's pulse and respiratory rates appear to be decreasing. Are these positive or negative signs? Why?

Answer: Somnolence and a decreasing respiratory rate in a patient in respiratory distress is an ominous sign. Breathing rapidly and using accessory muscles for both inhalation and exhalation take a tremendous amount of energy. A falling respiratory rate indicates that the patient is becoming too tired to keep up, and decreases in the level of consciousness indicate that the carbon dioxide level in the blood is rising. The patient is experiencing a life-threatening asthma attack.

Question 5: What other interventions might you consider now?

Answer: With the impending loss of airway patency, it is becoming necessary to utilize advanced airway management procedures, such as oral or nasal intubation.

Question 6: In retrospect, you suspect that the patient should have received ventilation assistance earlier. What respiratory parameters would you more closely assess next time?

Answer: Critical evaluation of the patient's respiratory rate, tidal volume, and effort is imperative to making accurate clinical decisions. Additional assessment techniques can shed more light on the clinical picture. Blood gases will show respiratory acidosis; the SpO_2 will be falling. Physical exam findings will likely include use of accessory muscles for both inspiration and expiration and the patient will have absent or severely diminished breath sounds due to poor alveolar ventilation.

Question 7: Can you explain how changes to the patient's condition during the incident are related to the hemoglobin dissociation curve?

Answer: As carbon dioxide accumulates within the patient's body tissues, acidosis increases. This increase shifts the oxyhemoglobin curve to the right, causing the red blood cells to lose oxygen more quickly, decreasing the efficiency of the transportation system.

Question 8: Is the patient's condition progressing positively or negatively? Why?

Answer: With the endotracheal intubation tube in place, the patient's condition appears to be improving fairly dramatically. Your skills in identifying and treating the early warning signs of impending respiratory failure can be lifesaving.

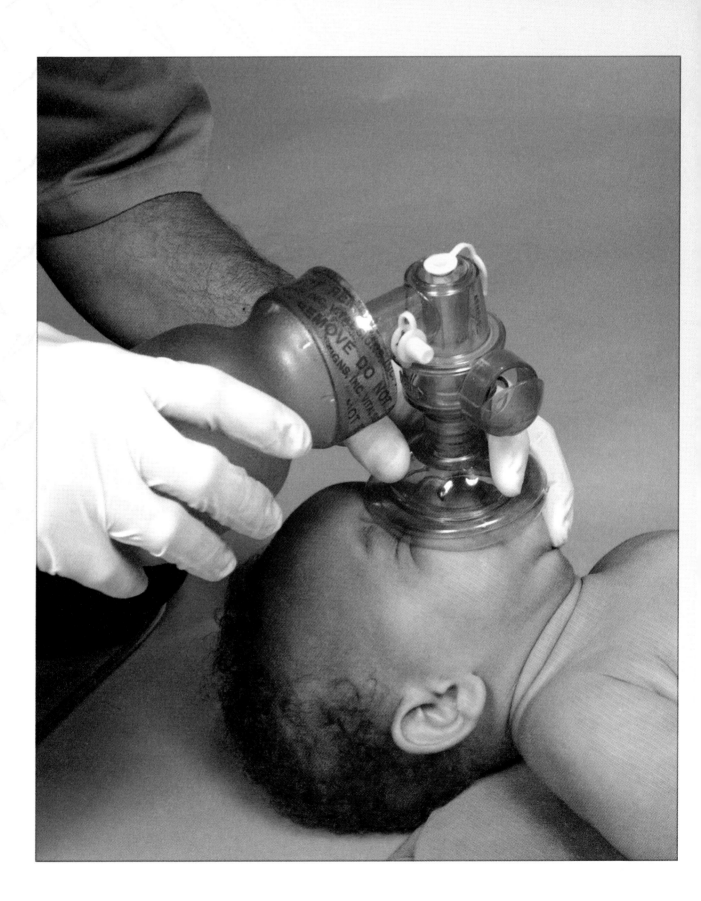

Evaluating Airway Patency and Ventilatory Efficiency

4

Objectives

Cognitive Objectives

2-1.6	Define gag reflex. (p 47)
2-1.9	Describe the measurement of oxygen in the blood. (p 65)
2-1.10	Describe the measurement of carbon dioxide in the blood. (p 66)
2-1.11	Describe peak expiratory flow. (p 58)
2-1.12	List factors that cause decreased oxygen concentrations in the blood. (p 48)
2-1.13	List factors that increase and decrease carbon dioxide production in the body. (p 69)
2-1.20	List factors that affect respiratory rate and depth. (p 60)
2-1.22	Define pulsus paradoxus. (p 60)
2-1.23	Define and explain the implications of partial airway obstruction with good and poor air exchange. (p 55)
2-1.24	Define complete airway obstruction. (p 51)
2-1.25	Describe causes of complete airway obstruction. (p 48)
2-1.26	Describe causes of respiratory distress. (p 60)
2-1.29	Describe complete airway obstruction maneuvers. (p 51)

Affective Objectives

2-1.77	Defend the need to oxygenate and ventilate a patient. (p 46)
2-1.78	Defend the necessity of establishing and/or maintaining patency of a patient's airway. (p 47)

Psychomotor Objectives

2-1.81	Perform pulse oximetry. (p 67) (Skill Drill 4-7)
2-1.83	Perform peak expiratory flow testing. (p 59) (Skill Drill 4-6)
2-1.87	Perform complete airway obstruction maneuvers, including:

- Heimlich maneuver (p 50) (Skill Drills 4-1, 4-2, and 4-4)
- Finger sweeps (p 50) (Skill Drills 4-1, 4-3, and 4-4)
- Chest thrusts (p 52) (Skill Drill 4-3)
- Removal with Magill forceps (p 56) (Skill Drill 4-5)

2-1.102	Perform retrieval of foreign bodies from the upper airway. (p 56) (Skill Drill 4-5)

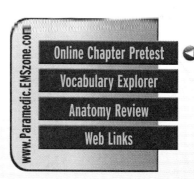

www.Paramedic.EMSzone.com

TECHNOLOGY

- Online Chapter Pretest
- Vocabulary Explorer
- Anatomy Review
- Web Links

Chapter FEATURES

- Case Studies
- Skill Drills
- Teamwork Tips
- Documentation Tips
- Paramedic Safety Tips
- Special Needs Tips
- Vital Vocabulary
- Prep Kit

The importance of following the ABCs (airway, breathing, and circulation) when managing emergency patients cannot be overemphasized. This approach is crucial because threats to the airway or breathing are among the most rapid—yet the most potentially correctable—threats to life. Failure to address a compromised airway or breathing immediately can lead to death or permanent disability. Unfortunately, poor patient outcome or deterioration from hypoxia often occurs hours or days after the period of hypoxia; patient survival through the emergency phase of treatment therefore does not mean that you have adequately addressed the patient's airway or ventilatory needs.

In reality, ensuring an adequate airway and breathing is often more difficult than it may seem. Although each end of the spectrum of breathing is fairly straight-forward (from normal, unlabored breathing to apnea), there is a large area in-between, in which knowing what to do is very challenging. The conditions of most patients fall within this area, and it is not always clear how to proceed.

The most difficult and stressful parts of airway management and ventilatory interventions are deciding what to do and when to do it. Once you decide what to do, the rest is only a matter of executing the plan. Airway management and ventilatory decisions are among the most time-critical and high-stakes decisions that you make in emergency situations. The consequences of being either too aggressive or not aggressive enough can be significant. You have to assess, decide, and intervene quickly and efficiently. Your decisions will be based on assessment findings and experience. This chapter reviews the assessment of airway patency and the effectiveness of ventilation. This information in combination with your

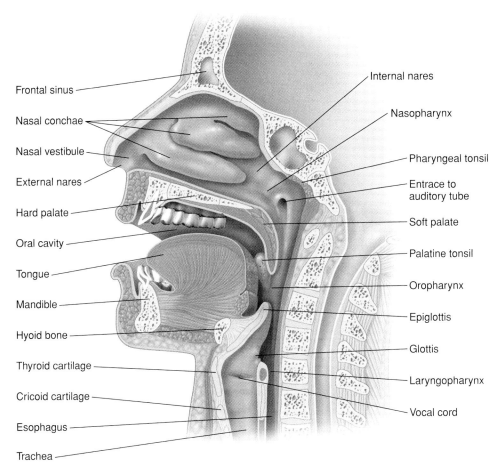

Frontal sinus

Nasal conchae

Nasal vestibule

External nares

Hard palate

Oral cavity

Tongue

Mandible

Hyoid bone

Thyroid cartilage

Cricoid cartilage

Esophagus

Trachea

Internal nares

Nasopharynx

Pharyngeal tonsil

Entrace to auditory tube

Soft palate

Palatine tonsil

Oropharynx

Epiglottis

Glottis

Laryngopharynx

Vocal cord

Figure 4-1 Illustration of the airway.

experience is necessary for airway and ventilation problem solving.

Airway Patency

For air to flow from the external environment to the functional level of gas exchange, the airway must be free and unobstructed. When the entire airway (from the lips/nostrils to the alveoli) is clear and free of obstruction, the airway is said to be **patent**.

Protecting the Upper Airway

The body has a number of protective reflexes that normally protect the patency of the airway (◄ Figure 4-1).

The Gag Reflex

Gagging is a forceful muscular contraction of the pharyngeal muscles and the glottis. This reaction is automatic when something touches an area deep in the oral cavity. A **gag reflex** helps protect the lower airway from **aspiration**, or entry of fluids or solids into the trachea, bronchi, and lungs, by expelling objects from the upper airway. An intact gag reflex is essential to protecting the airway from obstructions and aspiration.

Although everyone has a gag reflex, gag sensitivity varies in individuals, with some people being more prone to gagging than others. The main trigger point for the gag reflex is stimulation of the posterior pharyngeal wall. The reflex is mediated by the glossopharyngeal (IX) and vagus (X) nerves. As a person's level of consciousness decreases, the gag reflex weakens. Patients in deep coma may have no gag reflex or an inadequate gag reflex and therefore cannot protect their airway.

Although you can test for the presence of a gag reflex by touching the posterior pharyngeal wall with a tongue blade, in emergency care the gag reflex is usually evaluated during insertion of an oropharyngeal airway. If an unconscious patient gags, the device is removed and you can conclude that the patient is able to protect his or her airway. If the patient accepts the oropharyngeal airway without gagging, he or she will most likely require more aggressive airway management because the gag reflex necessary to prevent aspiration is not intact.

Stimulating the gag reflex causes retching and may cause vomiting. Both actions increase intracranial pressure, and, in the unconscious patient, vomiting severely threatens the patency of the airway. A good estimation of whether the patient has an intact gag reflex is the **eyelash reflex** (► Figure 4-2). If the patient's lower eyelid contracts when you gently stroke the upper eyelashes, the patient probably has a gag reflex. Try to elicit the eyelash reflex in an unresponsive patient before inserting an oropharyngeal

Case Study

Case Study, Part 1

An unusually quiet Saturday evening shift is interrupted by a report of a "man down" at an upscale nightclub in the theater district. You are led to the men's bathroom in the rear of the building and find a male in his 20s sprawled out on the floor with his head between the wall and the toilet. He is covered in vomit and appears to have bitten his lip. An initial assessment of the patient finds the following conditions:

Initial Assessment

Recording time
0 minutes

Appearance
Other than the cut on his lip, no obvious trauma is seen.

Level of consciousness
Unresponsive to physical stimulation

Airway
Gurgling can be heard as he breathes.

Breathing
His respiratory rate appears normal, but his chest wall shows little movement.

Circulation
He is pale, with a present radial pulse.

Question 1: What are some of the threats to your patient's airway patency?

Question 2: What are your initial management steps?

CASE STUDY

airway if you are concerned that the patient might vomit. If the patient has an eyelash reflex, be cautious about any stimulation of the upper airway.

Occasionally, airway maneuvers must be performed on patients with an intact gag reflex. In such cases use of a topical or systemic medication may suppress the gag reflex. These medications are very useful when you need to manage the airway of conscious or semiconscious patients. Although local anesthetics applied topically to the mucous membranes of the upper airway may make it easier to

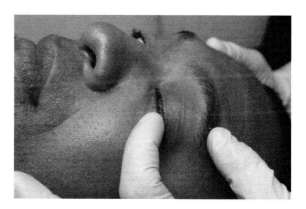

Figure 4-2 The eyelash reflex.

manage, such medications reduce the patient's ability to protect his or her own airway. Sedatives and analgesics given systemically also suppress the gag reflex and are used in conscious patients undergoing airway maneuvers or intubation. Local nerve blocks, frequently used during planned intubations for surgery, are rarely indicated in emergency situations.

Sneeze and Cough Reflex

Sneeze and __cough reflex__ also protect the airway. A __sneeze reflex__ is generally caused by irritation in the nose, whereas a cough is initiated by an irritation in the lower airway. A strong cough is initiated by stimulation of the carina and is called the carinal reflex. Both sneezes and coughs force a large volume of air to be exhaled to expel the cause of the irritation.

Threats to the Upper Airway

Anything that interferes with the free flow of air into the lungs represents an immediate threat to the patient. Unfortunately, many things can cause partial or complete obstruction of airflow through the airways.

The Tongue and Epiglottis

The tongue and epiglottis represent the most common threats to airway patency. In the unconscious patient, the positions of the tongue and epiglottis depend on gravity. If a patient in a supine position loses muscular control of the jaw, the mandible, submental tissue, and the hyoid bone all fall back toward the posterior pharyngeal wall. The flaccid jaw and all of the attached soft tissues are drawn posteriorly. As the base of the tongue comes in contact with the posterior pharyngeal wall, the airway becomes occluded (▼ Figure 4-3). This partial obstruction causes snoring, and in healthy patients with normal respiratory drives and strong inspiratory muscles, it

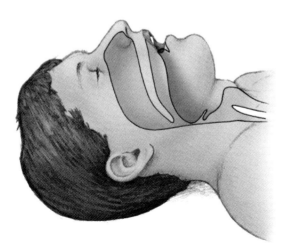

Figure 4-3 Occluded airway.

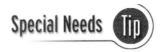

Special Needs

Infants "Back to Sleep!"

Infants present unique airway and respiratory challenges. Their tongues are larger in proportion to their mouths and jaws, making soft-tissue airway obstructions more of a threat. Infants also have a less developed respiratory drive and weaker inspiratory muscles. This increases the threat of apnea and sudden infant death syndrome (SIDS) if the infant is placed prone to sleep. Although SIDS is a multifactorial phenomenon, the immature respiratory drive combined with body weight on the chest and diaphragm are thought to be major contributors to the syndrome. For this reason, all infants should be placed flat on their backs for sleeping ("back to sleep"), with no pillows or objects under their heads (▼ Figure 4-4). When you treat infants, try to place them on their backs, and be very careful to control their head and jaw positions to prevent the tongue from obstructing the airway.

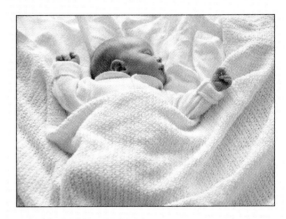

Figure 4-4 Infants should always be placed on their backs to sleep.

is rarely a problem. If a patient's respiratory drive is depressed and inspiratory muscles weakened, however, this obstruction can be fatal.

The epiglottis varies in size and cartilaginous support from person to person. In some people, the length and relative size of the epiglottis can partially or fully obstruct the airway when the patient is supine. Fortunately, the epiglottis is attached to the hyoid bone by the hyoepiglottic ligament, so that controlling the tongue also tends to control the epiglottis. Individual anatomic variations make controlling the airway easy in some people and difficult in others. With practice you will be able to identify anatomic clues that suggest that a patient may be a challenge for airway management.

Foreign Bodies

The tongue and epiglottis are anatomic threats to the airway, but foreign bodies can also interfere with the free flow of air into the lungs. **Foreign body airway obstruction** can occur in a number of ways. In adults and children, incompletely chewed food can block the airway, usually just above the glottic opening (▶ Figure 4-5). Eating while intoxicated dramatically increases the risk of foreign body airway obstruction.

Although aspiration of foreign objects can be a direct cause of airway obstruction, an obstruction may also result in association with diminished consciousness, especially if a patient has something in his or her mouth at the time consciousness is lost. Gum, candy, dentures, and chewing tobacco become potentially lethal threats to the airway in patients who experience a sudden decrease in their level of consciousness.

Vomitus

Vomitus in the airway is a serious problem. Not only does vomitus threaten the patency of the airway, it causes tremendous damage if it is aspirated into the lungs. Fully conscious patients who are not intoxicated typically protect their airways during vomiting in two important ways. They contract their abdominal muscles, which makes them lean forward to let the vomit drain from the mouth. They also close the glottic opening, which reduces the likelihood of airway obstruction and aspiration of vomitus.

Patients with a depressed gag reflex or decreased level of consciousness are at great risk for airway obstruction and aspiration if they vomit. The problem is greater in unconscious patients who are in a supine position and in patients being stabilized because of the possibility of a spinal injury.

Secretions

People constantly secrete and swallow saliva and mucus, which normally does not create an airway problem. When a patient is unable to swallow, these secretions accumulate and can cause a partial airway obstruction. Other patients, such as those with a stoma, some patients who are dependent on mechanical ventilation, and patients who receive certain medications, either have excessive secretions or have difficulty managing secretions. Vigilant monitoring and periodic suctioning of the airway are therefore necessary in patients with a decreased level of consciousness.

Blood

The mucous membranes of the mouth, nose, lips, and tongue are highly vascular and easily traumatized. Injuries in the mouth and nose tend to bleed profusely and can be hard to control. Blood, like any fluid, can make it impossible to inspire air into the lungs but unlike most fluids, blood gets thicker the longer it remains there. As the blood begins to clot, it can be difficult to remove by suctioning, manual extraction, or positioning.

Even in conscious patients, bleeding in the airway can create an airway problem. There is a natural tendency to swallow fluids that accumulate in the mouth. Blood irritates the stomach lining and quickly causes vomiting. Always suction blood from the mouth or have the patient spit it out.

Nosebleeds require specific attention. Many nosebleeds occur spontaneously, usually caused by dry or weakened blood vessels in the nasal mucosa, or by local and isolated trauma (digital nasal probing). In these cases, cervical spine injury is not a concern. These patients need to lean forward to drain the blood from the nostril; tilting the head back

Paramedic Safety Tip

Thousands of deaths per year occur from airway obstruction following acute alcohol intoxication or drug overdose. Generally, these patients vomit while lying on their backs and cannot protect their airway because of a severely decreased level of consciousness. Never leave anyone who has passed out unattended. If the person cannot be continually monitored, place the person prone or on their side, not supine.

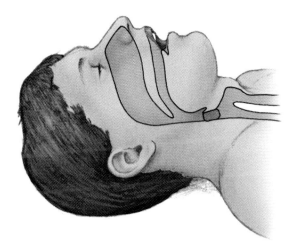

Figure 4-5 Food can block the airway.

Skill Drill

4-1 Managing Complete Airway Obstruction in the Unconscious Adult

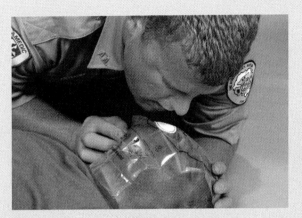

1 Open the airway and attempt ventilation.

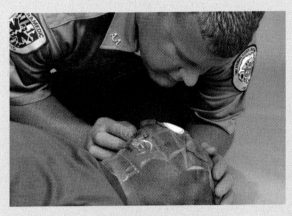

2 Reopen the airway and reattempt ventilation.

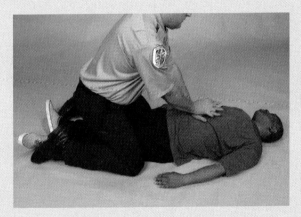

3 Perform the Heimlich maneuver up to five times.

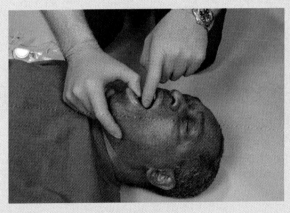

4 Open the patient's mouth with a tongue-jaw lift and perform a finger sweep to remove the object.

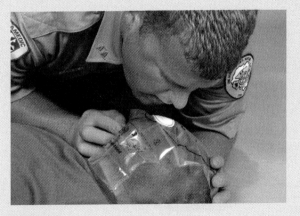

5 Attempt to ventilate.

Repeat steps 3 through 5 until successful or until help arrives.

Skill Drill

4-2 *Managing Complete Airway Obstruction or Incomplete Airway Obstruction with Poor Air Exchange in a Conscious Adult or Child*

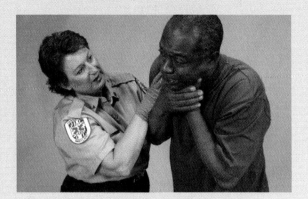

 Determine if the patient is choking by asking, "Are you choking?" If the patient is unable to answer, but indicates that he or she is choking, ask, "Do you want help?"

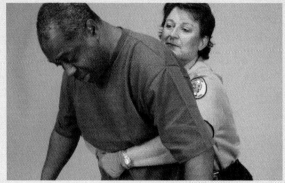

 Perform the Heimlich maneuver until the object is expelled or the patient becomes unresponsive.

causes the blood to drain down the throat. In patients who are bleeding from the nose secondary to blunt trauma to the face or head, you will need to take cervical spine precautions and stabilize the patient on a backboard. This forces the blood down the back of the patient's throat and will cause vomiting. Try to encourage the patient to spit out as much of the blood as possible, consider placing the board on the side, and/or consider packing the nose (following local protocol).

Recognizing Threats to the Upper Airway

In general, an airway obstruction is characterized as partial or complete; it can be caused by soft tissue, solids, or liquids. These classifications make it easier to recognize airway obstructions.

Complete or Incomplete Obstruction

In a **complete airway obstruction**, no air flows into or out of the lungs. Complete airway obstruction is one of the most rapidly fatal conditions and therefore must be recognized and treated quickly (◄ Skill Drills 4-1 through 4-4). Because no air is being moved, a patient with complete airway obstruction is silent. Complete airway obstructions are almost always caused by solid objects.

A conscious patient with a complete airway obstruction is anxious and may clutch at the throat

Paramedic Safety Tip

Fluids that create airway obstructions are potentially infectious. Be sure to protect yourself by wearing gloves, mask, and eye protection. Consider wearing a gown or apron on particularly messy cases.

Did You Know ?

If a patient is fully conscious and stabilized in a supine position (or in another position but reluctant to spit out blood), allow him or her to hold the suction catheter to remove the blood "just like in the dentist's office."

Skill Drill

4-3 Managing Complete Airway Obstruction in an Unconscious Infant

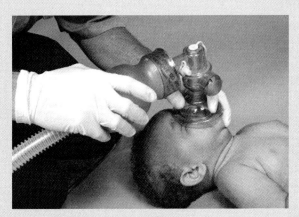

1 Open the airway and attempt ventilation.

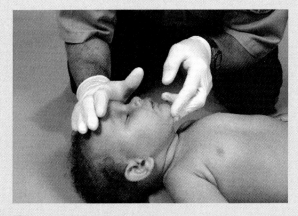

2 Reopen the airway and reattempt ventilation.

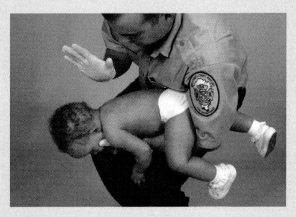

3 Perform up to five back blows.

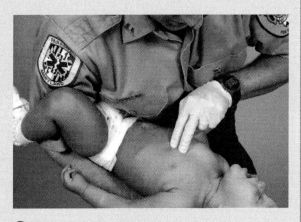

4 Perform up to five chest thrusts.

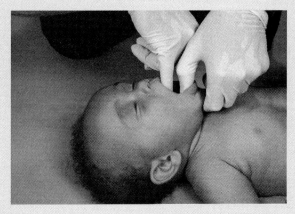

5 Open the patient's mouth with a tongue-jaw lift and look for an object in the pharynx. If the object is visible, perform a finger sweep to remove it.

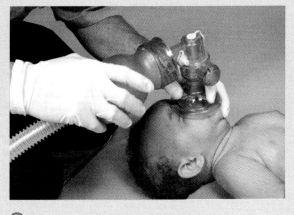

6 Attempt to ventilate.

Repeat steps 3 through 6 until successful or until help arrives.

Skill Drill

4-4 *Managing Complete Airway Obstruction in an Unconscious Child*

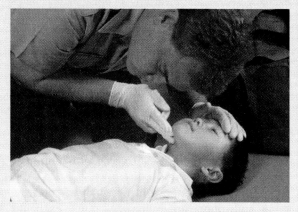

1 Open the airway and attempt ventilation.

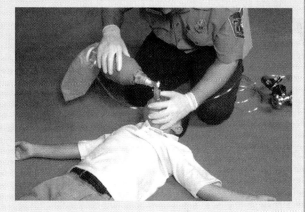

2 Reopen the airway and reattempt ventilation.

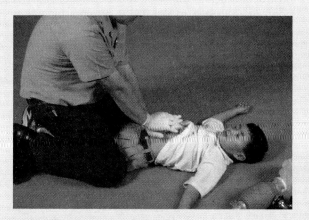

3 Perform the Heimlich maneuver up to five times.

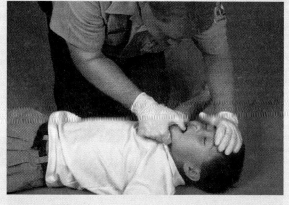

4 Open the patient's mouth with a tongue-jaw lift and look for an object in the pharynx. If the object is visible, perform a finger sweep to remove it.

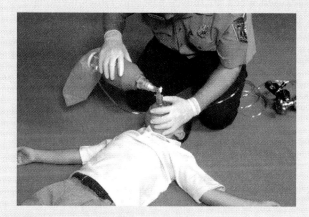

5 Attempt to ventilate.

Repeat steps 3 through 5 until successful or until help arrives.

Skill Drill

4-5 Removal of an Upper Airway Obstruction with Magill Forceps

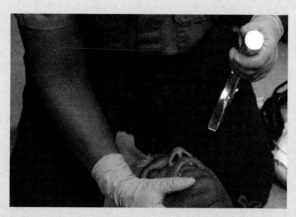

1 With the patient's head in the sniffing position, open the patient's mouth and insert the laryngoscope blade.

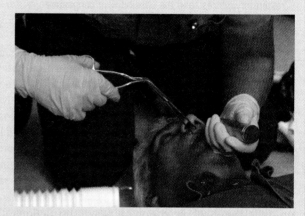

2 Visualize the obstruction and retrieve the object with the Magill forceps.

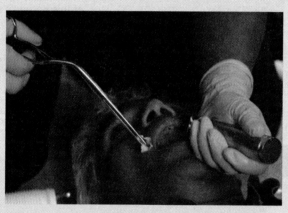

3 Remove the object with the Magill forceps.

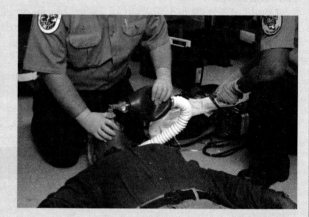

4 Reattempt to ventilate the patient.

In some patients with complete airway obstruction, the basic attempts previously described may prove unsuccessful. In cases such as this, if the patient is unconscious, the use of direct laryngoscopy and Magill forceps to retrieve the foreign body may be the only way of removing the obstruction and preventing death (◄ Skill Drill 4-5). The curvature of the Magill forceps allows the EMT-P to maneuver them in the airway and, after visualizing the obstruction, retrieving it from the upper airway (▼ Figure 4-7).

Threats to the Lower Airway

Laryngospasm

Laryngospasm is the forceful contraction of the vocal cords to prevent the aspiration of materials into the trachea. Laryngospasm plays an important role in protecting the lungs. You may have experienced a brief laryngospasm if you have accidentally aspirated water deep into the back of your throat while eating. In an extreme case, laryngospasm can completely occlude the airway and cause a total airway obstruction. The signs of laryngospasm are similar to partial airway obstructions caused by solid objects, including crowing, neck muscle tugging, and retractions.

Typically, laryngospasm resolves itself after a few seconds. Intravenous lidocaine (0.5 to 1.0 mg/kg) or 2% lidocaine applied directly to the vocal cords may help in relieving the spasm. Never try to force an airway device, such as an endotracheal tube, through vocal cords in spasm. The procedure will not be successful and will probably cause trauma and possible bleeding.

Laryngeal Edema

The mucosal tissue of the larynx is susceptible to swelling, which may partially or completely occlude the upper airway. The most common causes of laryngeal edema include burn injuries, allergic reactions, and some infections. The biggest threats to airway patency occur where the airway narrows (such as the glottic opening and the cricoid ring), and where there are areas of loose connective tissue (such as the epiglottis). In general, laryngeal swelling is progressive and early intervention is lifesaving. In cases where the patient's condition is stable, reassessment is necessary to identify airway threats early enough for nonsurgical intervention to be successful.

In the case of allergic reactions, epinephrine is given to treat the underlying problem. In cases such as burns or infections, you will have to intervene by intubating the patient before the swelling progresses to complete airway obstruction. If laryngeal edema progresses to this point, usually the only option is surgical or pseudosurgical access to the airway below the level of the obstruction.

Laryngeal Fracture and Penetrating Injuries to the Neck

Blunt, penetrating injuries to the neck are highly lethal, in large part because of the likelihood of airway compromise. Direct blows, seat belt injuries, striking the neck on the steering wheel or dashboard in motor vehicle crashes, and hangings can cause blunt injuries to the laryngeal structures. Extreme deceleration events can cause laryngeotracheal separation. Many patients with these injuries are typically found dead at the scene. If a patient survives, it is usually because airway structures are being held in close approximation by the connective tissue and muscles around the trachea. As long as the patient continues negative pressure ventilation, the airway is usually held together. Once spontaneous ventilations cease, or an endotracheal intubation is attempted, the severed ends separate and the airway is completely lost. Therefore, you should not attempt to intubate breathing patients with blunt trauma to the neck.

Penetrating injuries to the neck often involve the airway structures (▼ Figure 4-8). Mechanisms of injury typically include gunshot wounds and stabbing

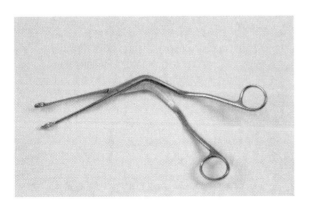

Figure 4-7 Magill Forceps

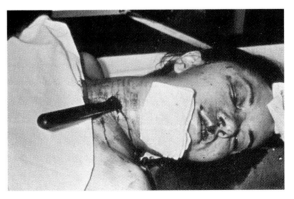

Figure 4-8 A penetrating injury to the neck.

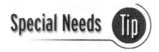

Obesity

Soft-tissue airway obstruction is a threat for all patients, but a much bigger problem for obese patients. Obesity increases the volume of upper airway soft tissue and subcutaneous fat, which lacks the rigidity and turgor of other tissue. This amorphous mass of tissue can easily threaten the airway.

injuries. In addition, foreign body airway obstruction, bleeding into the airway, hematoma formation, and subcutaneous emphysema complicate the management of these patients. In general, the management of penetrating airway injuries involves getting a cuffed endotracheal tube below the level of the injury. In some cases, it is possible to do so directly through the point of injury. In other cases, an oral approach is possible. The last resort is surgical access to the trachea below the injury.

Lower Airway Obstruction

A solid object aspirated into the trachea will continue down the bronchial tree until it becomes lodged in a bronchus or bronchiole. Tracheal obstructions are rare because an object small enough to pass through the glottic opening in adults, which is narrower than the trachea, or the cricoid ring in children usually does not become lodged in the trachea. Depending on the object's size and shape, a foreign body lower airway obstruction can affect a significant portion of the lung. Typically, these objects must be removed under direct visualization with a bronchoscope. In addition to the history, the signs include acute **dyspnea**, wheezing, cyanosis, low oxygen saturation, and diminished breath sounds in an isolated area.

Mucous plugs that become lodged in small and intermediate-sized bronchioles can also cause lower airway obstruction. Cystic fibrosis and chronic obstructive pulmonary diseases such as emphysema or asthma tend to increase mucus production in the lining of the bronchial tree and are associated with a decrease in the ciliary action that removes mucus. These diseases place patients at greater risk for lower airway obstruction. Chronic diseases that require patients to stay in a supine position for a prolonged period of time place them at an increased risk for mucous plugging.

Bronchoconstriction

The trachea and the bronchi are fairly rigid structures made primarily of cartilage. Swelling that decreases their diameter cannot be reversed by muscle movement. The bronchioles are flexible and contain a layer of smooth muscle. **Bronchoconstriction** occurs when contraction of the smooth muscle decreases the internal diameter of the bronchiole and dramatically decreases the airflow to a portion of the lungs. Bronchoconstriction is an important defense mechanism against the inhalation of toxins, but widespread bronchoconstriction can be life threatening. Many chronic and acute diseases cause bronchoconstriction, including asthma, emphysema, chronic obstructive pulmonary disease, bronchitis, and allergic reactions. Signs of bronchoconstriction include wheezing, dyspnea, decreased tidal volume, tachypnea, cyanosis, and decreased oxygen saturation. Bronchoconstriction is usually treated with sympathomimetic drugs.

Quantifying Bronchoconstriction

The amount of lung tissue affected by bronchoconstriction is evaluated by measuring the peak rate of a forceful exhalation with a peak expiratory flow monitor. **Peak expiratory flow** is a good approximation of the extent of bronchoconstriction and is used by many patients at home to monitor their disease. It can also be used to determine whether patients are improving with therapy (▶ **Skill Drill 4-6**).

Peak expiratory flow is measured by having the patient breathe as deeply as possible and exhale forcefully into a peak expiratory flow monitor. This pattern is repeated three times and the best value is recorded. Unfortunately, "normal" peak flow rates are hard to determine and vary tremendously. The peak expiratory flow rate is most useful as a relative value by comparing it to the same patient over time.

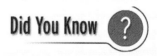

Bronchoconstriction occurs when contraction of the smooth muscle decreases the internal diameter of the bronchiole and dramatically decreases the airflow to a portion of the lungs. Bronchoconstriction is an important defense mechanism against the inhalation of toxins, but widespread bronchoconstriction can be life threatening.

Skill Drill

4-6 Peak Expiratory Flow Measurement

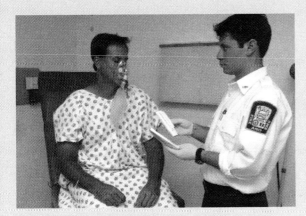

1 Place the patient in a seated position with legs dangling. Assemble the flowmeter and make sure that it reads zero.

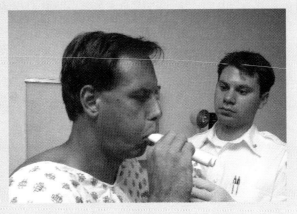

2 Ask the patient to take a deep breath, place the mouthpiece in his or her mouth, and ask the patient to exhale as forcefully as possible. Make sure that no air leaks around the device or comes from the patient's nose. Peak expiratory flow varies based on sex, height, and age. Normal adults have a peak expiratory flow rate of 350 to 750 L/min.

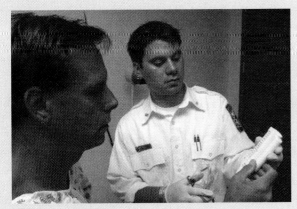

3 Perform the test three times, and take the best rate of the three.

An increasing peak expiratory flow rate suggests that the patient is responding to therapy. A decreasing peak expiratory flow rate may be an early indication that the patient's condition is deteriorating.

Identifying Threats to the Lower Airway

Patency of the lower airway is assessed most commonly by **auscultation**. Generally, wheezes indicate localized or widespread bronchoconstriction. Diminished or absent breath sounds in a specific location indicate that a portion of the lung is not being ventilated, often because of a lower airway obstruction. Unilaterally decreased breath sounds may suggest an obstruction at the level of the bronchi or a pneumothorax. Bilaterally diminished or absent breath sounds may indicate widespread severe bronchoconstriction or **hypoventilation**. Crackles or rales indicate fluid accumulation in the alveoli and small airways. A chest radiograph often provides additional information helpful in decision making. Unfortunately, this information is not available to you in the prehospital setting.

Ventilatory Efficiency

Ventilatory efficiency is a subjective assessment of the work of breathing. Normal breathing is extremely efficient and requires no conscious effort. As breathing becomes labored, its efficiency decreases, and more energy must be expended to meet the body's needs. Assessing the efficiency of ventilation is of primary importance for every patient and is often misunderstood or oversimplified. Unfortunately, no single variable or assessment technique provides a complete picture of ventilatory efficiency. You have to consider all of the signs, symptoms, and data available to you. You must place all of this information into the clinical context and consider the patient's complaints, presentation, and history.

Effective ventilation requires a patent airway and a well-functioning respiratory system. Ventilatory effectiveness is assessed in terms of **respiratory rate**, ventilatory depth, regularity, and effort. The complete assessment of ventilatory function includes visualization, auscultation, **palpation**, and quantitative data.

Respiratory distress is a term used to indicate some degree of difficulty breathing, although its determination is somewhat subjective. Patients in respiratory distress, unlike those in **respiratory failure**, are able to maintain near-normal blood gas levels and oxygenation. Respiratory distress is sometimes caused by upper or lower airway obstruction. All airway problems may cause some degree of respiratory distress, but not all respiratory distress is caused by

an airway problem. Other causes include inadequate ventilation, impairment of the respiratory muscles, heart failure, impairment of the nervous system, pneumonia, trauma, and cancer. Respiratory distress can also occur anytime that the body's need for oxygen exceeds its ability to deliver oxygen.

Most patients with ventilatory insufficiency have dyspnea. Patients often feel short of breath or say "I can't catch my breath." Dyspnea usually involves changes in the rate, regularity, depth, and/or effort of breathing. It may either result from or cause hypoxemia and tissue hypoxia. Recognizing and treating dyspnea are critical to the patient's survival because the brain and myocardium are sensitive to hypoxia.

Pulsus Paradoxus

Pulsus paradoxus is defined as a drop in systolic blood pressure during inspiration of more than 10 mm Hg. It is an important physical examination finding. Intrathoracic pressure normally changes during the respiratory cycle, and these changes in pressure typically have a small effect on blood pressure. In pathologic conditions in which a considerable increase in intrathoracic pressure occurs (such as in asthma, chronic obstructive pulmonary disease, severe congestive heart failure, or tension pneumothorax) or venous return is impeded (such as in cardiac tamponade, pericarditis, or superior vena cava syndrome), the systolic blood pressure may have more fluctuation during the respiratory cycle.

It is easiest to assess pulsus paradoxus when the patient's blood pressure is being monitored invasively, but it can be done with a sphygmomanometer and a stethoscope. First, obtain a baseline blood pressure. Reinflate the blood pressure cuff slightly higher than the initial systolic measurement and slowly deflate the cuff while observing the respiratory pattern. Note the first Korotkoff sound heard on expiration. Continue to deflate the cuff slowly and determine the first systolic sound on inspiration. A difference of more than 10 mm Hg is considered to be abnormal.

Essential Respiratory Parameters

Rate

Respiratory rate is the number of breaths taken in 1 minute. The normal respiratory rate for adults is 12 to 24 breaths/min. Children and infants breathe faster, primarily because of their higher metabolic rate. Although tachypnea or bradypnea do not necessarily indicate an underlying problem, either should be evaluated for a possible cause. Often these alterations in respiratory rate are caused by fear, anxiety, pain, stress, or exercise; however, you must seriously consider the possibility of impending respiratory distress or respiratory failure.

Depth

The normal resting tidal volume is 5 to 7 mL/kg with inhalation and exhalation. Exchanging this volume of air does not require the use of **accessory muscles** during inspiration or expiration. Hypoventilation is associated with smaller chest movements. **Hyperventilation** results in larger chest wall and abdominal wall excursion and may involve accessory muscle use.

The rate and depth of breathing are closely related. Both are important criteria for assessing the efficiency of breathing. Within limits, minute volume (the product of both tidal volume and respiratory rate) is more important than considering rate or depth independently (see Chapter 3 for a more complete discussion of minute volume).

Minute volume, however, does not take into account the energy expended to move the air. It is important to keep in mind that deep slow breathing is more efficient than rapid shallow breathing because the amount of anatomic dead space is the same regardless of the tidal volume. In shallow breathing, dead space accounts for a larger percentage of the inspired air. Because the normal reaction to "air hunger" is to breathe more quickly and less deeply, it is often necessary to coach patients who are panting to increase the depth of their breathing. Greater depth will decrease the respiratory rate, increase the percentage of inspired air that reaches the lungs, and increase ventilatory efficiency. ▼ **Table 4-2** provides details about different rates and depths of breathing.

Case Study

Case Study, Part 3

With no witnesses to report how the patient fell to the floor and because of the injury to his lip, you decide to stabilize him to protect his cervical spine. You perform this procedure, keeping a close watch on his ventilatory status. Your partner continues to "bag" the patient, although it becomes clearly difficult to do so as the cervical collar is applied. You quickly reassess the patient's vital signs as follows:

Vital Signs

Recording time
9 minutes after patient contact

Skin signs
Remains pale, diaphoretic

Pulse rate/quality
98 beats/min, regular

Blood pressure
132 mm Hg by palpation

Respiratory rate/depth
12 breaths/min, shallow; assisted with a BVM device at 20 breaths/min

Pupils
Dilated, sluggish to react, equal

SpO$_2$
90% on 100% oxygen

Electrocardiogram
Sinus rhythm

Question 4: Are you satisfied with the patient's condition?

Question 5: What would you consider your next treatment options?

CASE STUDY

Table 4-2 Characteristics of Different Rates and Depths of Breathing							
	Tidal volume	Respiratory rate (breaths/min)	Volume per minute (L)	Dead space	Alveolar air per breath (mL) = tidal volume − dead space	Alveolar air/tidal volume (%)	Alveolar air per minute (L/min)
Rapid, shallow breathing	250	40	10	150	100	40	4
Normal breathing	500	18	150	150	350	70	6.3
Slow, deep breathing	1,000	12	150	150	850	85	10.2

Regularity

Normal breathing has a steady, even pattern. Any breathing pattern that is not regular is considered to be abnormal. Speech and pain can interrupt the regularity of breathing and should not be interpreted as pathologic. Once these causes have been ruled out, any irregularity in the breathing pattern should be considered significant until proven otherwise. ▼ **Table 4-3** describes common irregular patterns of respiration and their causes.

It is often difficult to determine the cause of a particular respiratory pattern because the underlying pathologic condition is unknown. For example, it is almost impossible to differentiate between Kussmaul respirations and central neurogenic hyperventilation by rate, regularity, and depth alone in an unresponsive

Table 4-3
Patterns of Respiration

Name	Description	Common causes
Normal	Regularly spaced breaths of the same depth	Normal
Cheyne-Stokes	Crescendo-decrescendo breathing with periods of apnea	Anoxia
		Increased intracranial pressure
		Infection
		Edema
		Hydrocephalus
		Tumor
		Cerebrovascular accident
		Diastolic hypotension
		Cardiac failure
		Normal sleep in infants and the elderly
Kussmaul	Rapid, deep, regular breathing caused by metabolic changes	Diabetic ketoacidosis
		Uremia
		Shock
		Sepsis
		Pneumonia
Central neurogenic hyperventilation	Rapid breathing caused by neurologic changes	Brain stem dysfunction
		Transtentorial herniation
Apneustic	Irregular, slow breathing, often involving breath holding	Pontine level dysfunction
		Basilar artery occlusion
		Anoxia
		Meningitis
		Incipient herniation
Cluster	Intermittent periods of breathing	Cerebral hemorrhage
		Pontine hemorrhage
		Acute demyelination illnesses
		Poisonings (narcotics, barbiturates)
		Incipient herniation
Ataxic	Cluster breathing caused by dysfunction of the medullary respiratory centers	Medullary dysfunction
		Medullary tumor
Shallow	Regular breathing with minimal chest wall movement	Coma
		Narcotics overdose
Biot's or agonal respiration	Infrequent weak, irregular, chest wall movement	Terminal event
		Sudden cardiac death

patient with an unknown condition. However, combined with other assessment and history clues (history of diabetes, breath odor, medical identification device [tag or card], history of trauma), the breathing pattern can provide additional information about the underlying problem.

Effort

A strong indication of respiratory difficulty is the effort needed to breathe. Normal breathing is effortless. When breathing requires effort, you should search for a cause. One of the best ways to assess respiratory effort is to note how well the patient breathes while talking. Normally a person can talk easily while breathing. As breathing occupies the patient's thoughts, however, the need for oxygen outweighs the need to communicate. The patient becomes reluctant to speak and uses only short sentences. "One-word dyspnea" is a phrase for the situation in which a patient can only speak one word before pausing to breathe. One- or two-word dyspnea suggests severe respiratory distress.

Visualization

Much information about a patient's respiratory efficiency can be gained by simple observation. The first clue to respiratory function is body position. Patients experiencing respiratory difficulty seek a position in which breathing is easier. Patients in respiratory distress generally avoid being supine. They sit upright or lean forward in the tripod position (▼ Figure 4-9). Patients experiencing respiratory difficulty secondary to pulmonary edema may experience orthopnea, which is dyspnea that occurs in a supine position. A telltale sign of congestive heart failure is **paroxysmal nocturnal dyspnea**, which occurs when pulmonary edema causes hunger for air after the patient has been asleep for a few hours. These patients often sleep with several pillows to breathe more easily and avoid being awakened.

Deoxygenated blood is darker than oxygenated blood. As the amount of deoxygenated blood increases, the patient's skin, nail beds, and mucous membranes turn bluish, which is called cyanosis. Cyanosis is a late sign of hypoxia and indicates the condition is profound. Never wait for cyanosis to occur before identifying hypoxia, and if you notice cyanosis, you should realize that hypoxia is profound. Patients with chronic hypoxemia may have clubbing of the fingers and toes. Clubbing is a broadening and thickening of the fingers or toes with increased curvature of the finger and the tip of the nail (▼ Figure 4-10).

A good measure of the level of respiratory distress in patients is the amount of work required for them to breathe. In normal conditions, breathing only uses the external intercostal muscles and the diaphragm. As breathing becomes more difficult,

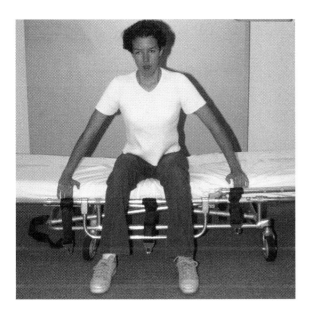

Figure 4-9 The tripod position.

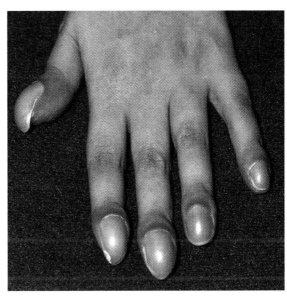

Figure 4-10 Clubbing of the fingers and toes.

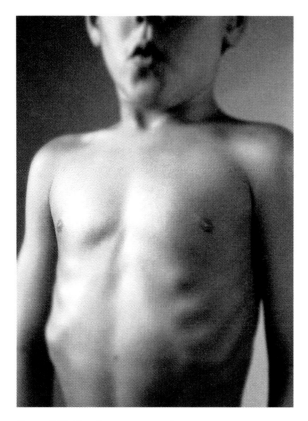

Figure 4-11 Use of accessory muscles.

additional muscles must be used. The use of the abdominal and neck muscles during inspiration and the internal intercostal muscles during expiration is called accessory muscle breathing and suggests a substantial increase in respiratory effort (▲ Figure 4-11).

The increased negative intrapulmonic pressure resulting from using accessory muscles may cause a retraction of the tissue overlying the thoracic cavity. Look for retraction between the ribs (intercostal retractions), just above the clavicle (supraclavicular retraction), and at the suprasternal notch during inspiration. It is much easier to see retractions in thin patients and children.

Observing a patient's face also provides important information. In addition to observing cyanosis of the lips, a patient's expressions may indicate anxiety related to the level of respiratory distress. Flaring of the nostrils, which occurs as an involuntary attempt to decrease the resistance to airflow, suggests severe respiratory distress. Some patients may exhale through pursed lips in order to create back pressure; this helps maintain lower airway and alveolar patency in patients with chronic obstructive pulmonary disease.

Auscultation

Your sense of hearing provides a tremendous amount of information about a patient's level of respiratory distress. If you hear a patient gasping for air, consider that a sign of significant respiratory difficulty. If a patient is unconscious, place your ear next to the mouth and nose. If the patient is breathing, you should be able to hear air moving in and out.

Auscultation of all lung fields is important for patients who complain of respiratory difficulty (▼ Figure 4-12). Wheezing usually suggests bronchoconstriction, while crackles suggest pulmonary edema or congestion. Diminished or absent breath

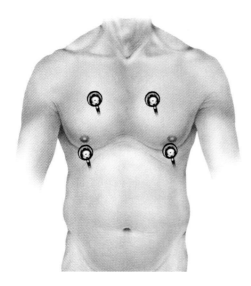
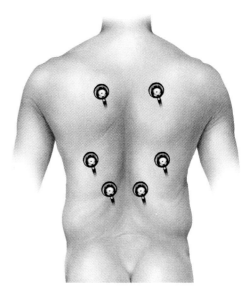

Figure 4-12 Auscultation of lung fields.

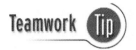

Teamwork Tip

As you will learn, preventing obstructions from entering the upper airway is the best approach to airway management. For example, the use of the Sellick maneuver during basic airway management of unconscious, near-apneic patients will simultaneously reduce the possibility of vomiting while increasing ventilatory volumes. To perform this procedure effectively requires practice among team members.

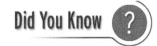

Did You Know ?

Widespread absent or diminished breath sounds are an ominous sign and often are a precursor to respiratory failure or arrest.

sounds result from inadequate airflow or pneumothorax and can be caused by severe bronchoconstriction, lower airway obstruction, or simply not breathing with an adequate tidal volume. Diminished breath sounds may also result from lung surgery or removal of a lung.

Percussion

Percussion involves tapping the fingertips against the surface of the skin to determine the characteristics of the underlying tissue (▼ Figure 4-13). Percussion provides additional valuable information, especially if breath sounds are diminished or absent. Normal resonance indicates that the underlying lung tissue is in contact with the inside of the thoracic cage and that the problem is most likely due to decreased airflow caused by an obstruction, bronchoconstriction, or hypoventilation. Hyperresonance suggests that air rather than lung tissue is in contact with the internal chest wall, suggesting a pneumothorax. Hyporesonance indicates that fluid (usually blood or exudate) or a solid mass of tissue (usually a tumor) is in contact with the internal chest wall.

Palpation

Palpation is the process of placing your hands on parts of the body in order to feel abnormalities (▼ Figure 4-14). Chest wall expansion is normally equal bilaterally. By spreading your fingers over the chest wall you can feel how much the chest wall is moving and whether its expansion is bilaterally equal. Asymmetric chest expansion indicates a unilateral obstruction, injury to one lung, or lung surgery.

If a patient has multiple ribs broken in more than one place, a free-floating section of chest wall may move in opposition to the normal chest expansion and relaxation. This paradoxical chest wall motion is relatively uncommon but occurs with flail chest segments. Paradoxical motion makes it difficult to generate enough negative pressure to ventilate normally and can represent a serious emergency.

Quantitative Information

Pulse Oximetry

Oxygen saturation (SpO_2) is the measure of the percentage of hemoglobin molecules that are bound in arterial blood. The oxyhemoglobin dissociation curve describes the relationship between oxygen saturation and the partial pressure of oxygen dissolved in the plasma (PaO_2). Because hemoglobin delivers 97% of the oxygen delivered to the body's tissues,

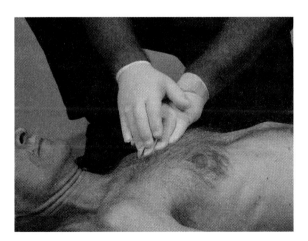

Figure 4-13 Percussion.

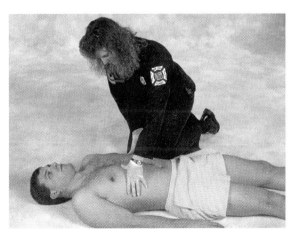

Figure 4-14 Palpation.

oxygen saturation is an excellent indication of the amount of oxygen available to the end organs. Remember that the **pulse oximeter** does *not* measure blood gases (partial pressures of oxygen or carbon dioxide dissolved in plasma) but provides an indirect but useful indication of the oxygenation of the blood.

The pulse oximeter (▼ Figure 4-15) measures oxygen saturation noninvasively. Hemoglobin saturation as measured by a pulse oximeter is abbreviated as SpO_2. The principle of the pulse oximeter is based on the fact that oxygenated blood is a different color (bright red) from deoxygenated blood (deep red). The pulse oximeter passes two wavelengths of light (red and infrared) through a vascular tissue. A photodetector determines the amount of each light wave that is absorbed by the tissue and uses this information to calculate the relative percentages of oxygenated and deoxygenated hemoglobin present in the blood passing through the arterioles. The pulse oximeter thus computes the arterial hemoglobin oxygen saturation and displays that value as a percentage on its screen.

In the past few years the pulse oximeter has become standard equipment in the treatment of emergency patients (▶ Skill Drill 4-7). The pulse oximeter provides a rapid, highly reliable, noninvasive, real-time indication of respiratory efficiency. Although its results must not be followed blindly, the careful use of the pulse oximeter provides valuable information about a patient's respiratory status.

A pulse oximeter measures the percentage of hemoglobin saturation. Under normal conditions the SpO_2 should be 98% to 100% while breathing room air. Although no definitive threshold for normal values exists, an SpO_2 of less than 96% in a nonsmoker may indicate hypoxemia. An SpO_2 of 90% corresponds to a PaO_2 of 85 mm Hg and generally requires treatment unless the patient has a chronic condition causing a perpetually low oxygenation status. Pulse

oximeters are highly reliable above 85% SpO_2. Readings below that level are less reliable but certainly indicate profound hypoxemia.

Although an SpO_2 reading is reasonably specific and sensitive at identifying hypoxemia, a high percentage of SpO_2 does not rule out tissue hypoxia. To meet the metabolic demand for oxygen, there must be an adequate amount of hemoglobin in the blood. In cases of hypovolemia or anemia, the hematocrit level or hemoglobin value, or both, may be low. In these cases, the hemoglobin that is present may be fully saturated even though the total amount of hemoglobin is inadequate, resulting in tissue hypoxia.

Keep in mind that the pulse oximeter provides a measurement of functional hemoglobin saturation, which is the ratio of saturated hemoglobin to the total hemoglobin available for binding. Hemoglobin molecules that are not available for binding are called dysfunctional. Fractional hemoglobin saturation, which is determined by laboratory instruments, is the ratio of hemoglobin molecules bound to the total number of hemoglobin molecules present. Fractional hemoglobin and functional saturation are the same if there are no dysfunctional hemoglobin molecules.

The two most common forms of dysfunctional hemoglobin molecules are carboxyhemoglobin and methemoglobin. Carbon monoxide has an affinity for hemoglobin that is 200 to 250 times greater than that of oxygen. When carbon monoxide is present in the inspired gas, it displaces oxygen from the hemoglobin, forming a molecule known as carboxyhemoglobin. Because of the ability of carbon monoxide to bind with hemoglobin, significant amounts of carboxyhemoglobin can result from small amounts of carbon monoxide in the breathing mix.

Therefore, in cases of carbon monoxide poisoning, the SpO_2 can be normal in the context of hypoxia. Methemoglobin is a hemoglobin molecule whose iron molecule has undergone oxidation; normally, less than 1% of methemoglobin is present in the bloodstream because the body has an enzyme that prevents its buildup. Methemoglobinemia (a buildup of methemoglobin in the blood) can result, however, from certain medications such as nitrates, nitrites, phenacetin, phenazopyridine (Pyridium), sulfonamides, and aniline dyes. Just as with carbon monoxide poisoning, methemoglobinemia can produce severe hypoxia with normal SpO_2 values.

To function properly, the pulse oximeter must find a pulsation in the selected tissue. The most commonly used site is a finger. In cases of significant vasoconstriction or very low perfusion states (including cardiac arrest), there may not be enough peripheral perfusion to be detected by the sensor. In these cases, move the sensor to a more central location (bridge of

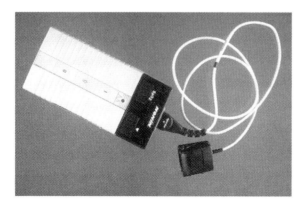

Figure 4-15 A pulse oximeter.

Skill Drill

4-7 Performing Pulse Oximetry

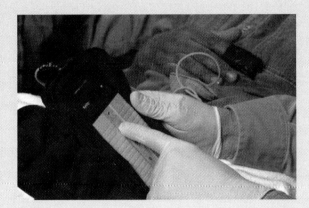

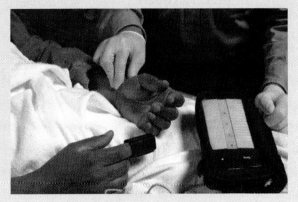

1 Clean finger and remove nail polish as needed. Place index or middle finger into pulse oximeter probe. Turn pulse oximeter on and note LED reading of SpO$_2$.

2 Palpate radial pulse to ensure that it correlates with the LED display on the pulse oximeter.

the nose or ear lobe). Inaccurate pulse oximetry readings may be caused by the following:

- Hypovolemia
- Anemia
- Severe peripheral vasoconstriction (chronic hypoxia, smoking, or hypothermia)
- Dark or metallic nail polish
- Dirty fingers
- Methemoglobinemia
- Carboxyhemoglobinemia

The pulse oximeter is a valuable adjunct to decision making, but it is not a panacea. Because of many factors, the pulse oximeter may give falsely high or low readings. Consider using pulse oximetry readings as one part of a complete patient assessment, *not* a single determination that provides all the comprehensive information you need.

Blood Gases

The most accurate static assessment of ventilatory effectiveness is a laboratory analysis of a sample of arterial blood. For practical reasons, there are limitations to the use of blood gases in emergency situations. A sample of arterial blood must be obtained, usually by inserting a needle into an artery; this takes time and is an invasive procedure. Some chronically ill patients have arterial catheters, which make taking a blood sample faster and easier, but these are not available in the prehospital setting.

Arterial blood gas analysis traditionally requires that the blood sample be sent to a laboratory for analysis, which even in the best situations takes a few minutes. For patients whose conditions are relatively stable, this short delay rarely presents a problem. This delay may be a factor for unstable patients because they may be undergoing rapid physiologic changes and a mechanical ventilator may not yet be controlling their ventilations.

Did You Know ?

The pulse oximeter provides a measurement of functional hemoglobin saturation, which is the ratio of saturated hemoglobin to the total hemoglobin available for binding. Hemoglobin molecules that are not available for binding are called dysfunctional. Fractional hemoglobin saturation, which is determined by laboratory instruments, is the ratio of hemoglobin molecules bound to the total number of hemoglobin molecules present. Fractional hemoglobin and functional saturation are the same if there are no dysfunctional hemoglobin molecules.

Despite the practical limitations, <u>arterial blood gas analysis</u> provides the most comprehensive quantitative information about ventilatory effectiveness. The arterial blood gas analysis includes the pH, the partial pressure of oxygen (PaO_2), the partial pressure of carbon dioxide ($PaCO_2$), and the bicarbonate (HCO_3^-) concentration. Because each of these variables reflects an aspect of respiration ventilation, arterial blood gas analysis is a useful barometer of the effectiveness of plumonary function.

Fortunately, new technology is making arterial blood gases and other laboratory values available at the bedside, virtually in real time. These values may prove to be of tremendous importance in emergency situations, in both in-hospital and out-of-hospital settings. New analyzers use a few milliliters of venous blood placed in a cartridge and can provide values for arterial blood gases, hemoglobin and hematocrit, and several electrolytes.

The pH is a direct measurement of the acidity of the plasma. The PaO_2 and the $PaCO_2$ are direct measurements of the amount of oxygen and carbon dioxide dissolved in the blood plasma. The HCO_3^- concentration is mathematically calculated using these known values.

Acid-base balance is a complex concept, and a comprehensive explanation is beyond the scope of this book. An overview of blood gas interpretation, however, can serve as a part of clinical decision making and a foundation for further study.

Acid-Base Balance

The rate of chemical reactions is greatly affected by the characteristics of the fluid in which these reactions occur. Variables such as temperature and acidity profoundly affect the rates of the biochemical processes in the body. The body must maintain its pH within a very narrow range for all biochemical reactions to occur at the proper rates. Even small alterations in the pH have serious consequences.

Hydrogen Ion Concentration and pH

Acidity is a measure of the concentration of hydrogen ions in a fluid. In general, pH ranges from 0 to 14. As the number of hydrogen ions increases, the pH drops. Chemically, a pH of 7.0 is defined as neutral—a pH less than 7.0 is an acid, a pH greater than 7.0 is a base. The body is usually slightly basic, having a normal pH of 7.35 to 7.45. <u>Acidosis</u> in the body is defined as a serum pH less than 7.35, and <u>alkalosis</u> is a serum pH greater than 7.45.

The by-products of chemical reactions in the cells produce more acids than bases. If not for buffers, which are chemical combinations that resist changes in pH, the serum would tend to become more and more acidic. Obviously, the body must prevent this from happening or all body cells would eventually become poisoned.

Buffer systems

Much body energy is expended maintaining the pH within the narrow range of acceptability. Buffer systems involve combinations of chemicals that resist changes to pH. Buffer systems prevent dramatic shifts in the pH by responding to excesses in acids or bases. The three most important buffers are the carbonic acid-bicarbonate buffer, the respiratory buffer, and the renal buffer. Different buffers are important in different situations. The carbonic acid-bicarbonate buffer is very fast and responds instantaneously to changes in serum pH. It constantly fine tunes the pH but usually cannot make big changes. The respiratory buffer usually takes a few minutes to respond, and the renal buffer is the slowest, taking minutes to hours. Both buffer systems, however, are able to make big changes in pH.

Carbonic Acid-Bicarbonate Buffer

Carbonic acid and bicarbonate in the plasma form an effective buffer system. Carbonic acid, which is a weak acid, and bicarbonate, a base, are both present in plasma. The kidneys control the level of bicarbonate. The level of carbonic acid is controlled indirectly by controlling the amount of carbon dioxide in the blood. This level is affected by respiratory rate; if the amount of carbonic acid decreases, the respiratory rate slows to retain more carbon dioxide.

Anytime that the concentration of hydrogen ions increases, they quickly combine with the bicarbonate ions, resulting in little sustained effect on the pH. Hydrogen ions in the carbonic acid combine with a base, reducing its effect on pH. These chemical reactions occur instantaneously and reduce short-term fluctuations in pH.

Water, carbon dioxide, carbonic acid, hydrogen ion, and bicarbonate ion are in equilibrium throughout the body. If there is excess of one component, an imbalance results that requires mitigation to maintain pH within normal range. For example, if the hydrogen ion concentration increases, it will combine with more bicarbonate ions, increasing the carbonic acid concentration. In the lungs, the carbonic acid will dissociate into water and carbon dioxide, which is eliminated by exhalation.

For this buffering system to be effective there must be about 20 times more bicarbonate ion than carbonic acid. This relationship is often expressed as a 20:1 ratio of bicarbonate to carbonic acid. As long as the body is able to keep this ratio constant, the pH will remain stable. If the serum concentration of carbonic acid rises only a little, however, there has to be a large increase in bicarbonate to keep it in balance. Any change in this ratio will result in a change in pH.

The Respiratory Buffer

The respiratory system plays a vital role in stabilizing the pH. Changes in the concentration of hydrogen ions will increase the amount of carbonic acid. If the respiratory rate increases, the carbonic acid will be eliminated from the lungs as carbon dioxide and water. If the pH of the plasma increases (becoming more alkaline), the respiratory system can return the pH to normal by decreasing the respiratory rate and thereby increasing the carbon dioxide level, which will combine with water to form carbonic acid.

The Renal Buffer

Finally, the kidneys play another important role in preventing changes in the pH. In addition to controlling the level of bicarbonate in the circulating plasma, the kidneys can excrete both hydrogen and bicarbonate in the urine. The pH of urine can vary between 4.5 and 8.0 to respond to changes in plasma acidity.

Acid-Base Imbalances

Acid-base imbalances are alterations in the pH, partial pressure of carbon dioxide, and/or bicarbonate ion concentration. Even though these buffers attempt to prevent changes in pH, fluctuations do occur (▶ Figure 4-16). In many diseases and conditions the amount of acidic or basic stress put on the body is simply too great for the buffer systems to completely correct. Even small changes in pH are dangerous and have many severe physiologic consequences.

Acid-base imbalances include acidosis and alkalosis. If the pH is too low (less than 7.35), the imbalance is defined as acidosis. If the pH is too high (greater than 7.45), the imbalance is defined as alkalosis. The two basic causes of acid-base imbalances are respiratory and metabolic. Therefore, there are four types of acid-base imbalances: respiratory acidosis, respiratory alkalosis, metabolic acidosis, and metabolic alkalosis. Respiratory acidosis and alkalosis, respectively, are pH changes caused by too much carbon dioxide or not enough elimination of carbon dioxide. Metabolic acidosis and alkalosis, respectively, are pH changes caused by too many bicarbonate ions or not enough bicarbonate ions.

Respiratory Acidosis

Carbon dioxide is continuously being produced as a by-product of cellular metabolism and must be constantly removed from the body. Respiratory acidosis results when the respiratory system does not eliminate enough carbon dioxide. When this happens,

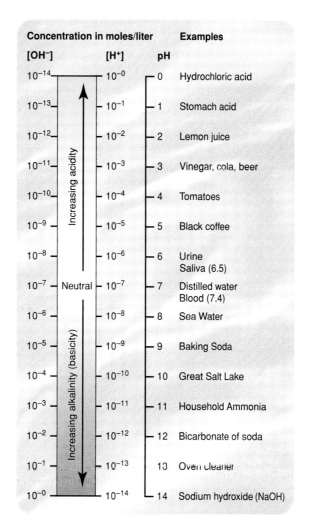

Figure 4-16 Acid-base imbalance.

carbon dioxide combines with water, forming carbonic acid, which increases the hydrogen ion concentration in the plasma. An interruption of breathing for just a few minutes can cause a profound change in pH.

Although many causes of respiratory acidosis exist, they all involve the failure of the lungs to rid the body of carbon dioxide adequately. Examples include bradypnea (which may be caused by a drug overdose), respiratory arrest, airway obstruction, pneumonia, chest injuries, pulmonary edema, asthma, and chronic obstructive pulmonary disease.

Respiratory Alkalosis

If you breathe too quickly, your lungs give off too much carbon dioxide. You may have noticed the effects of hyperventilation when you get dizzy from a few rapid deep breaths. Breathing too quickly causes more carbonic acid to dissociate, removing hydrogen ions and leaving bicarbonate ions. A decrease in hydrogen ion concentration and an increase in pH results in a condition known as respiratory alkalosis.

Although several causes of respiratory alkalosis exist, they all involve increased respiratory rates. Examples include hyperventilation caused by stress, some types of head injury or brain tumors, and a high fever.

Metabolic Acidosis

Metabolic acidosis results from an inadequate supply of bicarbonate in the body that causes the hydrogen ion concentration to increase and the pH to decrease. It may be caused by reduced production of bicarbonate ion in the kidney, as in renal failure, or by excessive elimination during severe diarrhea. Finally, an inadequate supply of bicarbonate may occur when a large influx of acid cannot be eliminated by the lungs. The most common acids include lactic acid and ketoacids. Lactic acid, produced as a result of incomplete metabolism of sugar, accumulates when the energy demand of the cells exceeds the ability to deliver oxygen (such as during exercise, seizures, respiratory failure, or heart failure). Because lactic acid cannot be eliminated through the lungs, it uses up the body's stores of bicarbonate. Because patients with diabetes are not able to burn sugar, they use proteins instead of carbohydrates as an energy source, which forms a ketoacid by-product that cannot be eliminated in the lungs but must be neutralized by bicarbonate ions.

Metabolic Alkalosis

Metabolic alkalosis, the least common acid-base imbalance, results from excess bicarbonate in the body. The bicarbonate ions combine with hydrogen ions, decreasing the concentration of hydrogen ions in the serum and increasing the pH. This imbalance can follow severe vomiting, where hydrochloric acid is lost from the stomach, an overdose of antacid medication, or hypokalemia.

Compensation

Even a small change in the pH of body fluids can dramatically affect the body's metabolism. If the pH changes too much, cells are directly damaged. Cell death can occur if the pH falls below 6.8 or rises above 7.8. For this reason, the body has a mechanism that compensates for the buffer systems when they cannot adequately stabilize pH within normal ranges. It takes a few minutes for these compensatory systems to take effect, but they can restore homeostasis temporarily and sometimes mean the difference between life and death.

Compensation is the body's attempt to return the pH to normal range. The respiratory system compensates for metabolic causes of pH change, and the metabolic system compensates for respiratory causes of pH change. As long as the body can maintain the 20:1 ratio of bicarbonate to carbonic acid the pH will remain normal and the imbalance will be compensated. If this ratio cannot be maintained, the pH will change, and the imbalance will be decompensated.

Blood Gas Analysis

Blood gas analysis gives you important information about acid-base balance in the body. Understanding the basic concepts of blood gases will help you understand many of your clinical situations even when you do not have blood gas readings available.

Most arterial blood gas measurements are derived from a sample of arterial blood usually taken from the radial or femoral artery. The sample is collected in a glass tube and kept on ice until laboratory analysis. The most important values obtained from blood gas analysis are the PaO_2, the $PaCO_2$, the serum pH, and the HCO_3^- (▼ **Table 4-4**). The levels of PaO_2 and $PaCO_2$ indicate the amount of the gas dissolved in the plasma.

The PaO_2 is an important variable, but it does not affect acid-base balance. For a quick analysis of acid-base balance, three variables need to be obtained—the $PaCO_2$, the serum pH, and the HCO_3^-. Although a thorough blood gas analysis can provide more useful information than the simplistic approach presented here, this information can help you understand some of the clinical situations you will encounter involving acid-base imbalance.

To understand this concept better, follow these steps:

- Evaluate the serum pH to determine whether it is normal (7.35 to 7.45), acidotic (<7.35) or alkalotic (>7.45)
- Evaluate the $PaCO_2$ to determine whether it is normal (35 to 42 mm Hg), low (<35 mm Hg), or high (>42 mm Hg)
- Evaluate the HCO_3^- to determine whether it is normal (20 to 28 mEq/L), low (<20 mEq/L), or high (>28 mEq/L)

Table 4-4
Normal Arterial Blood Gas Levels

PaO_2	80–100 mm Hg
$PaCO_2$	35–42 mm Hg
pH	7.35–7.45
HCO_3^-	22–26 mEq/L

Then apply the following rules:

- pH determines acidosis or alkalosis:
  - Normal pH is either normal or compensated.
  - Normal pH with normal carbon dioxide and HCO_3- is normal.
  - Normal pH with abnormal carbon dioxide or HCO_3- is compensated.
  - Low pH indicates acidosis.
  - High pH indicates alkalosis.
- Carbon dioxide represents the respiratory involvement:
  - Normal carbon dioxide with abnormal pH indicates an acute metabolic acid-base change without compensation.
  - High carbon dioxide with abnormal pH indicates respiratory acidosis or respiratory compensation for metabolic alkalosis.
  - Low carbon dioxide with abnormal pH indicates respiratory alkalosis or respiratory compensation for metabolic acidosis.
- HCO_3- represents the metabolic involvement:
  - Normal HCO_3- with an abnormal pH indicates acute respiratory acid base changes without compensation.
  - High HCO_3- with an abnormal pH indicates metabolic acidosis or metabolic compensation for respiratory acidosis.
  - Low HCO_3- with an abnormal pH indicates metabolic alkalosis or metabolic compensation for respiratory alkalosis.

These situations are summarized in ▶ **Table 4-5**. Notice that the rules are mutually exclusive: only one interpretation is possible for each set of blood gases. It is more important to understand the rules that lead to the values, rather than simply memorizing the table. In this way you can analyze blood gas problems rather than relying on memorized rules that you may forget.

Partial Pressure of Oxygen

Most blood gas analyses report the PaO_2 in the arterial gas sampled. The PaO_2 does not affect the acid-base balance, but provides valuable clinical information. Remember that PaO_2 represents the amount of oxygen dissolved in the plasma, which only represents a small percentage of the oxygen delivered to the body's tissues, but it is an important indication of respiratory effectiveness. A healthy patient breathing 21% oxygen (room air) should have a PaO_2 of 80 to 100 mm Hg. If the PaO_2 is less than 80 mm Hg, the patient is hypoxemic and

Table 4-5
pH, CO₂, and HCO₃- Changes in Acid-Base Imbalances

	pH	CO₂	HCO₃-
Normal	Normal	Normal	Normal
Respiratory acidosis	Low	High	Normal
Compensated respiratory acidosis	Normal	High	High
Respiratory alkalosis	High	Low	Normal
Compensated respiratory alkalosis	Normal	Low	Low
Metabolic acidosis	Low	Normal	Low
Compensated metabolic acidosis	Normal	High	Low
Metabolic alkalosis	High	Normal	High
Compensated metabolic alkalosis*	Normal	High	High

*The ability of the respiratory system to fully compensate for metabolic alkalosis is limited by the fact that you cannot decrease the respiratory rate infinitely or hypoxia will develop. Because hyperventilation is tiring and respiratory rates of more than 40 breaths/min are difficult to maintain for any significant period of time, patients with severe metabolic acidosis are also rarely able to compensate with respiratory mechanisms.

should be given supplemental oxygen immediately and closely monitored.

Expect a higher PaO_2 in a patient receiving supplemental oxygen or ventilatory support. Remember that a patient who is receiving 50% oxygen and who has a PaO_2 of 100 mm Hg would be severely hypoxic if breathing room air.

Clinical Decision Making

The decision to intervene is usually more difficult than the actual intervention. Many pieces of assessment data need to be integrated in order to see the "big picture." No single piece of information can determine the effectiveness of ventilation. Rather, you must look at all the information and make a thoughtful decision about the most appropriate course of action.

In general, you must integrate all the assessment findings to make a judgment about the level of respiratory difficulty. This takes practice. After seeing many patients with respiratory complaints, you will become skilled at evaluating distress. Think of respiratory difficulty as a continuum ranging from one extreme of no respiratory difficulty through respiratory distress to respiratory failure and respiratory arrest.

Respiratory distress is often categorized as mild, moderate, or severe. Unfortunately, no single assessment finding makes it easy to distinguish among these levels. ▼ **Table 4-6** provides a general guide for categories of respiratory distress, but you should be careful not to apply it rigidly.

Increasing respiratory effort requires a lot of energy, and eventually the patient will become fatigued. Unresolved, untreated respiratory distress will progress to respiratory failure as the patient can no longer compensate by increasing respiratory function. Respiratory failure is a transitional phase leading to respiratory arrest and death, and therefore it must be identified and treated aggressively.

The distinction between severe respiratory distress and respiratory failure is somewhat subjective. In general, the patient is clearly in respiratory failure if his or her level of consciousness begins to decrease as a result of respiratory distress. At this point, the patient has severe hypoxia and hypercapnia, and blood gas levels are no longer consistent with consciousness. This ominous sign requires immediate action.

Decision Making: The Risk Versus Benefit Ratio

Decision making involves balancing the risks and benefits of treatment. This balancing is important for airway interventions. Noninvasive tests and interventions, such as pulse oximetry and manual positioning, involve little risk but great opportunity to gain valuable information or provide therapeutic benefit. They can therefore be initiated quickly and require little deliberation. Invasive interventions, such as arterial blood gas sampling, intubation, and cricothyrotomy, have the potential both to help and

Table 4-6
Categories of Respiratory Distress

	Mild	**Moderate**	**Severe**
Respiratory rate	Increased	Significantly increased	Dramatically increased
Depth	Usually deep	Usually deep	May be shallow and panting
Effort	Slightly anxious, usually able to converse and answer questions	Increased anxiety, usually able to answer questions in short phrases	Very anxious, completely fixated on breathing, one- or two-word dyspnea
Position	Usually upright, but may not have a positional preference	Upright, lies down for a few seconds, but will immediately move back to upright position	Bolt upright
Skin color	Normal	Pale	Cyanotic
Respiratory effort	Increased	Significantly increased	Dramatically increased
Accessory muscle use	Not usually	Some	Usually
Retractions	Not usually	Occasionally some slight intercostal or supraclavicular retractions	Usually seen, especially in thin or young patients
Nasal flaring	Rarely	Occasionally	Often
Pulse oximetry	>96%	90%–96%	<90%
Blood gases	Usually normal	Some hypoxemia	Hypoxemia and hypercapnia

to do harm. They typically involve more risk, take more time, and are more costly and therefore require more consideration and evaluation in order to determine if the risks are outweighed by potential benefits for the patient.

Beware of the Technical Imperative

Decision makers sometimes fall into a trap called the technical imperative, which is to perform an intervention because it is possible rather than because it is indicated. An example in airway management is the decision to intubate a patient when effective ventilation is possible without an endotracheal tube. If you need only to support ventilation for a short period of time and can manage the airway and ventilate effectively with a simple technique, the risks of intubation may not outweigh its benefits.

Beware of the Low Self-Efficacy Reluctance Syndrome

The opposite of the technical imperative is called the low self-efficacy reluctance syndrome. Self-efficacy is the confidence that you have in your ability to implement your plan successfully. Although you should not perform a procedure in which you lack confidence, questioning your ability can lead to the rationalization that the procedure is not indicated. Whenever you decide not to perform a procedure, ask yourself, "Why did I make this decision?" If you are intimidated by the skill or reluctant to perform it on this patient, be honest with yourself and your colleagues. Manage this patient with the best of your ability with the skills in which you have confidence, and get backup help immediately. Do not complicate the problem by convincing yourself or others that "It was not really necessary." Such rationalization deprives the patient of needed care and can lead to future mistakes. When the situation resolves, make every effort to practice the skill and improve your confidence.

Case Study

Case Study, Part 4

After orally intubating the patient while maintaining cervical spine precautions, you and your partner load the patient into the ambulance for transport to the emergency department. There is little change in the patient's condition, although his vital signs appear to have improved as follows:

Vital Signs

Lung sounds
Equal bilaterally

Skin signs
Remains pale

Pulse rate/quality
86 beats/min, regular

Blood pressure
132/74 mm Hg

Respiratory rate/depth
Assisted at 20 breaths/min; spontaneous at 12 breaths/min

Pupils
Midrange, sluggish to react, equal

SpO₂
98% on 100% oxygen

Electrocardiogram
Sinus rhythm

At the hospital, you provide a short report to the resuscitation team, who take over care of the patient. Because the patient is unconscious and has no gag reflex, the attending physician elects to keep the patient intubated with a ventilator to manage the mechanics of breathing. Several hours later, you find out that the patient has improved dramatically; surprisingly, there appears to be minimal aspiration trauma to the lungs. A toxicology screen later reveals that the patient had ingested a significant amount of alcohol and GHB ("liquid X"), a common (and potentially dangerous) club "cocktail."

CASE STUDY

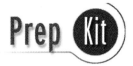

Chapter Summary

The ability to evaluate the effectiveness of ventilation and respiration quickly and accurately is critical to making appropriate intervention decisions. Unfortunately, no single sign, symptom, or test provides enough information to make good decisions.

EMT-Ps need to integrate all of the available information to make safe, effective decisions.

Patency of the airway from the nose and mouth to alveoli is essential for effective air exchange.

The body uses a variety of mechanisms to protect airway patency, including the gag reflex, coughing, and sneezing.

Loss of one or more of these protective mechanisms may allow unusual conditions such as excessive secretions or vomiting to threaten this patency.

The identification of these threats to airway patency is essential to the management of the patient's condition.

The ability to assess the ventilatory status of a patient quickly yet accurately is the hallmark of a good EMT-P.

The rate, depth, and effort of breathing are key parameters to measure both qualitatively and quantitatively.

Although the concepts of acid-base balance, acidosis, and alkalosis can be confusing and difficult to grasp, doing so may lead to a greater understanding of the patient who experiences respiratory distress.

Your choice of treatment must be appropriate for the patient's condition—not too aggressive, and not too timid.

Vital Vocabulary

accessory muscles Muscles other than the diaphragm and external intercostal muscles, which are used in times of increased respiratory demand. They include the sternocleidomastoid muscle, abdominal muscles, and the internal intercostal muscles.

acidosis In the body, a pH of less than 7.35.

alkalosis In the body, a pH of greater than 7.45.

arterial blood gas analysis A test using a sample of arterial blood that provides a quantitative assessment of the pH, bicarbonate ion concentration, and the partial pressures of oxygen and carbon dioxide.

aspiration The entry of fluids or solids into the tracheo-bronchial passages, causing partial or complete lower airway obstruction and/or damage to bronchial or lung tissue.

auscultation The process of listening to sounds in the body, usually with a stethoscope.

bronchoconstriction A condition in which the smooth muscles in the bronchioles constrict, causing decreased air-flow to some portion of the lung.

complete airway obstruction Condition in which a foreign object or soft tissue completely occludes the flow of any air into the lungs.

cough reflex A reflex action that causes the patient to cough when part of the airway is stimulated.

crowing A high-pitched sound on inspiration caused by an incomplete airway obstruction with poor air exchange.

cyanosis A bluish tint of the mucous membranes and nail beds, a late sign of hypoxemia.

dyspnea A feeling of difficulty breathing.

eyelash reflex A quivering of the lower eyelid when the upper eyelash is gently stroked.

foreign body airway obstruction An airway obstruction caused by a foreign body (ie, gum, dentures, blood, vomit, or broken teeth) in the airway.

gag reflex A protective reflex that attempts expulsion of foreign objects from the airway.

hyperventilation Minute volume greater than normal.

hypoventilation Minute volume less than normal.

incomplete airway obstruction Condition in which a foreign object or soft tissue partially occludes the flow of air into the lungs. Incomplete airway obstructions are classified as having either good or poor air exchange.

laryngospasm A protective reflex involving the spasmodic closure of the vocal cords that prevents the aspiration of foreign objects into the trachea.

palpation The process of placing your hands on parts of the body in order to feel abnormalities.

paroxysmal nocturnal dyspnea A condition in which pulmonary edema causes air hunger after the patient has been asleep (supine) for a few hours.

patent Open, clear of obstruction.

peak expiratory flow A measurement of the force of a patient's exhalation.

percussion The tapping the fingertips against the surface of the skin to determine the characteristics of the underlying tissue.

pulse oximeter A machine that uses infrared spectroscopy to determine the percentage of arterial hemoglobin bound with oxygen.

pulsus paradoxus A 10 mm Hg or greater drop in the systolic blood pressure during inspiration.

respiratory arrest The absence of respiration.

respiratory distress A condition in which the patient is having difficulty breathing but is able to maintain near-normal blood gas levels and oxygenation. Respiratory distress is subjectively divided into mild, moderate, and severe.

respiratory failure Condition in which a patient's respiratory distress has progressed to the point of severe alterations in blood gases, oxygen saturation, and/or decreased level of consciousness.

respiratory rate The number of breaths taken in 1 minute.

retractions Concavity of the soft tissue overlying bone in the thoracic cage during inhalation; a sign of increased work of breathing.

sneeze reflex A sudden, forceful exhalation caused by irritation of the nose or nasal passages.

snoring The sound created by air passing a soft-tissue partial occlusion of the airway, usually the tongue.

Case Study Answers

Question 1: What are some of the threats to your patient's airway patency?

Answer: There are many threats to this patient's airway. The most immediate threat is any vomit, blood, or secretions in the mouth and airway. Aspiration pneumonia has a high mortality rate and occurs when vomit is aspirated into the lungs. In addition, the tongue and epiglottis are also threats because this patient lacks the muscular control necessary to keep the tongue off of the posterior pharyngeal wall.

Question 2: What are your initial management steps?

Answer: Creating and maintaining a patent airway are critical for this patient's condition. However, the need to simultaneously manage a potential cervical spine injury is also important. Therefore, manual in-line spine stabilization and a jaw-thrust maneuver will be most appropriate as the initial steps. Additionally, clearing the oral cavity of vomit will be necessary. A combination of finger sweeps and mechanical suction will be useful in accomplishing this task.

Question 3: What would be your next step(s) in the management of this patient's condition?

Answer: With the airway patent, now is the time to move ahead in the management process. Because this patient appears to be compensating poorly (shallow respirations, marginal oxygen saturation), the use of an assisted ventilation device such as a BVM with high-flow oxygen will be necessary to overcome ventilatory obstacles. Intubation becomes a strong possibility at this point because of the continuing danger of aspiration.

Question 4: Are you satisfied with the patient's condition?

Answer: Even though your partner is doing his best to ventilate the patient, the oxygen saturation remains low, and skin signs remain poor.

Question 5: What would you consider your next treatment options?

Answer: Intubation becomes necessary now. The use of in-line manual stabilization of the cervical spine and oral intubation using a straight-blade laryngoscope will be needed to complete this task. Suction equipment should be immediately available. Transport of the patient should be initiated as soon as possible.

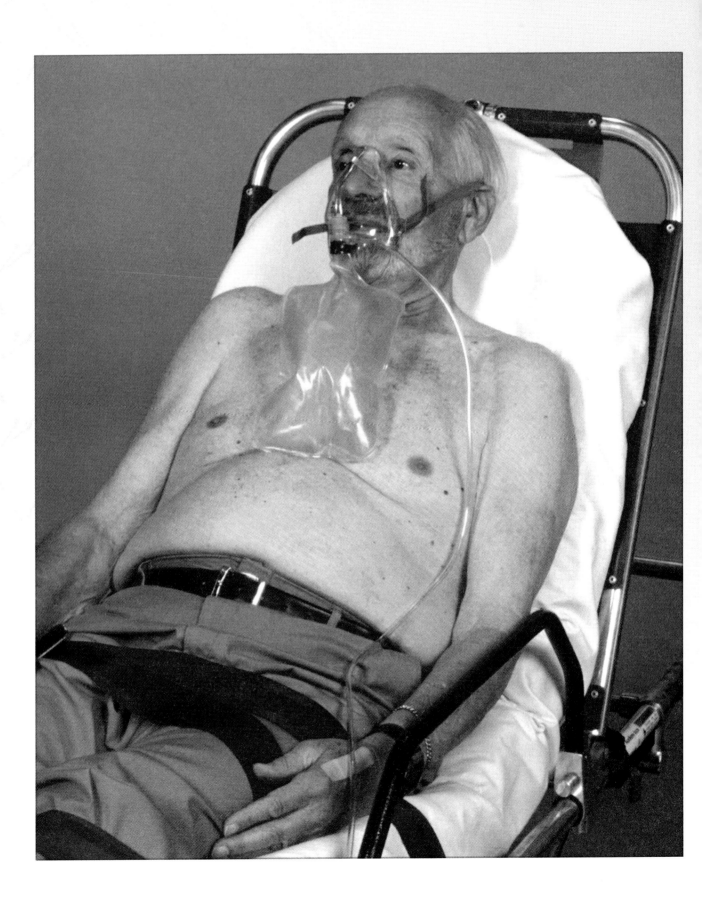

Objectives

Cognitive Objectives

2-1.14 Define atelectasis. (p 96)

2-1.15 Define FiO_2. (p 79)

2-1.47 Explain safety considerations of oxygen storage and delivery. (p 85)

2-1.48 Identify types of oxygen cylinders and pressure regulators (including a high-pressure regulator and a therapy regulator). (p 82)

2-1.49 List the steps for delivering oxygen from a cylinder and regulator. (p 86)

2-1.50 Describe the use, advantages, and disadvantages of an oxygen humidifier. (p 85)

2-1.51 Describe the indications, contra-indications, advantages, disadvantages, complications, liter flow range, and concentration of delivered oxygen for supplemental oxygen delivery devices. (p 86)

2-1.52 Define, identify, and describe a tracheostomy, stoma, and tracheostomy tube. (p 94)

Psychomotor Objectives

2-1.98 Perform oxygen delivery from a cylinder and regulator with an oxygen delivery device. (p 84) (Skill Drill 5-1)

2-1.99 Perform oxygen delivery with an oxygen humidifier. (p 87) (Skill Drill 5-2)

2-1.100 Deliver supplemental oxygen to a breathing patient using the following devices:

   a. Nasal cannula (p 87) (Skill Drill 5-2)

   b. Simple face mask (p 89) (Skill Drill 5-3)

   c. Nonrebreathing mask (p 90) (Skill Drill 5-4)

   d. Partial rebreathing mask (p 92) (Skill Drill 5-5)

   e. Venturi mask (p 93) (Skill Drill 5-6)

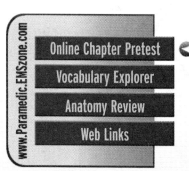

www.Paramedic.EMSzone.com

TECHNOLOGY

Online Chapter Pretest

Vocabulary Explorer

Anatomy Review

Web Links

Chapter FEATURES

Case Studies

Skill Drills

Teamwork Tips

Documentation Tips

Paramedic Safety Tips

Special Needs Tips

Vital Vocabulary

Prep Kit

The irreparable widespread tissue damage associated with hypoxia results in death. This simple fact emphasizes the importance of a constant delivery of oxygen to all body cells. The oxygen content of room air is approximately 21% (▼ **Table 5-1**). Under normal circumstances this provides enough oxygen to meet the metabolic demands of the body. In a medical or physiologic crisis, room air may no longer be able to provide enough oxygen to the body, and supplemental oxygen therapy is needed.

Every cell in the body needs oxygen. Oxygen is required for the conversion of glucose (fuel) into the energy needed for cells to perform their function. This process is analogous to a furnace burning wood (fuel) to generate heat (energy). If the furnace is deprived of oxygen, the fire goes out. If the oxygen supply is decreased, the fire may continue to smolder, but it will not be as efficient. When hypoxia occurs, the cell's "furnaces" are not as efficient at converting glucose into energy. Under these anaerobic conditions, toxins accumulate as a result of the incomplete combustion. By increasing the oxygen delivered to the cells, you can revive all of these tiny fires.

Supplemental Oxygen

Oxygen is the most common drug administered to emergency patients (▼ Figure 5-1). Although it should not be used indiscriminately, oxygen has few side effects and a great potential to benefit many patients. For this reason it should be and is used liberally with emergency patients. Air enriched with oxygen provides more oxygen to the body's cells and increases the body's ability to compensate for circulatory or respiratory compromise and can decrease systemic or local hypoxia. ▼ **Table 5-2** lists general guidelines for which patients should receive supplemental oxygen. As you can see, this list encompasses a large number of conditions. Although such guidelines are helpful, understanding how oxygen helps patients in crisis will help you better decide when to administer oxygen and how much to give.

Oxygen is transported in the body in two ways: bound to hemoglobin (SO_2) and dissolved in plasma (PaO_2). Increasing the percentage of oxygen in the inspired gas increases both SO_2 and PaO_2. If the SO_2 is decreased, an increase in the percentage of oxygen in the breathing gas will make more oxygen molecules available for transport by hemoglobin. This is particularly helpful in situations in which the perfusion exceeds ventilation. Dramatic increases in the hemoglobin saturation (SpO_2) often result from supplementing the breathing mix with oxygen. This can significantly affect the amount of oxygen available to the tissues.

Unfortunately, the pulse oximeter does not provide all of the information needed to make sound decisions about oxygen delivery. The SpO_2 represents

Table 5-1	
Composition of Air	
Nitrogen	78.08%
Oxygen	20.95%
Argon	0.93%
Carbon dioxide	0.03%

Table 5-2
Patient Conditions that Warrant Administration of Supplemental Oxygen
• Difficulty breathing
• Respiratory compromise from any cause
• Circulatory compromise
• Shock
• Decreased level of consciousness
• SpO_2 of less than 96%
• Any hypoxic/ischemic mechanism of cell damage

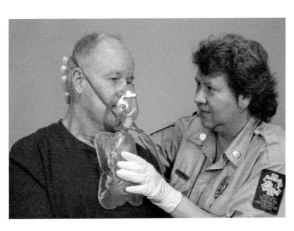

Figure 5-1 Patient receiving oxygen.

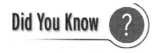

only the percentage of available hemoglobin that is saturated; it does not tell you whether the hemoglobin is saturated with oxygen. Additionally, the pulse oximeter does not tell you whether the oxygen is being adequately delivered to the tissues, which can be a problem in cases of poisoning. Oxygen saturation readings also can give a false sense of security in cases of anemia or hypovolemia in which there is an inadequate supply of hemoglobin. The saturation of hemoglobin may be high even while the patient remains hypoxic.

Supplemental oxygen is frequently indicated in patients with normal SpO_2 readings. Even with normal saturation, supplemental oxygen increases the amount of oxygen dissolved in the plasma (PaO_2). The more oxygen a patient inhales, the more oxygen is dissolved in plasma. This is why it can be valuable to treat any condition that involves a hypoxic or ischemic mechanism of tissue damage (eg, acute myocardial infarction or stroke) with a high percentage of oxygen, regardless of the pulse oximeter reading.

Oxygen Dosage

Clinical judgment and experience help determine how much oxygen to administer to a patient. The dosage of oxygen is typically measured in percentage of oxygen in the inspired gas. Room air contains approximately 21% oxygen; therefore, any supplemented breathing gas contains more than 21% oxygen. In general, dosages are categorized as low flow, medium flow, or high flow, depending on the resultant percentage of inspired oxygen.

Another way to describe the amount of oxygen being administered is to use the decimal equivalent of the percentage. In this case, the dosage is referred to as the **fraction of inspired oxygen** (**FiO_2**). Room air has an FiO_2 of 0.21. A patient receiving 60% oxygen has an FiO_2 of 0.6.

In emergency situations, it is generally better to risk giving too much oxygen rather than too little. Some physicians suggest that any emergency patient who needs oxygen needs a lot of oxygen until proven otherwise. For this reason, many protocols call for

Case Study

Case Study, Part 1

You are dispatched to a report of "difficulty breathing" at a nursing home in your district. At the home you are directed to a patient who is sitting straight up on the side of his bed with his legs dangling over the side. He is leaning forward on outstretched arms, and his head and neck are thrust forward slightly. He is wearing a nasal cannula that is attached to a squat oxygen cylinder. He is taking long inspiratory breaths with significant effort.

You make the following determinations on your initial assessment:

Initial Assessment

Recording time
0 Minutes

Appearance
Cachexic, obvious dyspnea with accessory muscle use evident

Level of consciousness
Appears alert

Airway
No audible sounds are heard

Breathing
His ventilations appear adequate in rate, although with great effort

Circulation
An irregular, rapid radial pulse is detected

Question 1: On the basis of your initial assessment findings, how would you classify the patient's condition?

Question 2: What is your initial treatment plan?

Question 3: What would be your next steps in assessing the patient?

CASE STUDY

high-flow oxygen, which typically provides percentages of oxygen of 60% to 95%. Although administering high-flow oxygen to all patients probably is not harmful, it may be wasteful and unnecessarily uncomfortable for the patient in some situations.

Another treatment approach is using the patient's level of respiratory distress as a guide for oxygen

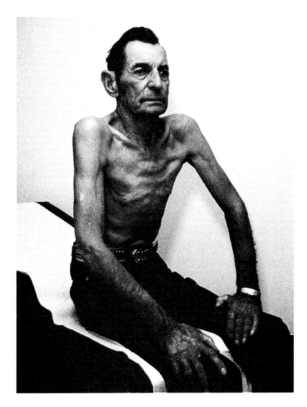

Figure 5-2 Patient in respiratory distress.

administration (▲ Figure 5-2). Unfortunately, this approach does not take into account situations such as stroke or acute myocardial infarction, which may not result in breathing difficulty but may be associated with profound tissue ischemia.

A more balanced treatment approach is to use a combination of information, experience, and knowledge of underlying pathophysiology to guide oxygen administration. Use high-flow oxygen in cases of ischemic injury, anemia, and respiratory or circulatory compromise. Use a combination of data obtained from the history and physical exam, the pulse oximeter, measurement of blood gases, and knowledge of the pathophysiology of the underlying problem to make thoughtful dosage decisions for all other situations.

Can Too Much Oxygen Hurt?

Unfortunately, some people think that oxygen can be harmful. Although this is sometimes true in the long-term management of patients, oxygen is not harmful in the resuscitation of the acutely ill or injured. Never withhold oxygen from patients who need it, regardless of the suspected cause or medical history.

The Hypoxic Drive

Normally, the stimulus to breathe is mediated by the acidity of the blood and cerebrospinal fluid, which are directly related to the concentration of carbon dioxide in the blood. Patients with chronic lung diseases, such as bronchitis or emphysema, tend to have elevated carbon dioxide levels all of the time. Eventually the sensitivity to the high partial pressure of carbon dioxide ($PaCO_2$) decreases and the body uses another feedback loop to control breathing. These patients develop a <u>hypoxic drive</u>, which regulates the respiratory rate based on the oxygen content of the blood. Theoretically, if a patient's only stimulus to breathe is a low PaO_2, providing supplemental oxygen might slow or stop the breathing. The following dilemma is therefore created: If you do not give the patient oxygen, the patient's condition may progress to respiratory failure, but if you increase the oxygen level, you may actually slow the patient's breathing.

The hypoxic drive is not a concern during acute resuscitation in life-threatening emergencies. It generally takes a few hours for a patient using the hypoxic drive to become bradypneic. Also, because emergency patients are closely monitored, it is unlikely that a slowdown in breathing would go unrecognized. Nevertheless, you should be aware of hypoxic drive and the theoretical risk of supplemental oxygen therapy in patients with chronic lung diseases. If the patient is in acute respiratory distress or has low oxygen saturation, you *must* provide a high concentration of supplemental oxygen or the patient's condition will quickly progress to respiratory failure and arrest. For patients with a history of chronic lung diseases, you must constantly monitor the respiratory rate and be prepared to coach the patient's breathing or intervene quickly if the elevated level of PaO_2 suppresses the stimulus to breathe.

The bottom line is that any patient in acute respiratory distress or hypoxia should receive a high concentration of oxygen *regardless of his or her medical history*. Closely monitor the respiratory rate, and, if it drops, provide ventilatory support; do not decrease the oxygen content. Once the patient is oxygenated, you can titrate the oxygen dosage in patients you suspect have a hypoxic drive.

Paramedic Safety 🕮

Always remember: In some circumstances a patient can be severely hypoxic and have pulse oximeter readings greater than 96%.

Hyperventilation Syndrome

Hyperventilation syndrome is common in emergency medicine. Often triggered by fear, anxiety, stress, or pain, this syndrome involves a vicious cycle of increasingly rapid breathing. As the respiratory rate increases, the $PaCO_2$ level decreases, resulting in respiratory alkalosis. Respiratory alkalosis causes a left shift of the oxyhemoglobin dissociation curve, in which the hemoglobin "holds on to" the oxygen molecules more tightly and does not unload them as effectively at the tissue level. The left shift results in tissue hypoxia, increasing air hunger, and anxiety, which further increase the respiratory rate, thus continuing the vicious cycle.

The key to breaking the cycle in hyperventilation syndrome is to allow the $PaCO_2$ level to rise by slowing the respiratory rate. It is difficult, however, to convince an anxious patient who is hungry for air to breathe more slowly, because this seems counterintuitive. The cycle is broken when the patient regains control of breathing or has a brief episode of syncope, during which time the respiratory rate slows and the $PaCO_2$ level rises.

It is important *not* to confuse hyperventilation syndrome with hyperventilation from a pathologic cause. Hyperventilation syndrome is a specific phenomenon in conscious patients that results in a cycle of increased respiratory rate caused by respiratory alkalosis. It is not a tachypneic response to some other pathologic process. Unfortunately, it can be difficult to distinguish between the two. A **carpopedal spasm** is a characteristic sign of respiratory alkalosis that strongly suggests hyperventilation syndrome. Carpopedal spasm involves tingling and contraction of the hands and feet caused by a temporary hypocalcemia secondary to acute hypocapnia. Respiratory alkalosis also causes light-headedness, a tingling sensation around the lips, and a metallic taste in the mouth. Hyperventilation syndrome never occurs in unconscious patients.

If you suspect a patient is experiencing hyperventilation syndrome, increase the patient's $PaCO_2$ level while maintaining the PaO_2 level. Remember that although the patient has a normal PaO_2 level, the end organs are hypoxic. Deaths have been reported from patients rebreathing their own expired air in an effort to increase the carbon dioxide level. Treatment of hyperventilation syndrome includes a combination of supplemental oxygen therapy and **coaching the breathing**.

The ideal treatment of hyperventilation syndrome involves a partial rebreathing mask (discussed in detail later) with an oxygen flow of 6 to 8 L/min. At this oxygen flow rate, the patient rebreathes a

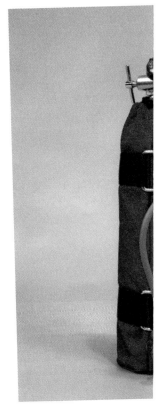

Figure 5-5 Portable oxygen ta

Did You Know

The most important part of syndrome is to decrease coach the patient to brea explaining to the patient too fast and too shallow. rapport, then mirror the p with the patient and tell you. As the patient begin pace, increase the depth your respiratory rate. A v cumbing to hyperventilat you are coaching a patie feel light-headed or dizzy decrease their respirator of their respirations with tions. If a patient does n at coaching, you should an underlying pathologic

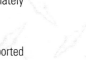

Case Study

Case Study, Part 2

After placing the patient on high-flow oxygen using a nonrebreathing mask, you turn your attention to history taking and focused physical assessment. Meanwhile, your partner enters the room with the patient's nursing home record. Your findings are recorded as follows:

Physical Examination

Recording time
2 minutes after patient contact

Level of orientation
Oriented to place and time

Head
Nasal flaring

Neck
Accessory muscle use

Chest
Appears abnormally large

Lung sounds
Diminished in all fields, scattered wheezing noted throughout

Abdomen
Distended, soft and nontender

Pelvis
Unremarkable

Extremities
Thin, moves all extremities

Back
Unremarkable

History

Age, sex, weight
72-year-old male, 70 kg

Signs and symptoms
Patient complains of increasing chest tightness and shortness of breath

Allergies to medications
No known allergies

Medications taken
Inhaled corticosteroid
beta$_2$-agonist daily
supplemental oxygen (1.5 L/min)
antihypertensive
Digoxin (Lanoxin)
Acetaminophen (Tylenol)

Past pertinent medical history
Emphysema, hypertension

Last food/fluid intake
Lunch served approximately 2 hours ago

Events prior to onset
No sentinel events reported

Onset of symptoms
Patient states being at rest when episode began

Provoking/palliative factors
Nursing home reports a 48-hour history of fever and cough

Quality of discomfort
"My chest is very tight."

Radiating/related signs/symptoms
Dry, nonproductive cough upon deep inspiration

Severity of complaint
Respiratory distress has become increasingly worse since it began

Time
The episode began 20 minutes ago

Vital Signs

Skin signs
Pale, warm, dry

Pulse rate/quality
96 beats/min, irregular

Blood pressure
140/82 mm Hg

Respiratory rate/depth
22 breaths/min, with effort

Pupils
Equal, reactive

SpO_2
85% (room air)

Electrocardiogram
Atrial fibrillation

Question 4: On the basis of your assessment findings, what treatment steps are next?

Question 5: Name a few possible causes of the patient's complaints.

sm
of
of

til
an
Be
br
cc
in
br
yc
bı
ca
d
b
ca
aı
n
d
s
F

$

N
f
t

Skill Drill

5-5 Oxygen Administration with a Partial Rebreathing Mask

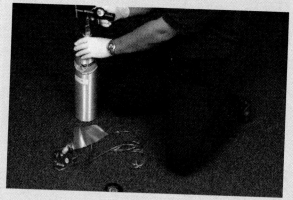

1 Gather the appropriate equipment (oxygen tank already assembled and partial rebreathing mask).

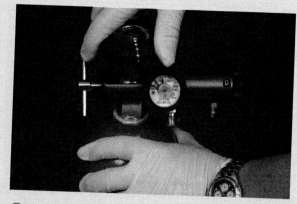

2 Turn on the oxygen tank.

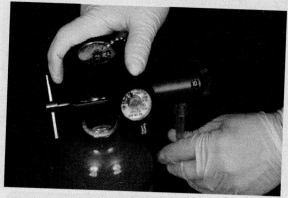

3 Attach partial rebreathing mask to the regulator and adjust the flowmeter to 10 L/min.

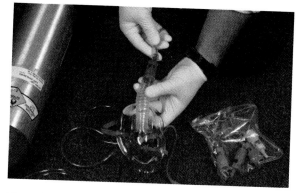

4 Secure the oxygen mask to the patient and tighten the straps.

Venturi Mask

A Venturi mask has a number of attachments that enable you to vary the percentage of oxygen delivered to the patient while a constant flow is maintained from the regulator (▶ Figure 5-12) (▶ Skill Drill 5-6). This is accomplished by the Venturi principle, which causes air to be drawn into the flow of oxygen as it passes a hole in the line. The Venturi mask is a medium-flow device that delivers 24% to 40% oxygen, depending on the manufacturer.

The main advantage of the Venturi mask is in the long-term management of physiologically stable patients. The Venturi mask allows the clinician to

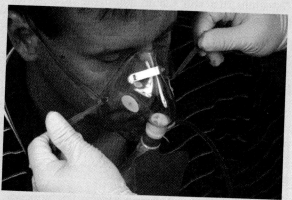

Figure 5-12 The Venturi mask.

Skill Drill

5-6 Oxygen Administration with a Venturi Mask

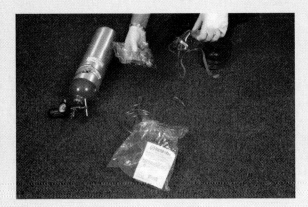

1 Gather the appropriate equipment (oxygen tank already assembled and Venturi mask with variety of oxygen concentration fittings).

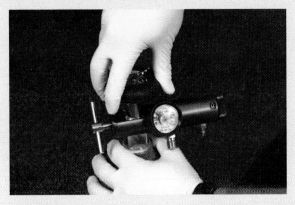

2 Turn on the oxygen tank.

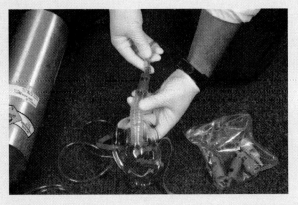

3 Attach the appropriate colored oxygen delivery fitting.

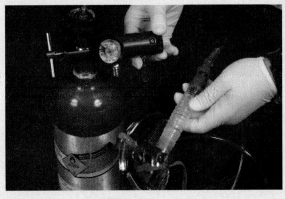

4 Attach the Venturi mask to the regulator and adjust the flowmeter to 10 L/min.

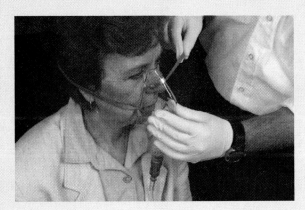

5 Secure the oxygen mask to the patient and tighten the straps.

Table 5-9
Venturi Mask

Indication
- Desire to deliver exact percentages of oxygen

Contraindications
- Apnea
- Poor respiratory effort

Advantage
- Fine control of the FiO_2 at a constant flow rate

Disadvantages
- Expensive
- Cannot deliver extremely high-concentration oxygen

Table 5-10
Flow-Restricted, Oxygen-Powered Ventilation Devices

Indication
- Need for 100% oxygen

Contraindications
- Apnea
- Poor respiratory effort

Advantages
- Provides the highest percentage of oxygen possible
- Efficient use of oxygen

Disadvantages
- Expensive
- Masks are typically not disposable
- Must be disinfected following each use

finely adjust the FiO_2 level, usually based on blood gas analysis or other laboratory data. In emergency situations, such fine control of the percentage of inspired oxygen is rarely needed. When you need to adjust the oxygen concentration in an emergency, it is typically done by adjusting the flow rate or changing the delivery device. ▲ **Table 5-9** lists the indications, contraindications, advantages, and disadvantages of using a Venturi mask.

Flow-Restricted, Oxygen-Powered Ventilation Devices

Flow-restricted, oxygen-powered ventilation devices (FROPVDs), also referred to as manually triggered ventilations devices, or MTV's, are mainly used to assist ventilation in apneic or hypoventilating patients, although these devices can also be used to provide supplemental oxygen to breathing patients. The FROPVD has a "demand valve" that is triggered by the negative pressure generated by inhalation. This valve automatically delivers 100% oxygen as the

patient begins to inhale and stops the flow of gas at the end of the inspiratory phase of the respiratory cycle. Because the FROPVD makes an airtight seal with the patient's face, the gas that the patient inspires is almost 100% oxygen.

Generally, patients find it most comfortable if they hold the mask to their face themselves. The FROPVD is an efficient way to conserve oxygen because it delivers only the volume needed by the patient during inspiration, rather than wasting oxygen with a constant flow. These masks, however, are relatively expensive and typically not disposable. The entire unit should be disinfected following each use. ▲ **Table 5-10** lists the indications, contraindications, advantages, and disadvantages of using FROPVDs.

Tracheostomy Masks

A **tracheostomy** is a surgical opening into the trachea. The **stoma**, which is the resulting orifice through which the patient breathes, is generally located just above the suprasternal notch. Some patients have a plastic tube, called a **tracheostomy tube**, in place through the stoma. Most tracheostomy tubes have a 15-mm adapter that can be connected to a bag-valve-mask device or a ventilator.

Did You Know ?

Generally, a patient finds it most comfortable if he or she holds the mask to his or her face. If a patient is able to do so, allow the patient to hold the mask of the flow-restricted, oxygen-powered ventilation device. Make certain that the patient holds the mask to the face correctly. If a patient is unable to do so, you must hold the mask.

Special Needs **Tip**

Have the pediatric patient's parent hold the tubing close to the child's face. Parents are more trusted by the child and may have greater success in ensuring compliance.

Special Needs Tip

Emergency situations can be frightening for all patients but especially for children. Most pediatric patients are uncomfortable with an oxygen delivery device on their face during times of high stress. If you believe the oxygen mask is significantly increasing the patient's anxiety, it may be better to remove the mask but continue to provide as much supplemental oxygen as possible through the use of an oxygen tent or hood.

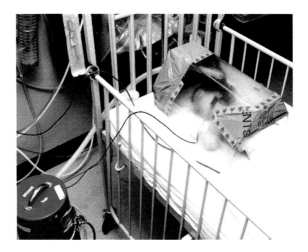

Figure 5-15 Oxygen tent or hood.

Patients with tracheostomies do not breathe through their mouth and nose. A face mask or nasal cannula therefore cannot be used to treat them. Masks designed specifically for these patients cover the tracheostomy hole and have a strap that goes around the neck. These masks are usually available in intensive care units, where many patients have tracheostomies, and may not be available in an emergency setting. If you do not have a tracheostomy mask, you can improvise by placing a face mask over the stoma. Even though the mask is shaped to fit the face, you can usually get an adequate fit over the patient's neck by adjusting the strap (▼ Figure 5-14).

Delivery of Supplemental Oxygen to Pediatric Patients

The general principles of supplemental oxygen therapy apply to patients of all ages. To be effective, however, oxygen masks need to fit the patient. All of the

oxygen delivery devices discussed above are available in sizes for pediatric patients. It is important to have a variety of sizes immediately available.

Emergency situations can be frightening for all patients but especially for children. Most pediatric patients are uncomfortable with an oxygen delivery device on their face during times of high stress. If you believe the oxygen mask is significantly increasing the patient's anxiety, it may be better to remove the mask but continue to provide as much supplemental oxygen as possible. One possible alternative is an oxygen tent or hood (▲ Figure 5-15). A hood covers the patient's entire head, and a tent is made of clear plastic to maintain an enriched oxygen atmosphere. The patient placed in a tent receives an increased FiO_2. Unfortunately, hoods and tents reduce access to the patient and often are not immediately available in emergency situations.

A quick alternative is to provide **blow-by oxygen**. Blow-by oxygen is administered by holding oxygen

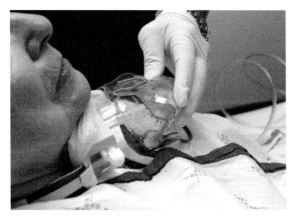

Figure 5-14 Using a face mask instead of a tracheostomy mask.

Teamwork Tip

Have you ever tried to administer oxygen to a critical patient only to find out that the tank was empty? This painful scenario is a reminder that someone needs to check the status of both the on-board and portable oxygen tanks at the beginning of each shift, as well as after the administration of oxygen.

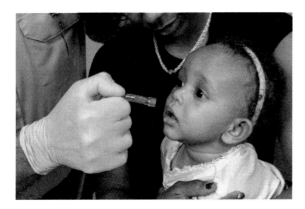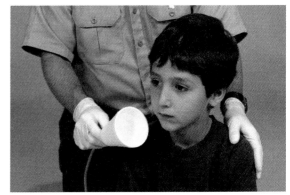

Figure 5-16 Two different methods of the blow-by method for infants and children.

tubing close to the patient's mouth and nose. Alternatively, you can place the tubing through a hole in the bottom of a paper cup and hold this above the patient's face (▲ Figure 5-16). Although the blow-by method cannot provide high-concentration oxygen, it is better than breathing unsupplemented room air.

Continuous Positive Airway Pressure

Continuous positive airway pressure (CPAP), a relatively new therapy, is proving to be tremendously valuable for some patients in acute respiratory distress and failure, especially when these conditions are caused by congestive heart failure. By definition, CPAP exists anytime that inspired pressure exceeds ambient pressure in the lungs and airway throughout the entire respiratory cycle. Traditionally, CPAP has been accomplished by maintaining pressure in an endotracheal tube following exhalation in a process called positive end expiratory pressure (PEEP).

CPAP improves patient ventilation by maintaining slight alveolar expansion between ventilations. This expansion is particularly useful in cases of atelectasis. Atelectasis is defined as collapsing of the alveolar sacs, which may be localized or widespread and can result in partial or complete collapsing of the lung. Common causes of atelectasis include deficiencies of pulmonary surfactant, mucous plugging of the alveoli, hypoventilation, or obstruction by tumors.

PEEP maintains pressure throughout the lungs at the end of exhalation, which recruits more lung tissue to participate in gas exchange and improves oxygenation. In the case of pulmonary edema, the positive pressure not only keeps the alveoli from collapsing, it also provides a mechanical force that drives pulmonary fluid from the lungs.

CPAP requires an airtight seal made between the ventilation device and the patient's airway. Until recently, CPAP was usually only performed in intubated patients during positive pressure ventilations. Most ventilators have a PEEP setting that maintains a constant pressure in the tube, even between expiration and inspiration. CPAP can also be accomplished by placing a PEEP valve between the endotracheal tube and the ventilation device.

New mask designs have made it possible to accomplish CPAP on breathing, nonintubated patients. CPAP for breathing patients requires that a tight-fitting mask make an airtight seal with the face. This can be difficult to accomplish on some patients (very large or small patients, or patients with beards), but new technology has made it possible and comfortable for most patients.

With an airtight mask, CPAP is accomplished by providing a constant flow of breathing gas in excess of the volume of air inspired. The simplest devices include a large volume, constant flow attachment to a 50-psi oxygen port (either on a portable oxygen tank or a wall-mounted unit). A replaceable valve controls the amount of PEEP. Provided that the seal is maintained and the gas flow is adequate, positive pressure is maintained throughout the entire respiratory cycle.

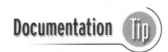

Documentation Tip

It is wise to document your efforts to administer oxygen to an uncooperative patient, especially when your attempt is unsuccessful.

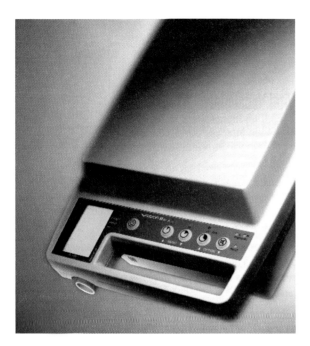

Figure 5-17 A bilevel positive airway pressure unit.

The exact mechanism whereby CPAP improves ventilation and oxygenation is unclear, but is probably due to a combination of therapeutic advantages. In addition to maintaining alveolar expansion and driving fluid from the lungs, CPAP reduces the work of breathing—a very important benefit in respiratory distress and failure. CPAP may recruit more alveoli in cases of obstructive pulmonary diseases and bronchoconstriction.

CPAP is not without some disadvantages. CPAP increases the work of exhalation. This problem is eliminated by bilevel positive airway pressure (BiPAP), which decreases the pressure during exhalation. Unfortunately, BiPAP requires a more sophisticated unit that is bulkier and more expensive than CPAP (▲ Figure 5-17). CPAP decreases preload and afterload, which generally has a positive effect in congestive heart failure, but can be detrimental in patients who are hemodynamically unstable. Because of the risk of pneumothorax and tension pneumothorax, CPAP should not be used in patients with chest trauma. Finally, CPAP should not be used in patients who are hypoventilating or apneic.

Case Study

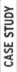

Case Study, Part 4

During patient transport to the community hospital, you administer a second dose of nebulized albuterol. The patient's condition continues to improve; in fact, he is able to provide you additional information about his medical history (smoked cigarettes from the time he was 17 until a few years ago when he quit after several severe emphysema attacks). Additionally, he is complaining about feeling claustrophobic from the nonrebreathing mask, he appears to tolerate a nasal cannula running at 6 L/min fairly well. At the emergency department, you report to the receiving nurse the patient's initial presentation, your treatment, and subsequent changes in the patient's condition. His last set of vital signs are noted below:

Vital Signs

Recording time
40 minutes after patient contact

Skin signs
Pink, warm, and dry

Pulse rate/quality
84 beats/min, irregular

Blood pressure
138/76 mm Hg

Respiratory rate/depth
18 breaths/min, full

Pupils
Equal and reactive

SpO$_2$
99% (on oxygen via nasal cannula)

Electrocardiogram
Atrial fibrillation

The patient is later admitted to the hospital, with test results suggesting an early stage of pneumonia.

CASE STUDY

Table 6-2
Head Tilt-Chin Lift Maneuver

Indications
- Soft-tissue upper airway obstruction
- Patient is unable to protect his or her own airway for any reason
- Noisy respirations

Contraindication
- Possible cervical spine injury

Advantages
- No equipment required
- Simple
- Safe
- Noninvasive

Disadvantages
- Head tilt hazardous to patients with cervical spine injury
- Does not protect patient from aspiration
- Is not equally effective in all patients

Complications
- Aspiration

Table 6-3
Jaw-Thrust Maneuver With Head Tilt

Indications
- Soft-tissue upper airway obstruction
- Unresponsive patient
- Patient is unable to protect his or her own airway

Contraindications
- Unable to open the patient's mouth
- Fractured jaw
- Patient is awake
- Dislocated jaw

Advantages
- May be used as an alternative airway technique for any patient without a suspected spinal injury
- Does not require special equipment

Disadvantages
- Cannot be maintained if patient becomes responsive or combative
- Difficult to maintain for extended period
- Does not protect against aspiration

Complications
- Posterior mandibular bruising

▲ **Table 6-2** lists the indications, contraindications, advantages, disadvantages, and complications of the head tilt-chin lift maneuver.

The Tongue-Jaw Lift Maneuver

The <u>tongue-jaw lift maneuver</u> is used most frequently to open a patient's airway and clear a foreign body airway obstruction using a finger sweep or suctioning. It cannot be used to ventilate a patient, as it will not allow for an adequate mask seal on the face. To grip on the jaw, place your thumb in the patient's

Special Needs (Tip)

Head Tilt in Children and the Elderly

The head tilt portion component of this skill may not be possible in patients with cervical spine stiffness, which occurs occasionally in the elderly. In children younger than 5 years, the cervical vertebrae are so flexible that hyperextension of the head causes the cervical spine to bow upward; elevating the posterior pharyngeal wall to the point that it may contact the tongue and epiglottis. Therefore, less of a head tilt is needed for young children. In fact, hyperextension of the head obstructs the young child's (< 5 years old) airway.

mouth and grasp the lower incisors or gums. The jaw is then lifted upward (▶ **Skill Drill 6-3**).

Jaw-Thrust Maneuver With Head Tilt

The <u>jaw-thrust maneuver with head tilt</u> is similar to the head tilt-chin lift maneuver, with a few exceptions. Kneel above the patient's head and place the meaty portion of the base of your thumbs on the zygomatic arches. Hook the tips of your index fingers under the angle of the mandible, in the indent below each ear. Lift the jaw upward and tilt the patient's head back (▶ Figure 6-4) (▶ **Skill Drill 6-4**). ▲ **Table 6-3** lists the indications, contraindications, advantages, disadvantages, and complications of the jaw-thrust maneuver with head tilt.

Jaw-Thrust Maneuver Without Head Tilt

The <u>jaw-thrust maneuver without head tilt</u> is particularly useful in patients with suspected spinal injuries. It uses the same forward displacement of the jaw from the angles of the mandible as used with the jaw thrust with head-tilt, but without tilting the head back (▶ Figure 6-5) (▶ **Skill Drill 6-5**). The jaw thrust without head tilt is slightly less effective than the head tilt-chin lift or the jaw thrust with head-tilt, because the muscle fibers between the jaw and hyoid bone remain lax in the neutral position. ▶ **Table 6-4** lists the indications, contraindications, advantages,

Skill Drill

6-3 Tongue-Jaw Lift Maneuver

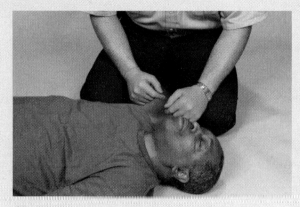

1 Position yourself at the side of the patient.

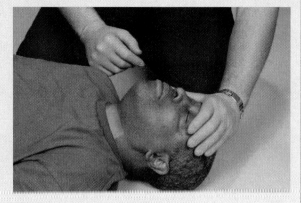

2 Place the hand closest to the patient's head on the forehead.

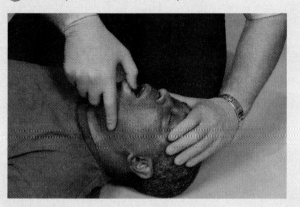

3 With your other hand reach into the patient's mouth and hook your first knuckle under the incisors at the gum line. While holding the patient's head and still keeping the hand on the forehead, lift the jaw straight up.

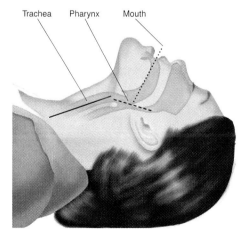

Trachea   Pharynx   Mouth

Figure 6-4 The jaw-thrust maneuver with head tilt is an effective way to open the airway.

Did You Know ?

You should be able to maintain an adequate airway without equipment in order to intervene in unexpected emergency situations. These situations usually involve family members or friends—situations in which you may want to assume the role of a Good Samaritan. Although it is important to be proficient in basic airway management for the role of first responder, more commonly manual airway maneuvers are used in the initial management of emergency patients. Even in the best circumstances it takes a few minutes to obtain and set-up adjunctive airway equipment. Meanwhile, the patient's airway should be opened with manual techniques.

Skill Drill

6-4 *Jaw-Thrust Maneuver with Head Tilt*

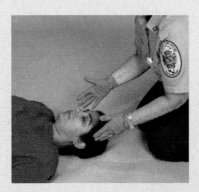

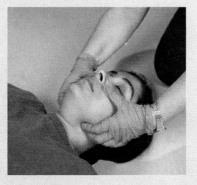

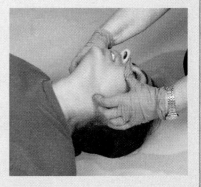

1 Position yourself at the top of the patient's head.

2 Place the meaty portion of the base of your thumbs on the zygomatic arches, and hook the tips of your index fingers under the angle of the mandible, in the indent below each ear.

3 Displace the jaw upward and tilt the head back.

Skill Drill

6-5 *Jaw-Thrust Maneuver without Head Tilt*

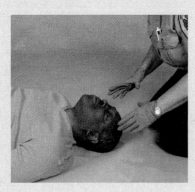

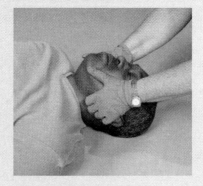

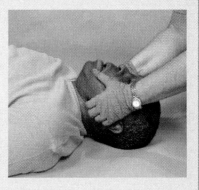

1 Position yourself at the top of the patient's head.

2 Place the meaty portion of the base of your thumbs on the zygomatic arches, and hook the tips of your index fingers under the angle of the mandible, in the indent below each ear.

3 While holding the patient's head still, displace the jaw upward and open the patient's mouth with your thumb tips.

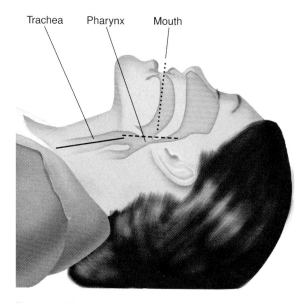

Trachea   Pharynx   Mouth

Figure 6-5 The jaw-thrust maneuver without head tilt is an effective way to open the airway without moving the head. It is particularly useful in patients with suspected spinal injuries.

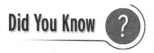

Did You Know

The jaw-thrust maneuver without head tilt is slightly less effective than the head tilt-chin lift because the muscle fibers between the jaw and hyoid bone remain lax in the neutral position. The primary use of the jaw-thrust maneuver without head tilt is for treating patients with possible cervical spine injuries. Although this maneuver is technically more difficult, it has the advantage of not requiring that you place your thumb in the patient's mouth. This is safer for you and makes it possible for someone else to ventilate the patient with positive pressure.

disadvantages, and complications of the jaw-thrust maneuver without head tilt.

The Triple Airway Maneuver

In some unconscious patients, none of the above procedures produces an acceptable airway. By combining three techniques—the head tilt, jaw lift, and mouth opening—the **triple airway maneuver** provides the best chance for achieving supralaryngeal airway patency (▶ **Skill Drill 6-6**). This maneuver is difficult to perform and maintain for an extended period of time but should be part of your repertoire of airway management skills for situations in which the previously described techniques are ineffective. The possibility

of a cervical spine injury is a relative contraindication to the triple airway maneuver. If you cannot establish an airway, you must still act despite the possibility of cervical injury or the patient will die. In that case, tilt the patient's head as little as possible to achieve a patent airway. ▶ **Table 6-5** lists the indications, contraindications, advantages, disadvantages, and complications of using the triple airway maneuver.

Airway Adjuncts

While manual airway maneuvers are quick and relatively easy to perform, they require both of your hands. When a patient requires resuscitation, many

Table 6-4
Jaw-Thrust Maneuver Without Head Tilt

Indications
- Unresponsive patient
- Possible cervical spine injury
- Patient is unable to protect his or her own airway
- Patient is resistant to opening mouth

Contraindications
- Unable to open the patient's mouth
- Fractured jaw
- Patient is awake
- Dislocated jaw

Advantages
- Noninvasive
- Requires no special equipment
- May be used with cervical collar in place
- A second rescuer can ventilate the patient with positive pressure

Disadvantages
- Difficult to maintain for a long period of time
- Does not protect against aspiration

Complication
- Posterior mandibular bruising

Skill Drill

6-6 Triple Airway Maneuver

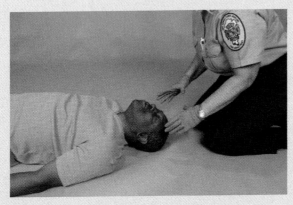

1 Position yourself at the top of the patient's head.

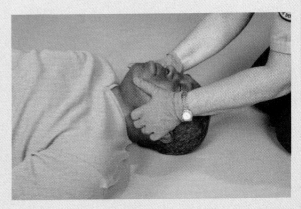

2 Place the meaty portion of the base of your thumbs on the zygomatic arches and hook the tips of your index fingers under the angle of the mandible, in the indent below each ear.

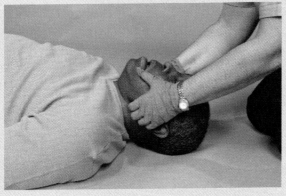

3 While tilting the patient's head back, displace the jaw upward and open the patient's mouth with your thumb tips.

things have to be accomplished simultaneously, and maintaining the airway with adjunctive equipment allows you to work more efficiently. Always remember that maintaining the airway is of the utmost importance. If you are able to maintain a patent airway with a manual technique and airway adjuncts prove ineffective, you must continue to employ the manual technique. In most cases, a combination of one of the manual techniques described above *and* the use of adjunctive equipment described below gives the best chance for success.

Oral Airways

The **oral airway** is a rigid curved device made from hard plastic or similar material (▶ Figure 6-6). It is placed into the unconscious patient's mouth and extends into the oropharynx. Oral airways either are hollow or have side channels that provide a passageway for air as the base of the tongue is kept away from the posterior pharyngeal wall. The oral airway is also known as an oropharyngeal airway, an OP airway, and a Guedel airway.

Table 6-5
Triple Airway Maneuver

Indications

- Unresponsive patient
- Other techniques are ineffective

Contraindication

- Possible cervical spine injury is a relative contraindication
- Patient is awake

Advantages

- Noninvasive
- Requires no special equipment
- A second rescuer can ventilate the patient with positive pressure

Disadvantages

- Extremely difficult to maintain for a long period of time
- Requires a second rescuer if the patient must be ventilated
- Does not protect against aspiration

Complication

- Posterior mandibular bruising

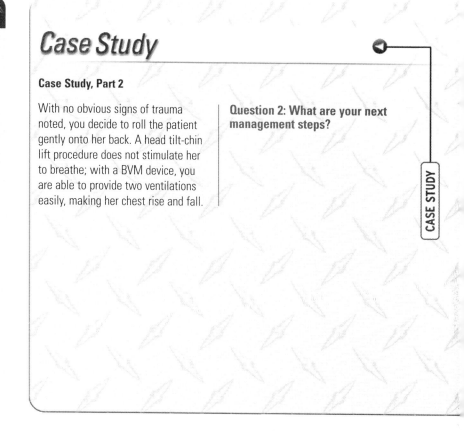

Case Study

Case Study, Part 2

With no obvious signs of trauma noted, you decide to roll the patient gently onto her back. A head tilt-chin lift procedure does not stimulate her to breathe; with a BVM device, you are able to provide two ventilations easily, making her chest rise and fall.

Question 2: What are your next management steps?

CASE STUDY

While one benefit of the oral airway is to reduce the contact of the base of the tongue with the posterior pharyngeal wall, the oral airway has another major advantage during resuscitation. When properly inserted, the oral airway keeps the patient's teeth and lips from closing during mask ventilation.

The oral airway is available in a variety of lengths. To select the proper size, place the airway at the corner of the patient's mouth. Alternatively, it can be sized from the corner of the mouth to the angle of the jaw. A device of the correct size will touch the earlobe (▼ Figure 6-7) An airway that is too small (or improperly inserted) can cause the base of the tongue to be pushed into the oropharynx, worsening airway patency.

You will typically use the insertion of the oral airway as a test of the patient's gag reflex. If the patient gags or retches upon insertion, remove the device immediately. Because the oral airway can stimulate the gag reflex and laryngospasm, it should be used only in

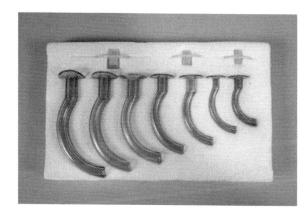

Figure 6-6 Oral airways.

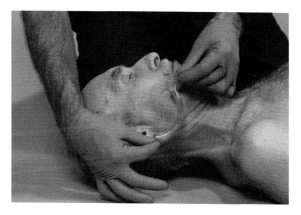

Figure 6-7 Proper sizing for the oral airway.

deeply unconscious patients. Technique 1, described later (▶ **Skill Drill 6-7**), should not be used in pediatric patients because delicate soft tissue can be lacerated by turning the device deep in the airway. Technique 2 (▶ **Skill Drill 6-8**) can be used for pediatric patients.

The oral airway does not extend below the oropharynx and therefore does not prevent the epiglottis from causing partial airway obstruction. For this reason you often need to maintain a head tilt to ensure an adequate airway, even after the oral airway has been inserted. ▼ **Table 6-6** lists the indications, contraindications, advantages, disadvantages, and complications of oral airways.

Nasal Airways

The <u>nasal airway</u> is a flexible rubber or silicone tube that is placed into the patient's nostril (▶ **Figure 6-8**) (▶ **Skill Drill 6-9**). When extended past the nasopharynx and into the oropharynx, the nasal airway provides a conduit for air inspired through its lumen. The nasal airway is also known as a nasopharyngeal airway, an NP airway, or a nasal trumpet.

The main advantage of the nasal airway is that it is much better tolerated in patients who have a functional gag reflex but who still are unable to maintain airway patency. This is often the case in intoxicated patients. When a nasal airway is properly sized and inserted, it is unlikely to cause retching, vomiting, or

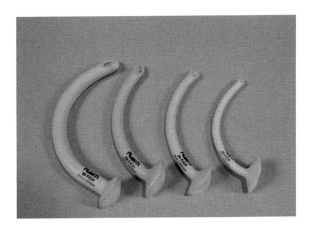

Figure 6-8 Nasal airways.

laryngospasm. A major disadvantage of a nasopharyngeal airway is the possibility of bleeding secondary to poor insertion technique, inadequate lubrication, or a patient's underlying coagulation abnormality.

The nasal airway is available in a variety of sizes. Since the diameter varies with the length, either of two methods of choosing the right size is acceptable. The proper length can be determined by placing one end of the device on the tip of the nose and the other on the earlobe. Alternatively, select the device with a diameter most closely approximating that of the nostril. A nasal airway that is too short will not provide an adequate airway.

The nasal airway should be inserted with its curvature following the contour of the airway and its bevel against the nasal septum. Because the right nostril is slightly larger and straighter than the left nostril in most people, nasal airways are designed to be placed on the right side. If you meet resistance on the right side, or if there is trauma or an anatomic obstruction on the right side, insert the device on the left side. In this case, keep the bevel toward the septum and rotate the airway 180° as the tip enters the nasopharynx.

Like the oral airway, the nasal airway does not control the epiglottis, and you may need to maintain a head tilt to ensure an adequate airway in some patients. ▶ **Table 6-7** lists the indications, contraindications, advantages, disadvantages, and complications of nasal airways.

Upper Airway Suctioning

Suction is used to clear the upper airway of partial obstructions caused by fluids (▶ **Skill Drill 6-10**). The basic indication for upper airway suctioning is the presence of fluids in the airway. Fluids can significantly decrease the flow of air and present a serious risk for aspiration into the lungs.

Table 6-6 Oral Airways

Indications
- Deeply unconscious patients
- Absent gag reflex

Contraindication
- Presence of a gag reflex

Advantages
- Noninvasive
- Easily placed
- Prevents blockage of glottis by tongue

Disadvantages
- Does not prevent aspiration
- Unexpected gag may produce vomiting and/or laryngospasm
- Still may require a head tilt

Complications
- Gagging and retching, which may cause vomiting, laryngospasm, and increased intracranial pressure
- Pharyngeal or dental trauma with poor technique

Skill Drill

6-7 Oral Airway Insertion Technique 1 for Adults Only

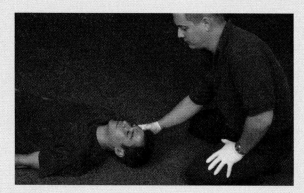

1 Approach the patient from the top of the head.

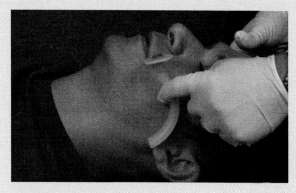

2 Select the correct sized airway for the patient.

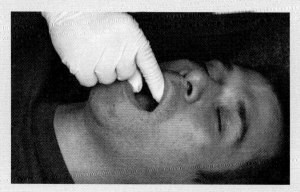

3 Using your nondominant hand, tilt the patient's head back and open the mouth. The latter can be accomplished by placing the side of your thumb just below the lower lip and pushing gently toward the feet, or by using the crossfinger maneuver, in which you cross your thumb and index finger and place the tip of your thumb on the lower incisors and the tip of your index finger on the upper incisors.

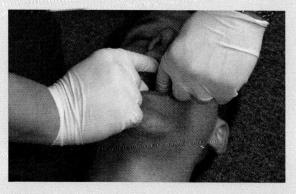

4 Remove any visible obstructions.

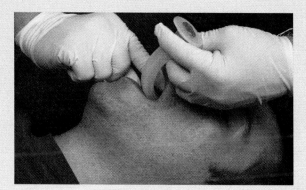

5 Insert the device with your dominant hand by placing its distal tip toward the palate (concavity cephalad) and inserting the device until you feel a slight resistance.

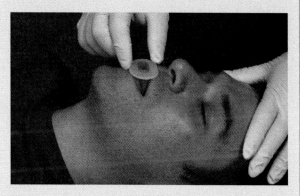

6 Turn the device 180° until the flange comes to rest at the patient's incisors.

Skill Drill

6-8 Oral Airway Insertion Technique 2 for Adults or Pediatric Patients

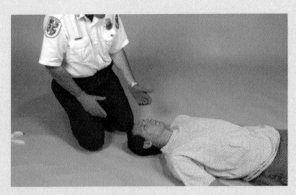

1 Approach the patient from the top of the head.

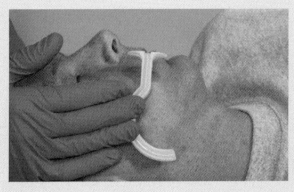

2 Select the correct sized airway for the patient.

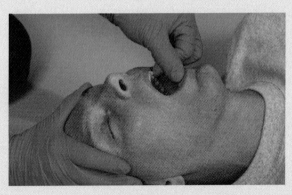

3 Tilt the patient's head back and open the patient's mouth with your dominant hand by placing the side of your thumb just below the lower lip and pushing gently toward the feet, or by using the crossfinger maneuver (cross your thumb and index finger and place the tip of your thumb on the lower incisors and the tip of your index finger on the upper incisors).

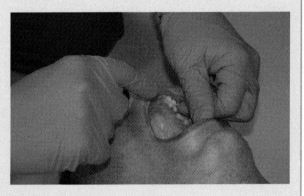

4 Remove any visible obstructions.

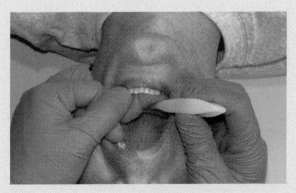

5 With your nondominant hand, lift the base of the tongue off the posterior pharyngeal wall with a tongue depressor.

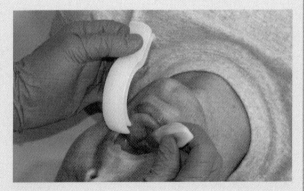

6 Using your dominant hand, place the distal tip of the device toward the tongue (concavity caudad) and insert it into place until the flange comes to rest at the patient's incisors.

Skill Drill

6-9 Inserting a Nasal Airway

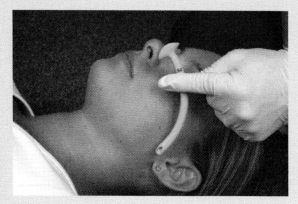

1 Select the correct sized airway for the patient

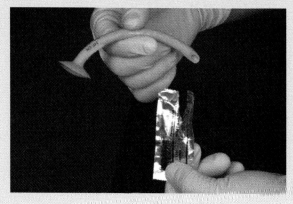

2 Lubricate the airway with a water-soluble lubricant.

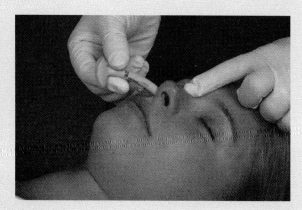

3 With the bevel towards the septum, gently insert the device straight back (toward the ear, not the eye) until the flange rests at the nostril.

Special Needs Tip

Inserting Oral Airways in Pediatric Patients

It is generally recommended that technique 2 be used for infants. Twisting the airway into position can cause damage to the tonsular and/or adenoidal tissue.

Documentation Tip

It is a good idea to document which nare holds the nasal airway, in case any soft-tissue damage or bleeding is noticed later by emergency department personnel.

Suction Equipment

Suction equipment includes the suction unit itself and the suction catheter.

Suction Units

The suction unit is the device that creates the vacuum necessary to remove fluids from the airway. Ideally, the suction unit should be capable of generating 300 mm Hg of negative pressure when occluded and an airflow of 30 L/min when open. The four basic types of suction units used in emergency situations are mounted vacuum-powered units, battery-operated units, hand-powered units, and oxygen-powered units. Each type of unit has its own set of advantages and disadvantages.

Mounted Vacuum Suction Devices

The most powerful and reliable suction units are permanently mounted on the wall in hospitals or ambulances (▼ Figure 6-9). These suction units provide a very strong, constant vacuum that is usually adjustable with a regulator to correspond to the needs of the patient. These units are generally powered by alternating current and therefore depend on a wall outlet or an inverter when mounted in an ambulance. The device consists of an electric motor that moves a piston to generate the vacuum, a collecting chamber, a regulator, and tubing. The collecting chamber is a disposable repository for the suctioned material. Unfortunately, mounted suction units are not portable and can be used only within the hose length of the unit.

Table 6-7
Nasal Airways

Indications
- Unconsciousness
- Altered mental status with suppressed gag reflex
- Patient is conscious but unable to maintain an airway
- Seizure

Contraindications
- Patient intolerance
- Nasal fractures
- Nasal airway occlusion
- Marked deviated septum
- Coagulopathy

Advantages
- Can be suctioned through
- Provides patent airway
- Better tolerated by patients with intact gag reflex who are awake
- Can be safely placed without direct visualization of oropharynx or nasopharynx
- Does not require the mouth to be open

Disadvantages
- Poor technique may result in severe bleeding, and resulting epistaxis may be difficult to control
- Does not protect from aspiration

Complication
- Bleeding

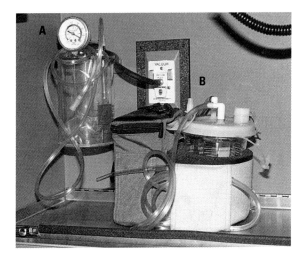

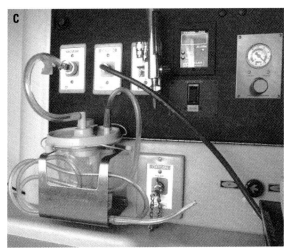

Figure 6-9 Vacuum suction devices. **A.** Wall-mounted unit in an ambulance. **B.** Portable unit in an ambulance. **C.** Wall-mounted unit in a hospital.

Special Needs Tip

The small-diameter airways of infants are particularly susceptible to complete occlusion by liquid obstructions. Early suctioning in pediatric patients can be lifesaving.

Battery-Operated Portable Suction Devices

To solve the portability problem, lightweight battery-powered, portable suction units have been developed (▼ Figure 6-10). In general, these modern battery-powered devices generate excellent suction power and perform well if properly maintained. Unfortunately, since portable units are sometimes jostled and occasionally dropped, they generally become less reliable over time. Therefore, be careful with portable suction equipment and check it frequently to ensure it is functioning properly.

Most battery-powered portable units use rechargeable batteries. Be sure that the unit is being charged when not in use. Over time, batteries usually lose strength and their ability to hold a charge. These units include an electric motor, which generates the suction, a collection chamber, and tubing. Some units have a disposable collection chamber; in others it is reusable and must be cleaned after each use. The negative pressure generated by portable units is generally not adjustable.

Improper maintenance of portable suction units can lead to unreliability and failure at the worst possible moment. Although such problems can often be fixed in the field at the time, this can result in a delay in patient care. Unfortunately, portable suction units are still relatively large and bulky and therefore are often not kept close enough to the patient to be used quickly in an emergency. *The major error in suctioning is not having it when you need it!*

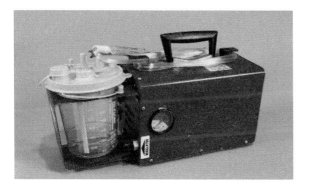

Figure 6-10 Battery-operated portable suction devices.

Case Study

Case Study, Part 3

As you begin to insert a correctly sized oropharyngeal airway, you recognize that the patient has a slight but present gag reflex. Afraid of potential vomiting, you withdraw the oropharyngeal airway and pick up a nasal airway instead. After lubricating it, you can easily insert it into the right nare. Picking the chin back up you begin to ventilate the patient with the BVM device. Your partner has attached oxygen tubing to the bag, allowing 100% oxygen to fill the reservoir.

Your first set of vital signs is as follows:

Vital Signs

Recording time
1 minute after patient contact

Skin signs
Cyanotic, diaphoretic

Pulse rate/quality
120 beats/min, regular and weak

Blood pressure
130/60 mm Hg

Respiratory rate/depth
Assisted with BVM device at 20 breaths/minute

Pupils
Pinpoint, equal, nonreactive

SpO_2
92% (100% oxygen)

Electrocardiogram
Sinus tachycardia

A rapid physical assessment provides the following information:

Physical Examination

Level of orientation
Remains unconscious to a sternal rub

Head
Atraumatic

Neck
No JVD noted

Chest
Equal chest expansion, no bruises

Lung sounds
Equal, clear, full

Abdomen
Soft, flat

Pelvis
Nontrauma

Upper extremities
Multiple needle tracks noted bilaterally

Lower extremities
Nontrauma

Back
Unremarkable

Question 3: What possible threats to your patient's airway might exist? How would you mitigate these threats?

CASE STUDY

Skill Drill

6-10 Suctioning

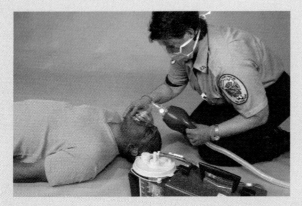

1 Apply a pulse oximeter and cardiac monitor, if possible and practical. Preoxygenate by ventilation with 100% oxygen for 2 to 3 minutes, *if possible*.

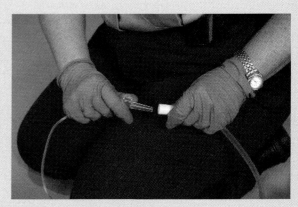

2 Select an appropriate catheter and attach it to the tubing.

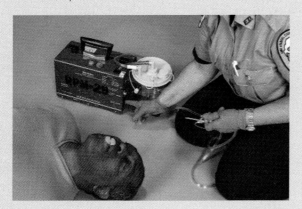

3 Turn on the suction unit.

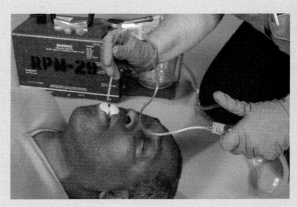

4 Insert the catheter into the oropharynx. Occlude the hole and apply suction as you withdraw the catheter in a sweeping motion (flexible catheter only).

Teamwork Tip

It is not the right time to check whether a suction device is working when the patient needs it! Checking all suction devices at the beginning of each shift is a prudent work habit.

Hand-Powered Suction Devices

Because of the drawbacks of the weight, bulk, and unreliability of portable battery-operated suction units, a number of hand-powered suction units have been developed (► Figure 6-11). These devices are relatively inexpensive, mechanically simple, and smaller and lighter than battery-powered units. The paramedic generally uses a pumping or squeezing action to generate the negative pressure necessary to create a vacuum. Hand-powered suction devices can suction large quantities of material very quickly. It can be difficult to control the amount of suction generated by these devices.

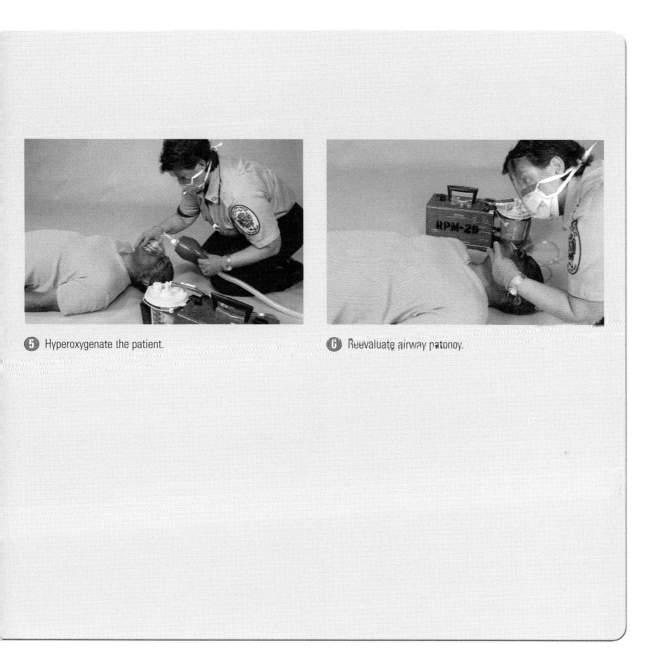

5 Hyperoxygenate the patient.

6 Reevaluate airway patency.

The major disadvantage of hand-powered devices is that the suction is intermittent, sustained only for a second or two without interruption. The negative pressure is created only during the pumping phase, with no suction created during the recovery phase. This fluctuation in negative pressure can make it difficult to suction thin liquids. Hand-powered units typically have small collection chambers and hold less volume than battery-powered units.

Oxygen-Powered Portable Suction Devices

Some older oxygen regulators have an attachment that uses the flow of oxygen to create negative pressure for

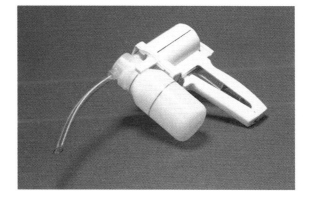

Figure 6-11 Hand-powered suction device.

suctioning the airway. These attachments are small and add little weight to the tank/regulator assembly. In theory, this is an ideal setup because most emergency or critical care patients being transported are receiving oxygen from a tank. Unfortunately, a high flow of oxygen is necessary to create a strong enough vacuum to be clinically useful, and this results in the rapid depletion of oxygen from the tank. For this reason, very few oxygen-powered devices are still in use.

Suction Catheters

Suction catheters direct the suction to the exact place needed. The design is important for minimizing the risk of trauma during suctioning. Suction catheters have multiple openings and side ports to prevent all of the force of negative pressure from being concentrated in one location. This decreases the risk that the catheter will create a concentrated suction injury at any single point of contact with soft tissue.

Although many types of catheters exist, the two most common in emergency medicine are rigid and flexible catheters.

Rigid Suction Catheters

Rigid suction catheters are also known as Yankauer or tonsil tip catheters (▶ Figure 6-12), are made of hard plastic, and can be easily maneuvered to the exact site where suctioning is needed. Most rigid catheters have a hole in the side. The operator covers the hole on the side of the catheter to increase the suction at the tip. If the catheter does not have a hole along its side, you must regulate the suction by turning the mask on and off. Rigid catheters have the advantage of being able to easily direct the tip to where you need it, and are generally preferred for oral suctioning.

Flexible Suction Catheters

Flexible, or soft suction, catheters are longer than rigid catheters and are made from a flexible tube with multiple openings at the distal tip. The primary advantage of flexible catheters is that they can be placed through or around other airway adjuncts. Flexible catheters therefore can be used more effectively than rigid catheters to suction the oropharynx and nasopharynx even with an airway adjunct in place. Flexible catheters are also used to suction the trachea and bronchi in intubated patients. As with rigid catheters, the operator must cover the hole on the side of the catheter to increase the suction at the tip. Flexible catheters are available in a variety of lengths and diameters.

Occasionally you need to remove large volumes of material, such as when a patient vomits. Vomitus usually contains bits of partially digested food that tend to clog the suction catheter. Therefore, with large volumes of vomit, it is best to turn the patient on his or her side.

Suctioning Technique

Although upper airway suctioning is often a life-saving intervention, improper technique can cause serious complications. When you suction the airway to remove secretions, you are also removing oxygen. This, combined with the fact that you cannot artificially ventilate the patient while suctioning, leads to a major complication of suctioning: hypoxemia.

Two strategies can be used to decrease the risk of hypoxemia caused by suctioning. First, preoxygenate patients before suctioning, *if possible*. Ideally, ventilate patients with 100% oxygen for 2 to 3 minutes prior to suctioning. This will enable them to withstand the brief period of apnea while suctioning. Unfortunately, it is not always possible to preoxygenate patients, especially if secretions are significantly interfering with ventilation. Use your judgment to decide whether ventilation is possible prior to suctioning. If ventilation is impossible or

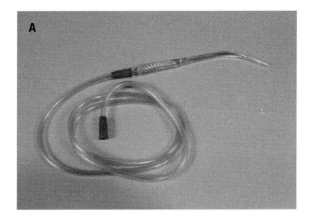

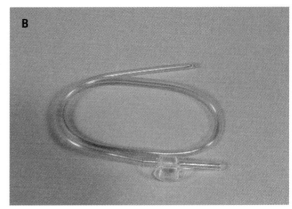

Figure 6-12 Rigid (**A**) and flexible (**B**) suction catheters.

ineffective, you will have no choice but to proceed with suctioning immediately. In this case, suction only as long as absolutely necessary to clear the obstruction.

The second way to decrease the risk of hypoxemia is to limit the amount of time that you suction. It is generally desirable to preoxygenate patients and to limit upper airway suctioning to 10 seconds at a time without pausing to ventilate. Again, this is not always possible, especially when large volumes of secretions or vomit are in the airway. In this situation you must balance the risk of aspiration against the risk of hypoxemia.

Some patients experience dysrhythmias during suctioning. The dysrhythmias may be caused by hypoxia, vagal stimulation, or a combination of both. If possible and practical, place patients on a pulse oximeter and cardiac monitor before suctioning the upper airway and stop if dysrhythmias occur.

Care of Patients With a Stoma

The paramedic must be able to manage the airway of patients with a stoma. A <u>stoma</u> is the hole created in the neck after a patient has had a laryngectomy (surgical removal of the larynx). You may encounter such patients who require suctioning of thick secretions from the stoma (▶ **Skill Drill 6-11**). Failure to recognize and identify these patients could result in hypoxia to the patient. It is not uncommon for the patient's stoma to become occluded with mucous plugs. Because patient's with laryngectomies possess a less efficient cough, they will clearly have difficulty in spontaneously clearing the stoma themselves.

Suctioning of the patient's stoma must be performed with extreme care, especially if laryngeal edema is suspected. Even the slightest irritation of the tracheal wall can result in a violent laryngospasm and complete airway closure. Additionally, to further minimize the risk of complications, specifically hypoxia, you should limit suctioning of the stoma to 10 seconds.

You may also be called upon to replace the <u>tracheostomy tube</u> in a patient if it becomes inadvertently dislodged (▶ **Skill Drill 6-12**). When the tracheostomy tube becomes dislodged, stenosis (narrowing) of the stoma occurs, which can significantly impair the patient's ventilatory ability. In such cases, you may not be able to replace the tracheostomy tube itself

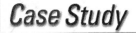

Case Study

Case Study, Part 4

Fortunately, the patient did not vomit during your ventilations. Suspecting a narcotic overdose, you decide to administer naloxone. A few minutes later she begins to breathe spontaneously. You remove the nasal airway without difficulty. En route to the hospital the patient reveals that she had recently tried to "kick" her habitual use of intravenous heroin with the use of oral methadone but was unable to control the urge to use today. Her vital signs on reassessment are as follows:

Vital Signs

Recording time
35 minutes after patient contact

Skin signs
Pale, warm, and dry

Pulse rate/quality
90 beats/min, regular, strong

Blood pressure
136/70 mm Hg

Respiratory rate/depth
16 breaths/min, regular, full

Pupils
Constricted (2 mm), reactive, equal

SpO₂
99% (6 L/min oxygen via nasal cannula)

Electrocardiogram
Sinus rhythm

You transfer her to the care of the emergency department, where she stayed for another 4 hours for observation before being discharged.

and may have to insert an endotracheal tube into the stoma before it becomes totally occluded. Regardless of whether or not the stoma requires suctioning or the tracheostomy tube needs to be reinserted, the paramedic must be prepared to take immediate action in order to minimize further compromise of oxygenation and ventilation. You must also consider the fact that the patient with the stoma has the device because of a significant medical problem (ie, brain injury, chronic respiratory insufficiency, etc), which means that they may be less tolerant of even brief periods of hypoxia.

Skill Drill

6-11 Suctioning of a Stoma

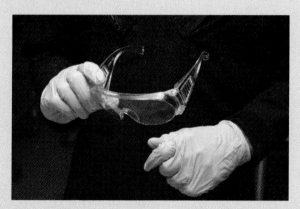

1 Take BSI precautions (gloves and face mask).

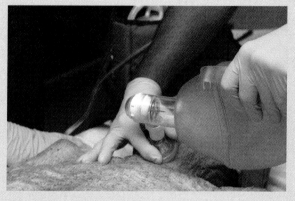

2 Preoxygenate the patient with a bag-valve mask and 100% oxygen.

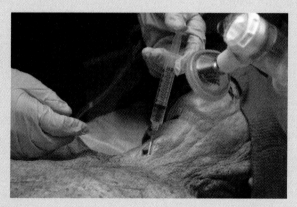

3 Inject 3 ml of sterile saline through the stoma and into the trachea.

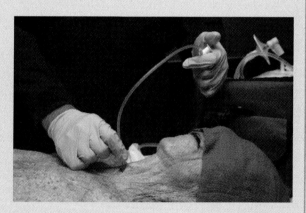

4 Instruct the patient to exhale and insert the catheter (without providing suction) until resistance is felt (no more than 12 cm).

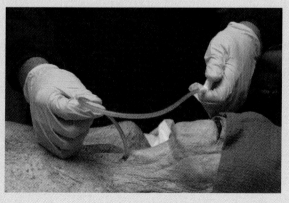

5 Suction while withdrawing the catheter as you instruct the patient to cough or exhale.

Skill Drill

6-12 *Replacing a Dislodged Tracheostomy Tube*

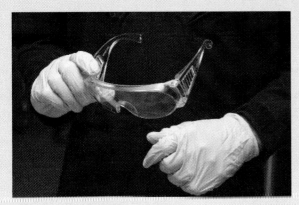

1 Take BSI precautions (gloves and face mask).

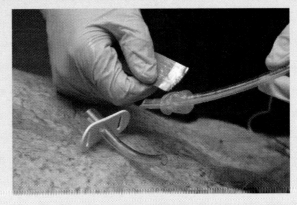

2 Lubricate the same sized tracheostomy tube or an endotracheal tube (at least 5.0 mm).

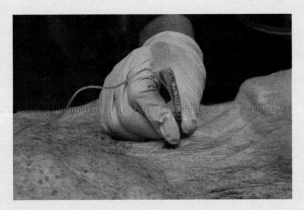

3 Instruct the patient to exhale and gently insert the tube approximately 1 to 2 cm beyond the balloon cuff.

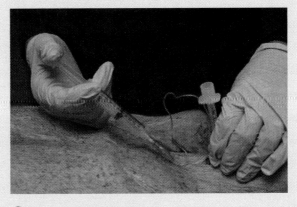

4 Inflate the balloon cuff.

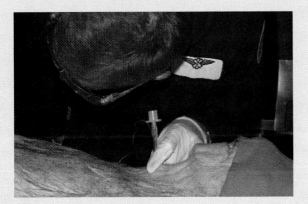

5 Ensure that the patient is comfortable and confirm patency and proper placement of the tube by listening for air movement from the tube and noting the patient's clinical status.

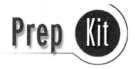

Chapter Summary

Basic airway management is critical in the initial management of patients. No level of proficiency in advanced techniques can substitute for strict attention to the fundamentals. In many situations close attention to airway basics will have a positive effect on patient outcome and may eliminate the need for more invasive intervention.

Although often overlooked, placing unresponsive but breathing patients on their sides can help to reduce a multitude of potential airway obstructions.

Regardless of the exact technique, it is necessary to elevate the hyoid bone away from the pharynx in order to adequately open the airway. This in turn will move the base of the tongue away from the glottic opening.

The use of a basic airway adjunct such as an oral pharyngeal airway or nasal airway can greatly help control the upper airway. It is often too easy to avoid bringing in suction equipment to a call. However, the ability to control the airway when fluid or vomitus is present in the oropharynx is greatly diminished, and is not worth the risk.

Proper management of patients with a stoma, to include suctioning and replacement of the device, requires key skills that the paramedic must possess. Clogging of the stoma or tracheostomy tube by mucous plugging can significantly decrease the patient's ability to effectively ventilate, thus resulting in hypoxia.

Vital Vocabulary

<u>aspiration</u> The process of foreign material, such as vomit, getting into the lungs.

<u>head tilt-chin lift maneuver</u> A manual technique involving tilting the head and lifting the jaw to open the airway.

<u>jaw-thrust maneuver with head tilt</u> A manual technique involving thrusting the jaw forward to open the airway.

<u>jaw-thrust maneuver without head tilt</u> A manual technique involving thrusting the jaw forward without tilting the head to open the airway.

<u>nasal airway</u> A flexible tube of rubber or silicone that is designed to be inserted into the nostril to provide assistance in maintaining a patent airway. This device is especially useful and better tolerated in patients with a gag reflex.

<u>oral airway</u> A rigid curved tube or channeled device designed to be inserted into the mouth to provide assistance in maintaining a patent airway. This device should only be used in unconscious patients with no gag reflex.

<u>recovery position</u> A position for nontrauma breathing patients that decreases the risk of aspiration and airway obstruction.

<u>stoma</u> The hole created by a laryngectomy.

<u>tongue-jaw lift maneuver</u> A manual technique used to clear a foreign body airway obstruction using a finger sweep or suctioning.

<u>tracheostomy tube</u> A tube that is placed into a tracheostomy. The tube has a standard 15-mm adaptor at its proximal end, which makes it compatible with all types of ventilation devices.

<u>triple airway maneuver</u> A manual technique involving tilting the head, thrusting the jaw forward, and opening the mouth to open the airway.

Case Study Answers

Question 1: What are your initial management priorities for this patient?

Answer: Moving the patient to a position where her airway status can be accurately assessed and managed is vitally important. This cannot be done with the patient lying on her side.

Question 2: What are your next management steps?

Answer: With airway patency established, the patient's breathing and circulatory status must be assessed. Simultaneously, some form of airway adjunct must be inserted to control the tongue and soft tissues of the upper airway, and high-flow oxygen must be administered.

Question 3: What possible threats to your patient's airway might exist? How would you mitigate these threats?

Answer: The threat of aspiration from vomiting is significant in this unconscious patient. Minimizing gastric distention by using careful ventilation technique and having suction immediately available will help to minimize this problem.

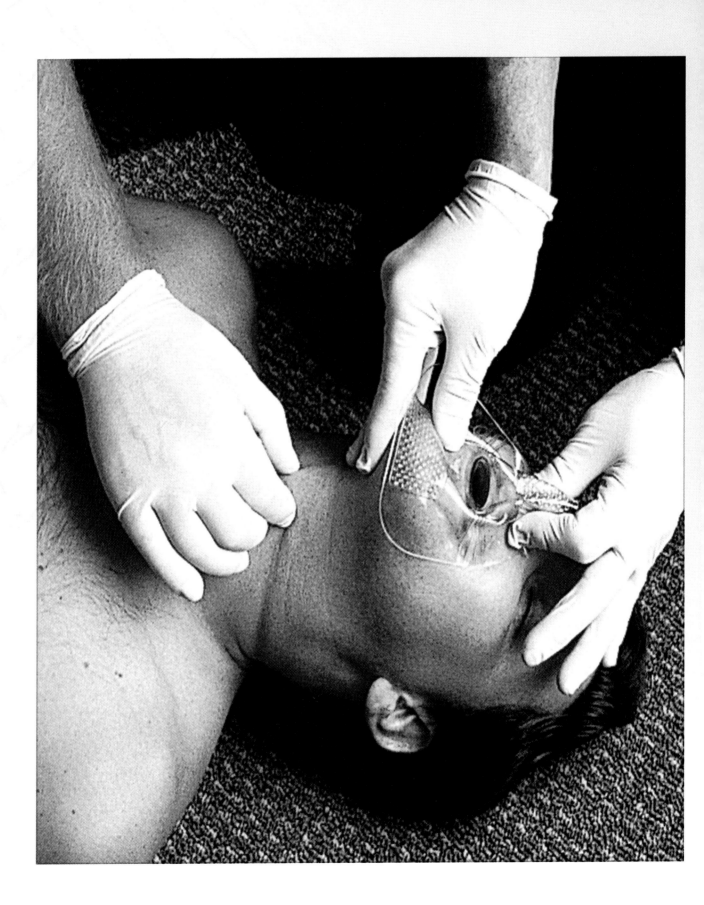

Objectives

Cognitive Objectives

2-1.28 Describe the Sellick maneuver. (cricoid pressure) (p 133)

2-1.39 Define gastric distention. (p 132)

2-1.40 Describe the indications, contraindications, advantages, disadvantages, complications, equipment, and technique for inserting a nasogastric tube and orogastric tube. (p 136)

2-1.41 Identify special considerations of gastric decompression. (p 135)

Psychomotor Objectives

2-1.86 Perform the Sellick maneuver. (cricoid pressure). (p 134) (Skill Drill 7-1)

2-1.90 Demonstrate insertion of the nasogastric tube. (p 138) (Skill Drill 7-2)

2-1.91 Demonstrate insertion of the orogastric tube. (p 140) (Skill Drill 7-3)

2-1.92 Perform gastric decompression by selecting a suction device, catheter, and technique. (p 142) (Skill Drill 7-4)

www.Paramedic.EMSzone.com

TECHNOLOGY

- Online Chapter Pretest
- Vocabulary Explorer
- Anatomy Review
- Web Links

Chapter FEATURES

- Case Studies
- Skill Drills
- Teamwork Tips
- Documentation Tips
- Paramedic Safety Tips
- Special Needs Tips
- Vital Vocabulary
- Prep Kit

pening the airway is only one of the challenges of managing the respiratory status of emergency patients. Once the patency of the airway has been ensured, the patient often must be ventilated. In emergency situations this is accomplished by positive pressure ventilation. Although positive pressure ventilation can be a life-saving intervention, its complications must be considered and minimized.

Introduction

Airway management and ventilation are closely related but they are two separate components of patient care. Both are necessary for respiration to occur. In some patients, once the airway has been secured, ventilation will begin with no intervention. Unfortunately, this does not occur often, and in most cases you will need to support ventilation artificially, with positive pressure ventilation techniques.

Negative Pressure Ventilation

Gas always flows from an area of higher pressure to an area of lower pressure. During normal ventilation, negative intrapulmonic pressure is created by the expansion of the thoracic cavity, which is caused by contraction of the external intercostal muscles and the diaphragm. Air flows in through the mouth and nose to correct the resultant pressure imbalance

(▼ Figure 7-1). During normal, negative pressure ventilations, the average tidal volume is 5 to 7 mL/kg at rest.

Positive Pressure Ventilation

When the chest is not moving or is moving inadequately, not enough air flows for effective ventilation to occur. When negative pressure ventilation is ineffective, positive pressure ventilation can be lifesaving. All of the methods of ventilation used in emergency situations employ positive pressure ventilation. Pos-itive pressure ventilation requires that the airway and lungs are isolated from the external environment by creating an airtight seal between the ventilation device and the patient's lungs. Initially, you will have to achieve an airtight seal of a mask around the patient's nose and mouth. When the pressure around the mouth and nose is increased, air is forced into the lungs (▶ Figure 7-2).

Numerous techniques are used for positive pressure ventilation, but they all have some important things in common. Positive pressure ventilation is

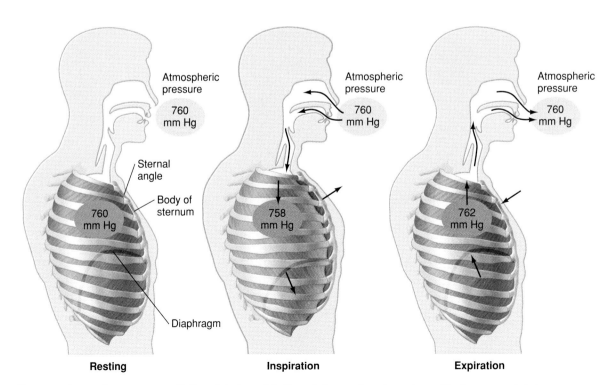

Resting   **Inspiration**   **Expiration**

Figure 7-1 In negative pressure ventilation, air is drawn into through the mouth and nose to equilibrate pressure imbalance between the lungs and the external environment.

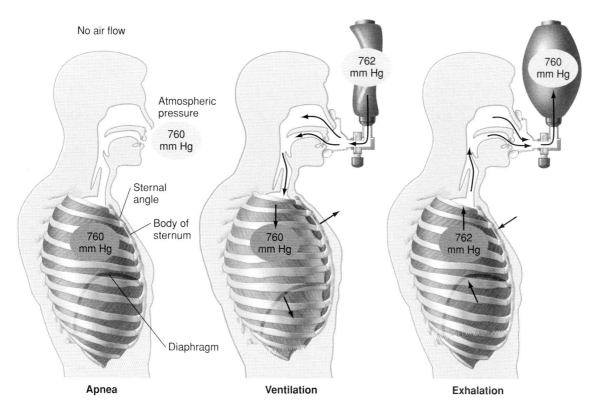

Figure 7-2 In positive pressure ventilation, air is forced into the lungs to equilibrate pressure imbalance between the lungs and the gas outside of the body.

indicated anytime a patient needs ventilatory support. The most common situations that require positive pressure ventilation in emergency medicine involve patients who are hypoventilating or apneic. Regardless of the specific technique used, positive pressure ventilation of a patient with an unprotected airway requires an airtight seal with the patient's face. Establishing this seal can be difficult and requires significant practice. Even a small mask leak can result in a dramatic decrease in ventilatory volume.

▶ **Table 7-1** lists the indications, contraindications, advantages, disadvantages, and complications of positive pressure ventilation.

During positive pressure ventilations it is necessary to overcome the distention of upper airway soft tissues (around the mouth and nose) and the inevitable loss of some air from an incomplete mask seal. When ventilating patients who are not breathing with a positive pressure technique and room air, the patients should be ventilated with 10 mL/kg of air to provide adequate oxygen to support life. As soon as possible, the patient should be ventilated with 100% oxygen. Once the patient is being resuscitated with oxygen, the ventilatory volume should be decreased to 6 to 7 mL/kg. This provides adequate ventilation because the supplemental oxygen overcomes the decrease in tidal volume due to distention and mask leak.

Table 7-1
Positive Pressure Ventilation

Indications
- Apnea
- Hypoventilation

Contraindications
- Conscious patient with adequate air exchange

Advantages
- Provides rapid lifesaving ventilation

Disadvantages
- Requires a mask seal, which can be difficult to achieve
- Can cause gastric distention
- Turbulent flow causes a decrease in deep lung ventilation
- Increased volume necessary to achieve adequate ventilation compared to negative pressure ventilation

Complications
- Hypoventilation resulting from poor mask seal and/or inadequate ventilatory volume
- Gastric distention
- Pulmonary barotrauma
- Hypoventilation from gastric pressure on the diaphragm
- Decreased cardiac output
- May not provide adequate ventilation for severe bronchoconstriction

During positive pressure ventilation a dramatic rise in intrapulmonic pressure occurs that makes it necessary to overcome the weight of the chest wall and the elasticity of the chest muscles with each ventilation. This is analogous to inflating a tire with the weight of the car on it. This high pressure increases the risk of **pulmonary barotrauma**. Pulmonary barotrauma can result in pneumothorax, tension pneumothorax, pneumomediastinum, and/or subcutaneous emphysema during positive pressure ventilation.

The Mechanics of Positive Pressure Ventilation

In many ways positive pressure ventilation is dramatically different than normal breathing.

Airflow Dynamics

Flow is the volume of a gas or liquid that moves in a unit of time. The flow of a gas though a tube or hose is either laminar or turbulent. In laminar flow, the gas molecules move in relatively straight, parallel lines. In a turbulent flow, they are chaotic, bounce into each other, and sometimes move in a manner that causes circular eddies. Laminar flow is very efficient, but turbulent flow wastes energy. The factors that determine whether a flow is laminar or turbulent include flow rate, viscosity of the gas, and the diameter and any obstructions within the tube through which the gas is flowing. Assuming the viscosity of the gas and diameter of the airway are constant, flow rate becomes the most critical factor determining whether the flow is laminar or turbulent.

At slow flow rates, gas molecules move in relatively straight lines with few disruptions—an efficient laminar flow. As the flow rate increases, or the diameter of the tube through which the gas is flowing decreases, the molecules can no longer move in parallel lines. As they bump into each other and the walls of the tube, the flow becomes turbulent. It takes more energy to move gas in turbulent flow. In the airway, flow is never entirely laminar or turbulent but rather a mix of both.

The negative pressure ventilation of normal breathing results primarily in laminar flow throughout the airways. The flow is laminar because air is pulled into the lungs at a modest flow rate. When air is pushed into the lungs, on the other hand, significant turbulence occurs, especially where the airways **bifurcate**. Turbulent flow results in increased airway pressure and a decreased proportion of gas reaching the alveolar-capillary interface (▶ Figure 7-3).

To decrease the amount of turbulence in the patient's lower airways, you must control the flow of the gas when providing ventilation. Generally, the flow rate for positive pressure ventilation should be less than 60 L/min. This rate reduces (but does not eliminate) the turbulence of the flow and results in increased gas delivery deep in the lungs. For practical purposes, the easiest way to control the flow rate is to deliver the ventilatory volume over 1.5 to 2 seconds. Slow inspiration provides a gentle, gradual rise in flow rate and significantly improves deep lung ventilation. This 2-second inspiratory time applies to all forms of positive pressure ventilation with or without intubation.

Hemodynamics

In normal breathing, the negative pressure caused by each breath increases the venous return of blood to the heart. Just as negative intrathoracic pressure sucks air into the chest through the airway, the same pressure also sucks venous blood into the chest from the head and abdomen. The superior and inferior vena cava, which return blood from the head, arms, and abdomen, are the vessels most affected by this phenomenon. When patients transition from negative pressure ventilation to positive pressure ventilation, however, they lose this stimulus for venous return, and some patients who are particularly susceptible may experience decreased cardiac output or hypotension as a result.

The increased intrathoracic pressure also creates a pressure gradient against which the heart must pump. This increases the **afterload**, which can further decrease cardiac output. The greater the pressure used to ventilate an apneic or hypoventilating patient, the greater the decrease in **preload** and increase in afterload and therefore the greater the possible resulting decrease in cardiac output.

Patients who are hypotensive, in shock, or hemodynamically unstable may experience profound changes in blood pressure as a result of the hemodynamic effects of positive pressure ventilation. The best way to limit these complications is to use as little pressure as necessary to achieve adequate deep lung ventilation. In practical terms this is achieved

Did You Know ?

When using a BVM device, or other ventilation device that does not measure volume quantitatively, you are going to have to estimate tidal volume based on chest rise. Typically, 6 to 7 mL/kg will cause minimal chest rise and fall with each ventilation; 10 mL/kg will cause more obvious chest rise and fall.

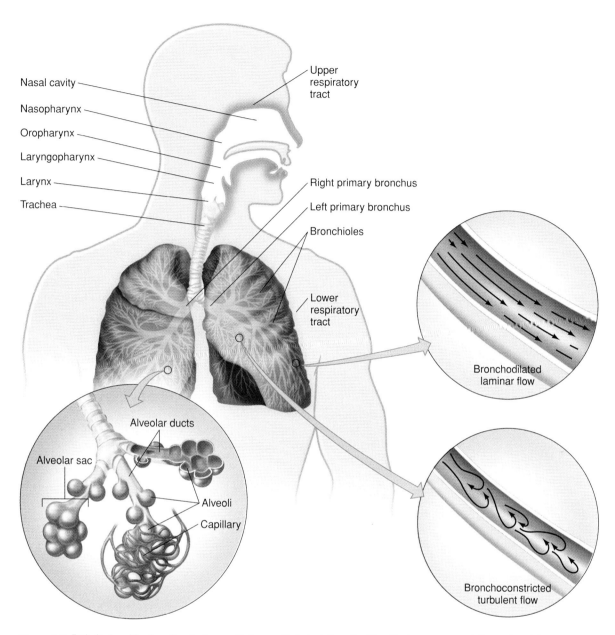

Figure 7-3 Turbulent and laminar flow in the small airways. Turbulent flow significantly decreases gas delivery deep into the lungs.

by using an inspiratory time of 2 seconds, limited chest rise, and/or a manometer (discussed later in this chapter).

Distention of Soft Tissues

Gases always flow from high pressure to low pressure. When air is pulled into the lungs by negative intrapulmonic pressure, the diameter of the airway remains relatively unchanged. In contrast, positive pressure ventilation pushes air into the lungs, and the entire upper airway must have higher pressure than the pressure at the capillary alveolar membrane. Increasing this pressure causes the patient's cheeks to puff out and

the entire upper airway to distend with each breath. This distention of airway and soft tissues results in a larger air space that needs to be filled.

In normal, relaxed negative pressure breathing, the tidal volume is approximately 6 to 7 mL/kg. To maintain deep lung ventilation and oxygenation, either the tidal volume must be increased or the oxygen concentration increased. Using any form of positive pressure ventilation, you should deliver 10 mL/kg if the patient is not intubated and not receiving oxygen-supplemented breathing gas. As soon as possible, the patient should be ventilated with 6 to 7 mL/kg with 100% oxygen. Once the patient is intubated, he or she can generally be adequately ventilated with 6 to 7 mL/kg because the endotracheal tube does not distend and there is less loss of gas volume than typically occurs with mask leakage.

Gastric Distention

Air drawn into the mouth and nose by negative pressure flows directly into the lungs. When air is forced under positive pressure into the mouth and nose, most of it goes into the lungs, but some of it may enter and become trapped in the stomach. The accumulation of air in the stomach leads to **gastric distention**. Gastric distention interferes with ventilation by pushing against the diaphragm and preventing complete lung expansion. Gastric distention causes a number of problems for airway management and ventilation and should be minimized as much as possible.

An understanding of how to prevent gastric distention is based on knowing why air accumulates in the stomach during artificial ventilation. The amount of air that goes into the stomach depends on the esophageal opening pressure and the pressure of the gas in the upper airway (▼ Figure 7-4).

The esophagus is a collapsible tube of tissue that is usually not open. The esophageal opening pressure is the amount of pressure required to force air though this flaccid tube. In unconscious patients, it takes about 15 to 25 cm H_2O pressure to open the esophagus. Unfortunately, the esophageal opening pressure decreases considerably as the patient remains unconscious and can fall as low as 0 to 5 cm H_2O in cardiac arrest.

When the pressure of the gas in the upper airway exceeds the esophageal opening pressure, air enters the stomach. The distended stomach pushing against the diaphragm makes ventilation more difficult. To

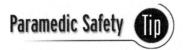

overcome this difficulty, greater pressure is required, creating a vicious cycle of increased gastric distention. Although hypoventilation due to gastric distention is a potential problem in all patients, it is particularly problematic in pediatric patients.

In addition to decreasing the effectiveness of ventilation, gastric distention significantly increases the risk of vomiting. The stomach is a distendable organ but can hold only so much volume. As gastric distention increases, the intragastric pressure increases. Eventually this pressure will exceed the esophageal opening pressure, causing **passive regurgitation**. Any time a patient regurgitates stomach contents, the patient is at a serious risk for aspiration of vomitus into the lungs. Patients with a suppressed gag reflex are at an even greater risk. Aspiration of stomach contents into the lungs causes aspiration pneumonitis, which has a high mortality.

Managing Gastric Distention

Gastric distention is one of the most significant and life-threatening complications of positive pressure ventilation. The risk of aspiration following regurgitation cannot be overemphasized. Aspiration pneumonitis has a good chance of developing in a patient who aspirates even a small amount of stomach contents into the lungs. The key to decreasing this risk is not to accept gastric distention but to manage it. There are two strategies for managing gastric distention during positive pressure ventilation: reduction and relief.

Reducing Gastric Distention

Controlling Upper Airway Pressure

The most effective way to reduce gastric distention is to keep upper airway pressure lower than the esophageal opening pressure. Again, the best way to do this is to deliver the ventilatory volume over 1.5 to 2 seconds. This limits peaks in the upper airway pressure. Monitoring of upper airway pressure can be accomplished by using a manometer attached to

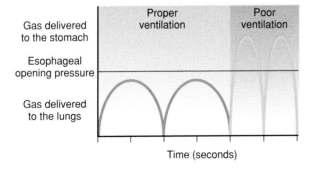

Figure 7-4 Any upper airway pressure that exceeds the lower esophageal opening pressure will cause gas to be delivered to the stomach, not the lungs, when ventilating the unprotected airway. Long, slow ventilations (1.5 to 2 second inspiratory rate) decrease the upper airway pressure and thereby decrease gastric distention.

the ventilation device (▼ Figure 7-5). Small, disposable manometers are becoming common options on BVM devices. You should ventilate in a manner that keeps peak inspiratory pressure as low as possible, ideally below 15 cm of H_2O.

Unfortunately, it is not always possible to keep the upper airway pressure below the esophageal opening pressure. In some conditions you must generate significant pressure to ventilate the patient. This is the case when the lungs are "stiff" (ie, have poor compliance), when there is high airway resistance (as occurs in bronchoconstriction), or when there is an airway obstruction. Large patients are another challenge. The larger the patient, the heavier the chest, and overcoming the weight of the chest with ventilation may require high pressures. All of these situations are true dilemmas. If you do not ventilate the patient with high enough pressure, you cannot effectively ventilate and hypoxemia will develop. As you ventilate the patient with sufficient pressure, the possibility of gastric distention increases.

Finally, the esophageal opening pressure is not a constant. Extensive research indicates that the esophageal opening pressure is generally between 15 to 25 cm H_2O in patients undergoing anesthesia. Unfortunately, the esophageal opening pressure has not been as extensively studied in emergency patients. While we do not know for certain, we must assume that alcohol, other drugs, food, and some diseases decrease the esophageal opening pressure. In cardiac arrest the esophageal opening pressure may fall as low as 0 to 5 cm H_2O. In such cases it is not possible to ventilate a patient who has not been intubated without exceeding the esophageal opening pressure.

Posterior Cricoid Pressure

Generally it is not possible to prevent all gastric distention, especially in cases of prolonged ventilation or cardiac arrest. An additional strategy is to apply posterior cricoid pressure to reduce the amount of

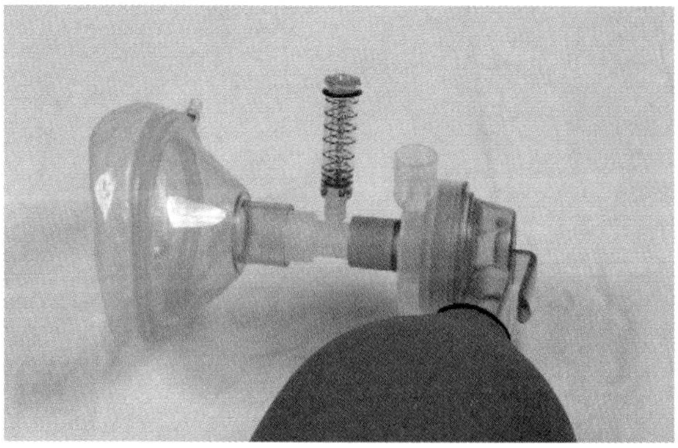

Figure 7-5 Manometer attached to a ventilation device.

Case Study

Case Study, Part 1

En route to a report of a "man down" you receive a report from the first responders on scene that "CPR is in progress." Your pulse quickens as you begin your mental checklist of equipment to bring onto the scene: paramedicbag, suction, medication kit, and monitor/defibrillator. You and your partner discuss role assignments; you jointly decide that you will manage the airway while she establishes an IV and operates the monitor.

Arriving at the scene, you can see the fire department first responders performing CPR on a middle-aged man lying on the sidewalk. The first responders report that a witness observed the patient stumble, sit down, and finally "pass out" as another bystander was dialing 9-1-1. Arriving on scene, the first responders found the patient pulseless and not breathing and began CPR. Using an AED, they delivered two shocks to the patient, with no return of spontaneous pulses, and continued CPR. It has been 3 minutes since they arrived on scene.

You quickly assess the patient's condition:

Initial Assessment

Recording time
0 minutes

Appearance
Cyanotic, with a pronounced distended abdomen

Level of consciousness
Unconscious, unresponsive to physical stimulus

Airway
Being managed by first respondor

Breathing
Not breathing spontaneously

Circulation
No carotid pulse

As you set up your airway kit you observe something peculiar. It appears that the patient's stomach is growing larger with each ventilation!

Question 1: What is causing this to happen?

Question 2: How might this affect the patient?

Question 3: What can you do to change this situation?

CASE STUDY

air entering the stomach. The technique was first described by Sellick in 1961 and is often referred to as the **Sellick maneuver**.

The Sellick maneuver is based on the fact that the esophagus lies between the cricoid cartilage, which is a complete ring, and the cervical vertebrae (▶ **Skill Drill 7-1**). Pressure applied to the anterior portion of the ring is transmitted to the posterior portion of the ring without decreasing the internal diameter of the airway. Posterior cricoid pressure therefore partially occludes the esophagus by pinching it between two hard objects, the cricoid cartilage and the cervical vertebrae (▶ Figure 7-6).

Skill Drill

7-1 The Sellick Maneuver

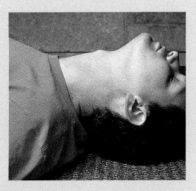 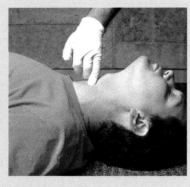 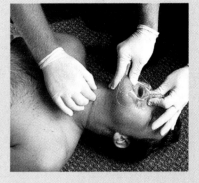

1 Visualize the cricoid cartilage.

2 Palpate to confirm its location.

3 Apply firm pressure on the cricoid ring with your thumb and index finger on either side of the midline. Maintain pressure until intubated.

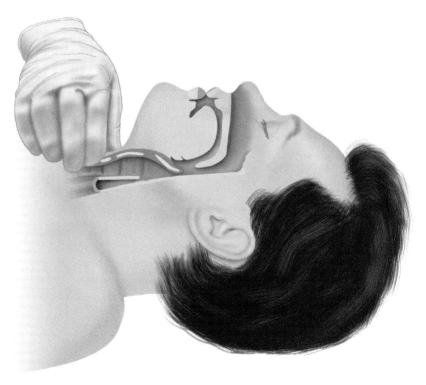

Figure 7-6 The Sellick maneuver. Posterior pressure applied to the cricoid cartilage partially occludes the esophagus between the cricoid ring and the cervical vertebrae, decreasing gastric distention and the possibility of passive regurgitation.

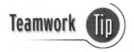

Like any other technique, the Sellick maneuver requires practice to be able to apply it properly and consistently. Remember, frequency matters. Plan on spending many hours practicing this skill until you can do it automatically.

In addition to decreasing the volume of air that enters the stomach during positive pressure ventilation, posterior cricoid pressure has another benefit. Occlusion of the esophagus increases the threshold at which intragastric pressure would lead to passive regurgitation. The Sellick maneuver therefore decreases the risk of vomiting during positive pressure ventilation. The decrease in gastric distention and reduced risk of regurgitation are both beneficial during positive pressure ventilation of patients with an unprotected airway. Unfortunately, many patients vomit immediately upon release of posterior cricoid pressure. Therefore, once you apply the Sellick maneuver, you should not release pressure until the patient's airway has been protected. If this is not possible, place the patient on his or her side and have suction immediately available.

Posterior cricoid pressure should never be used in an attempt to stop active regurgitation. Active regurgitation occurs when the brain signals the stomach to contract and expel its contents. This occurs in response to illness or the presence of irritants or poisons. Active regurgitation is different from the passive regurgitation that occurs when air is insufflated into the stomach causing the intragastric pressure to exceed the esophageal opening pressure. Never use the Sellick maneuver to stop active vomiting because it is unlikely to stop the vomiting and can result in esophageal rupture.

In theory, posterior cricoid pressure can cause movement of the cervical vertebrae. This movement could complicate an unstable cervical spine injury. Since the research findings on this theoretical risk are conflicting, the Sellick maneuver should be used with caution in patients with confirmed or suspected cervical injury.

Finally, use caution not to apply too much force. Laryngeal fracture and tracheal obstruction, while unlikely in healthy adults, is possible if anatomic landmarks are poorly identified or excessive force is used. ▶ **Table 7-2** lists the indications, contraindications, advantages, disadvantages, and complications of the Sellick maneuver.

Case Study

Case Study, Part 2

With your positive coaching, the responder opens the patient's airway with a head tilt-chin lift maneuver and creates an airtight seal around the patient's mouth and nose with the BVM device. You observe the chest beginning to rise and fall. With CPR under way, you assemble your airway equipment. The responder interrupts you, however, saying, "It seems a bit easier to bag the patient, but I am still having problems compressing the bag." You note that the patient's stomach looks almost like a basketball tucked under his shirt.

Question 4: What is happening now?

Question 5: What could you do change this situation?

CASE STUDY

Table 7-2
The Sellick Maneuver

Indications
- To decrease gastric distention during positive pressure ventilation
- Passive regurgitation is imminent or occurring

Contraindications
- Should not be used to stop active regurgitation
- Use with caution in cervical spine injury

Advantages
- Decreases gastric distention
- Decreases passive regurgitation
- Noninvasive

Disadvantages
- May cause extreme emesis if pressure is removed
- Additional rescuers are required

Complications
- Laryngeal trauma may occur with excessive force
- Esophageal rupture from active regurgitation
- Excessive pressure may obstruct the trachea in small children

One of the most common questions about posterior cricoid pressure is how hard to push. Although each patient is unique, you need to apply firm cricoid ring pressure to decrease gastric distention and the risk of passive regurgitation. You can approximate how hard to push on an adult patient's cricoid cartilage by practicing on the bridge of your nose. You need to push hard enough to cause slight discomfort.

Relieving Gastric Distention

Another strategy to decrease the effect of gastric distention is to remove air and other contents from the stomach, which is called <u>gastric decompression</u> and can be done invasively or noninvasively.

Invasive Gastric Decompression

Invasive gastric decompression involves inserting a tube, called a <u>gastric tube</u>, into the stomach and then sucking out the contents. In addition to decompressing the stomach, gastric tubes are also used for tube feeding, administering medications, and removing poisons from the stomach, but these other uses are not discussed.

A gastric tube is a very effective tool to remove air and liquid from the stomach, which decreases the pressure on the diaphragm and virtually eliminates the risk of regurgitation and aspiration. The gastric tube can be inserted into the stomach through either the mouth (if inserted through the mouth it is referred to as an <u>orogastric [OG] tube</u>) or through the nose (if inserted through the nose it is referred to as a <u>nasogastric [NG] tube</u>).

A gastric tube should be considered for any patient who will need ventilation for an extended period of time. Also, insert an NG or OG tube any time gastric distention is interfering with ventilating a patient. This occurs commonly when children are

receiving positive pressure ventilation or have gulped and swallowed air while breathing on their own.

Because both NG and OG tubes are inserted through the esophagus, they must be used with caution in any patient with known esophageal disease (eg, tumors or varices). They should never be used in a patient whose esophagus is not patent. After insertion, you must be sure that the tube has been placed into the stomach. Occasionally the tube may remain in the esophagus or may have been inadvertently placed into the trachea.

Nasogastric tube

An NG tube is a long tube inserted through the nose, into the nasopharynx, through the esophagus, and into the stomach (▼ Figure 7-7). For the purposes of airway management and ventilation, the tube is used to decompress the stomach, thereby decreasing pressure on the diaphragm and limiting the risk of regurgitation. Although an NG tube causes some discomfort, it is relatively well tolerated, even by patients who are awake. Patients can still talk with an NG tube in place, and after a few hours most patients get used to the feeling of having something in their nose and the back of their throat. For these reasons, the NG route of insertion is generally preferred for conscious patients.

During the insertion of an NG tube (▶ Skill Drill 7-2), most patients who are awake will gag and may even vomit. In a patient with a decreased level of consciousness, vomiting can seriously threaten the air-

Special Needs Tip

Occasionally, patients will pose difficult challenges to positive pressure ventilation. For example, patients with a significant episode of reactive airway disease such as asthma may be so "tight" or constricted in the bronchioles that a significant amount of positive pressure is needed to overcome it, resulting in decreased venous return and potential barotrauma. These patients are especially difficult to manage using only basic airway procedures; advanced airway management techniques and/or rapid transport to the hospital is necessary.

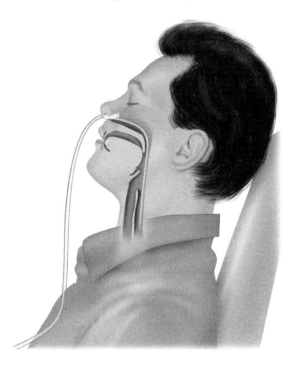

Figure 7-7 Nasogastric tube.

way. Insertion of an NG tube in patients with severe facial injuries, particularly midface fractures and basilar skull fractures, is contraindicated. While extremely rare, NG tubes have been inadvertently inserted into the cranial vault of patients with severe facial and basilar skull fractures. In these cases, use the OG route of insertion.

The NG tube in patients who are not intubated interferes with the mask's seal, which is a significant disadvantage. If you are unable to ventilate a patient because of serious gastric distention, however, you must make a difficult choice. You have to balance the benefit of gastric decompression against the risk of a poor mask seal, and judge which is the priority.

▶ **Table 7-3** lists the indications, contraindications, advantages, disadvantages, and complications of using a nasogastric tube.

Orogastric Tube

An OG tube is the same tube as a NG tube but is inserted through the mouth instead of the nose (▼ Figure 7-8). It works the same way and has most of the same advantages and disadvantages. The major differences include the lower risk of nasal bleeding and increased safety in patients with severe facial trauma. The OG tube, however, is less comfortable for conscious patients, causes gagging much more often, and increases the possibility of vomiting. Considering these advantages and disadvantages, the OG route is generally preferred when a gastric tube is needed in an unconscious patient without a gag reflex. Because these patients obviously need aggressive airway management, the OG tube is almost always inserted after the patient's airway is protected with an endotracheal tube (▶ Skill Drill 7-3).

Table 7-3
Nasogastric Tube

Indications
- Threat of aspiration
- Decrease the pressure of the stomach on the diaphragm

Contraindications
- Extreme caution in esophageal disease or esophageal trauma
- Facial trauma
- Esophageal obstruction

Advantages
- Tolerated by awake patients
- Does not interfere with intubation
- Mitigates recurrent gastric distention
- Patient can still talk

Disadvantages
- Uncomfortable for patient
- May cause patient to vomit during placement even if gag reflex is suppressed
- Interferes with BVM seal

Complications
- Nasal, esophageal, or gastric trauma from poor technique
- Endotracheal placement
- Supragastric placement
- Tube obstruction

Figure 7-8 The orogastric tube.

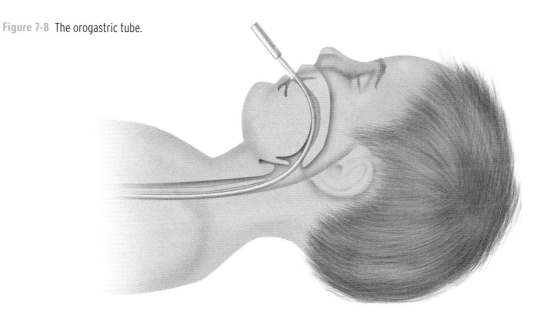

Skill Drill

7-2 Nasogastric Tube Insertion in a Conscious Patient

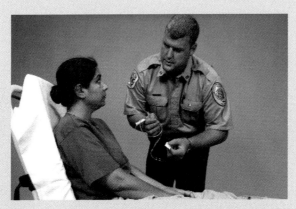

1 Explain the procedure to the patient and oxygenate the patient, if necessary and possible. Suppress the gag reflex with a topical anesthetic (such as viscous lidocaine).

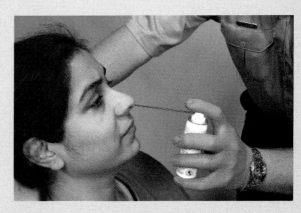

2 Constrict the blood vessels in the nares with a topical alphaagonist.

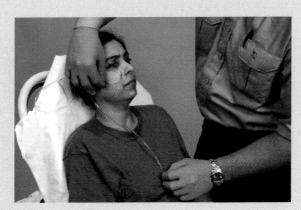

3 Measure the tube for the correct depth of insertion (nose to ear to xiphoid process).

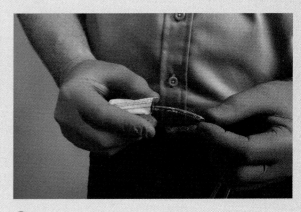

4 Lubricate the tube.

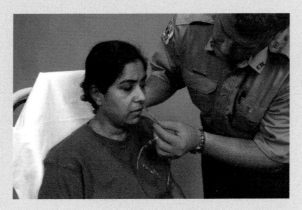

5 Advance the tube gently along the nasal floor.

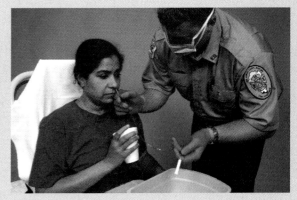

6 Encourage the patient to swallow or drink to facilitate passage of the tube.

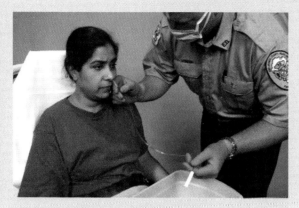

7 Advance the tube into the stomach.

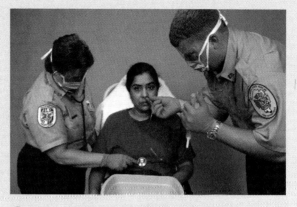

8 Confirm placement: auscultate while injecting 30 to 50 mL of air and/or note gastric contents through the tube.

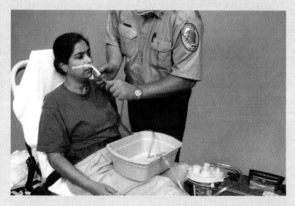

9 Apply suction to the tube to aspirate the stomach contents and secure the tube in place.

▶ **Table 7-4** lists the indications, contraindications, advantages, disadvantages, and complications of using an OG tube.

Noninvasive Gastric Decompression

Occasionally, you may have to decompress the stomach quickly and may not have time to get an NG or OG tube. This situation may occur with life-threatening gastric distention that prevents effective ventilation, which is more common in children than adults. Noninvasive gastric decompression involves applying epigastric pressure to force the patient to expel some air from the stomach (▼ **Skill Drill 7-4**). Unfortunately, this almost always causes vomiting as well. Although this action may seem extreme, it is better to have the

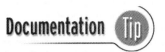

Documentation Tip

Be sure to document the need to manually decompress gastric distention. Because vomiting and therefore aspiration might occur, it will be important to document the justification of performing manual decompression. Remember, documentation serves as protection. If the need is not documented, you will not be able to prove that the need existed later if questions arise.

Skill Drill

7-4 Manual Gastric Decompression

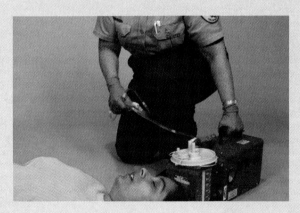

1 Prepare for large-volume suction.

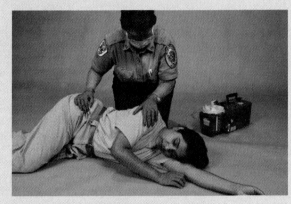

2 Position the patient on the left side.

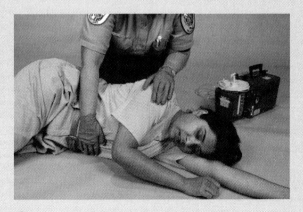

3 Slowly apply pressure to epigastric region.

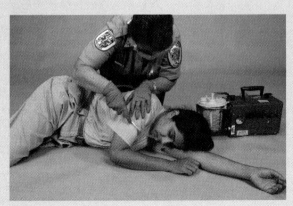

3 Suction as necessary.

Table 7-4
Orogastric Tube

Indications
- Threat of aspiration
- Decrease the pressure of the stomach on the diaphragm
- Patient is unconscious

Contraindications
- Use extreme caution with esophageal disease or esophageal trauma
- Esophageal obstruction

Advantages
- May use larger tubes
- Safe to pass in facial fracture

Disadvantages
- Uncomfortable for conscious patients
- May cause retching and vomiting in patients with a gag reflex

Complications
- Patient may bite tube

---

patient vomit when you can position him or her properly and have suction immediately available than for the patient to vomit unexpectedly

Fortunately, cases in which gastric distention completely prevents ventilation are rare. When it does occur, it poses an immediate life threat, and extreme situations sometimes call for extreme measures. You must carefully evaluate the risk of hypoventilation against the risk of aspiration.

▼ **Table 7-5** lists the indications, contraindications, advantages, disadvantages, and complications of using manual gastric decompression.

Table 7-5
Manual Gastric Decompression

Indications
- Severe gastric distention that is interfering with ventilation
- No gastric tube immediately available

Contraindications
- A gastric tube available
- Adequate ventilation possible despite severe gastric distention

Advantages
- Noninvasive
- Quick

Disadvantages
- Serious risk of aspiration

Complications
- Significant exposure risk
- Aspiration

Case Study

Case Study, Part 3

Although the patient vomits when you perform manual decompression for his gastric distention, a combination of the patient being positioned on his side and being suctioned immediately helps prevent the patient from aspirating stomach contents. After placing the patient supine, you reassess his condition.

Ongoing Assessment

Recording time
5 minutes after patient contact

Initial assessment
Airway is patent, no spontaneous respirations, faint carotid pulse

Intervention reassessment
Responder reports significantly better ventilatory efforts with the BVM device

Any other changes
An oral pharyngeal airway is successfully inserted

Vital Signs

Skin signs
Cyanotic, diaphoretic

Pulse rate/quality
70 beats/min, regular, increasing in strength

Blood pressure
80/60 mm Hg

Respiratory rate/depth
Assisted at 20 breaths/min

Pupils
Fixed, midpoint

SpO_2
86 (100% oxygen)

Electrocardiogram
Accelerated junctional rhythm

After controlling his airway with endotracheal intubation and establishing IV access, your crew loads the patient into the back of the ALS unit. The ride to the hospital is brief, yet you observe that the patient continues to improve, with spontaneous inspiratory efforts noted and increasing color to his skin. At the hospital the patient is further evaluated, eventually being transferred to the intensive care unit. He is discharged 1 week later, with no apparent permanent neurologic sequelae.

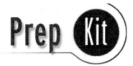

Chapter Summary

When a patient is not breathing or is breathing inadequately, intervention must be quick and decisive. Positive pressure ventilation provides a quick, lifesaving alternative to normal "negative pressure" ventilation. While positive pressure ventilation has saved countless lives, it can also cause complications. The incidence of complications can be decreased by careful attention to the details of the technique.

Although both negative and positive pressure ventilation seemingly end with the same result—air moving into and out of the chest—the ease of negative pressure ventilation contrasts sharply with the effort of positive pressure ventilation.

Under normal physiologic conditions, the body uses negative pressure to efficiently and effectively move air into and out of the lungs. We can approximate negative pressure ventilation using positive pressure techniques, but there are potential hazards such as gastric distention that we must be conscious of in order to ventilate the patient effectively.

Gastric distention caused by air entering the stomach can pose a significant barrier to effective ventilation. Although it is preferable to use invasive gastric decompression techniques to relieve stomach pressure, at times noninvasive procedures may be necessary to improve ventilatory techniques. Proper body positioning and immediate suctioning will minimize the risk of aspiration.

Vital Vocabulary

afterload The pressure gradient against which the heart must pump. Increasing the afterload can decrease cardiac output.

bifurcate Divide into two.

gastric decompression The removal of air and other contents from the stomach.

gastric distention The accumulation of air in the stomach.

gastric tube A tube placed into the stomach.

nasogastric (NG) tube A tube placed into the stomach through the nose.

orogastric (OG) tube A tube placed into the stomach through the mouth.

passive regurgitation Regurgitation that occurs passively when the intragastric pressure exceeds the esophageal opening pressure.

preload The pressure of blood that is returned to the heart (venous return). Until a critical point, an increase in preload causes an increase in cardiac output.

pulmonary barotrauma Lung tissue damage caused by pressure.

Sellick maneuver Posterior cricoid pressure used to decrease gastric distention and reduce the risk of passive regurgitation during positive pressure ventilation.

Case Study Answers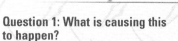

Question 1: What is causing this to happen?

Answer: Either there is some form of obstruction within the upper airway, or more likely the technical proficiency of the responder is not adequate to positively ventilate the patient, resulting in most of the volume entering the stomach.

Question 2: How might this affect the patient?

Answer: As gastric distention continues to build, the pressure within the stomach will cause it to expand, invading the space that the diaphragm normally occupies during inspiration. The resulting loss of expansion space may result in decreased air volumes entering the lung fields.

Question 3: What can you do to change this situation?

Answer: It is possible to assist the responder in his technique. Assess and provide feedback on the following areas:

Is his manual airway maneuver adequate?

Does he have an adequate seal between the face and the mask?

Are the ventilations slow enough to prevent upper airway overpressurization?

Question 4: What is happening now?

Answer: The changes in the responder's technique came a little too late; there is enough pressure within the stomach to prevent adequate expansion of the lungs.

Question 5: What could you do change this situation?

Answer: Although there is risk of aspiration, it is necessary to decompress the gastric distention in order to increase ventilatory volume in the lungs.

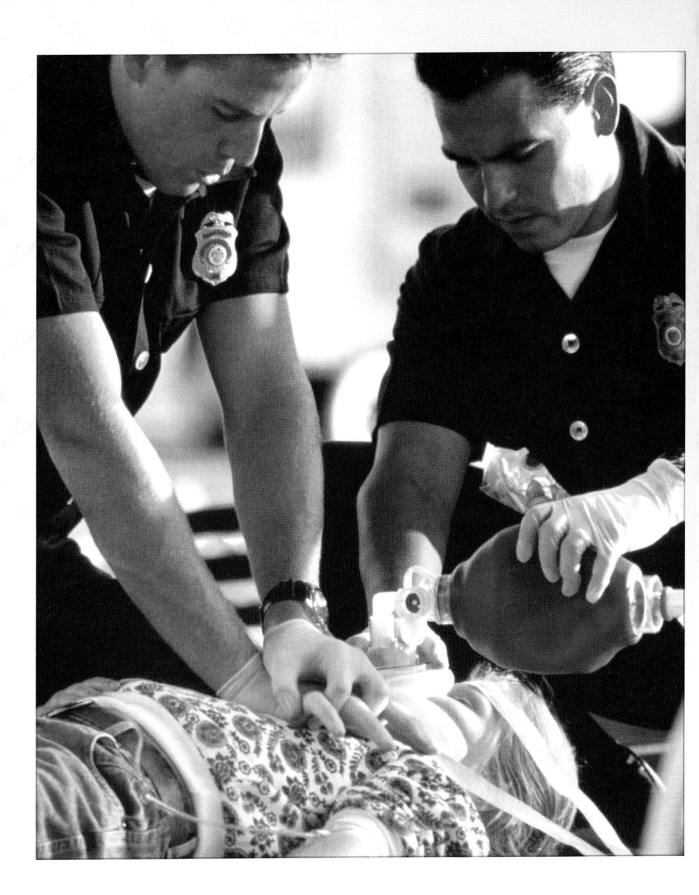

Objectives

Cognitive Objectives

2-1.43 Describe the indications, contraindications, advantages, disadvantages, complications, and technique for ventilating a patient by:

    a. Mouth-to-mouth (p 149)

    b. Mouth-to-nose (p 149)

    c. Mouth-to-mask (p 151)

    d. One-person bag-valve-mask (p 155)

    e. Two-person bag-valve-mask (p 157)

    f. Three-person bag-valve-mask (p 157)

    g. Flow-restricted, oxygen-powered ventilation device (p 160)

2-1.44 Explain the advantage of the two-person method when ventilating with the bag-valve-mask. (p 157)

2-1.45 Describe indications, contraindications, advantages, disadvantages, complications, and technique for ventilating a patient with an automatic transport ventilator (ATV). (p 163)

2-1.53 Define, identify, and describe a laryngectomy. (p 167)

2-1.54 Define how to ventilate a patient with a stoma, including mouth-to-stoma and bag-valve-mask-to-stoma ventilation. (p 167)

2-1.55 Describe the special considerations in airway management and ventilation in patients with facial injuries. (p 166)

Psychomotor Objectives

2-1.95 Demonstrate ventilating a patient by the following techniques:

    a. Mouth-to-mouth ventilation (p 150) (Skill Drill 8-1)

    b. Mouth-to-mask ventilation (p 152) (Skill Drill 8-2)

    c. One-person bag-valve-mask (p 156) (Skill Drill 8-3)

    d. Two-person bag-valve mask (p 159) (Skill Drill 8-5)

    e. Three-person bag-valve mask (p 160) (Skill Drill 8-6)

    f. Flow-restricted, oxygen-powered ventilation device (p 162) (Skill Drill 8-7)

    g. Automatic transport ventilator (p 164) (Box 8-3 and Table 8-8)

    h. Mouth-to-stoma (p 168) (Skill Drill 8-9)

    i. Bag-valve-mask-to-stoma ventilation (p 169) (Skill Drill 8-10)

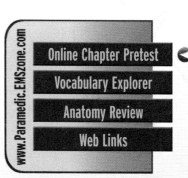

www.Paramedic.EMSzone.com

TECHNOLOGY

- Online Chapter Pretest
- Vocabulary Explorer
- Anatomy Review
- Web Links

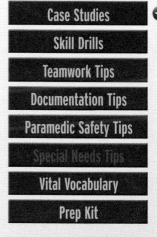

FEATURES

- Case Studies
- Skill Drills
- Teamwork Tips
- Documentation Tips
- Paramedic Safety Tips
- Special Needs Tips
- Vital Vocabulary
- Prep Kit

Chapter

Ill of the forms of ventilation used to support breathing in hypoventilating or apneic patients use some form of positive pressure. Each type of ventilation has advantages and disadvantages that you should carefully consider when deciding which is best in a given situation. No matter which technique that you use, everybody involved in the care of the patient should constantly evaluate the effectiveness of the ventilation (▼ **Table 8-1**). Remember, anything that interferes with the effectiveness of ventilation, even for a few seconds, can a have profoundly negative effect on patient outcome.

The level of difficulty in ventilating patients varies from easy to impossible. Some patients' airways are open and require little effort to ventilate (▼ **Box 8-1**). A very small percentage of patients cannot be ventilated by any means. Airway management and ventilation are dynamic and ever-changing. Some techniques work for some patients, whereas others do not. If one technique for ventilating is not effective, switch to another technique. You can also learn to anticipate certain difficulties when ventilating patients.

Some patients are simply more difficult to ventilate than others. Anticipating those patients who present challenges is an important airway management skill. Anticipate difficulty in the following situations:

- Facial hair
- Facial trauma
- Any foreign object, blood, or vomitus in the mouth
- Very large or obese patients
- Pediatric patients
- Patients with noncompliant lungs (such as those with asthma or cystic fibrosis or drowning victims)

Table 8-1
Evaluating the Effectiveness of Artificial Ventilation

Signs of Effective Ventilation
- Increasing SpO_2
- Improving skin color
- Increasing level of consciousness
- Adequate chest rise
- Quiet ventilation
- Improving blood gases
- Normalization of heart rate
- Good bilateral breath sounds

Signs of Ineffective Ventilation
- Falling or low SpO_2
- Poor skin color
- Decreasing level of consciousness
- Inadequate chest rise
- Noisy ventilation
- Low PaO_2 and/or high $PaCO_2$
- Abnormal heart rate
- Absent, diminished breath sounds

Box 8-1
How Much Volume?

Normally, with negative pressure ventilation, you exchange about 6 to 7 mL of air for each kilogram of body weight. When ventilating the unprotected airway with room air, the ventilation volume should be increased to 10 to 12 mL/kg of body weight due to inevitable mask leak and the distention of the airways during positive pressure ventilations. If you are ventilating manually, this is best gauged by full chest rise.

Unfortunately, this increased volume can lead to gastric distention, so it should be delivered slowly (over 2 seconds) and gently. Once the breathing gas has been supplemented

with oxygen, the ventilatory volume can be returned to 6 to 7 mL/kg. Even though you still will have mask leak and distention to deal with, increasing the oxygen concentration will generally result in adequate oxygenation. The ventilations should still be delivered slowly and gauged during manual ventilation by adequate chest rise.

Once the patient has been intubated, there will be virtually no air leak, airway distention, or gastric inflation. Aggressive, forceful, or excessive ventilations can cause barotrauma and result in hemodynamic complications. Positive pressure ventilations should be continued at 6 to 7 mL/kg delivered over 1.5 to 2 seconds.

- Patients with possible cervical spine injuries
- Patients stabilized with a cervical collar and backboard

Exhaled Breath Ventilation

In the simplest form of positive pressure ventilation, the air in the rescuer's lungs is the reservoir of gas for ventilation. The different techniques using this air are broadly classified as exhaled breath ventilation. These are the oldest forms of artificial breathing.

Exhaled air contains about 16% oxygen. Although this is enough oxygen to sustain life for a short time, it is less effective than the oxygen-enriched gas mixtures that can be given with other techniques. As well, it is difficult to increase the oxygen concentration in exhaled air.

Mouth-to-Mouth and Mouth-to-Nose Ventilation

Mouth-to-mouth ventilation has a long history of success in the resuscitation of apneic patients. It is one of the oldest forms of ventilation and has saved countless lives. The main advantage of mouth-to-mouth ventilation is the fact that no equipment is required. Everyone should practice mouth-to-mouth ventilation and be prepared for the possibility of needing to ventilate a family member or friend in a nonclinical setting. In general, most paramedics do not use mouth-to-mouth ventilation while on duty because of the risk of exposure to infectious diseases and because alternative ventilation methods are usually quickly available.

In mouth-to-mouth ventilation a seal is made directly between the mouths of the rescuer and the patient, and the patient's nostrils are pinched (▶ Figure 8-1) (▶ Skill Drill 8-1). An airtight seal is possible, with little leakage. Because of this and the fact that the lungs are a relatively large reservoir of air, mouth-to-mouth ventilation can deliver outstanding tidal volume. In fact, mouth-to-mouth ventilation delivers tidal volumes superior to those of most other forms of ventilation.

A variation of mouth-to-mouth ventilation is mouth-to-nose ventilation. Mouth-to-nose ventilation may be necessary in cases of oral trauma or any other factor that prevents obtaining an airtight seal with the patient's mouth. In mouth-to-nose ventilation, the patient's mouth is closed with one hand and an airtight seal is made around the patient's nose.

Because of the psychological barriers of using mouth-to-mouth ventilation on a patient whom you do not know and the fear of contracting a communicable disease, mouth-to-mouth ventilation is relatively rarely used in traditional patient care settings. Nonetheless, you should be familiar with mouth-to-mouth

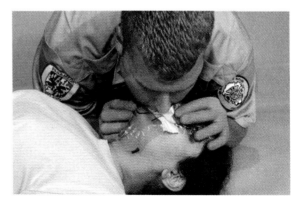
Figure 8-1 Mouth-to-mouth ventilation using a barrier device.

Skill Drill

8-1 Mouth-to-Mouth Ventilation with a Barrier Device

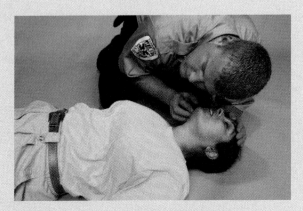

1 Open the patient's airway with a head tilt-chin lift maneuver.

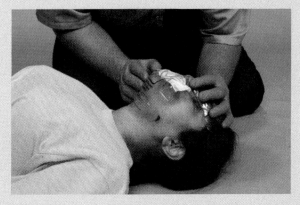

2 Inhale deeply.

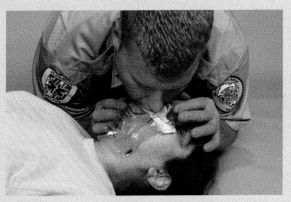

3 Seal your lips over the patient's mouth.

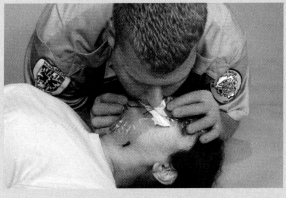

4 Pinch the patient's nose and exhale slowly (1.5 to 2 seconds) until you see the patient's chest rise.

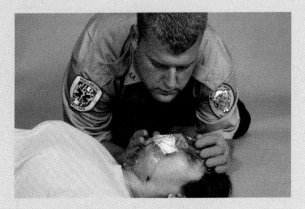

5 Remove your mouth and allow the patient to exhale passively.

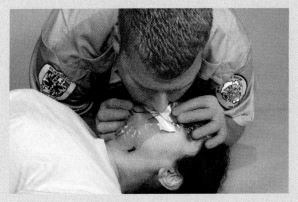

6 Continue ventilation to maintain an acceptable minute volume.

Paramedic Safety Tip

Carrying a small, inexpensive barrier device with you is a form of good insurance, even on duty! You never know when you might be called to deliver artificial respirations and no airway adjunct equipment is immediately available.

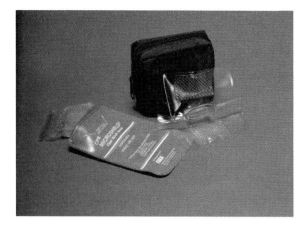

Figure 8-2 Barrier device.

ventilation to use in other situations, such as when a loved one requires ventilation, or as a possible option if other forms of ventilation fail. ▼ **Table 8-2** lists the indications, contraindications, advantages, disadvantages, and complications of mouth-to-mouth ventilation.

Barrier Device Ventilation

In order to decrease the psychological reluctance that people often have to perform direct mouth-to-mouth resuscitation, a number of devices have been developed that place a barrier between the mouth of the paramedic and the patient (◄ Figure 8-1). All of these devices continue to use exhaled breath as the

method of ventilation. They are typically small (designed to fit in a pocket or purse) and designed for single use. Many types and styles are available, with new styles being developed frequently (▲ Figure 8-2). Make sure you follow the manufacturer's directions for use because variations exist.

Unfortunately, the effectiveness of barrier devices, both in providing adequate ventilation and protecting the rescuer from communicable diseases, is difficult to study.

Resuscitation Mask Ventilation

A resuscitation mask is a simple device designed to serve as a barrier between the rescuer and the patient during exhaled breath ventilation (▼ Figure 8-3). In general, resuscitation mask ventilation retains the advantages of simplicity, convenience, and excellent tidal volume while decreasing the psychological barriers and risk of infectious disease transmission associated with mouth-to-mouth and mouth-to-nose ventilation.

Table 8-2
Mouth-to-Mouth Ventilations

Indications
- Apnea of any cause, when ventilation devices are not available

Contraindications
- Communicable disease risk

Advantages
- No special equipment required
- Delivers excellent tidal volume
- Delivers enough oxygen to sustain life

Disadvantages
- Psychological barriers
  - Sanition problems
  - Possible risk of contracting a communicable disease from direct blood or body fluid contact

Complications
- Hyperinflation of patient's lungs
- Gastric distention
- Blood or body fluid contact
- Hyperventilation of rescuer

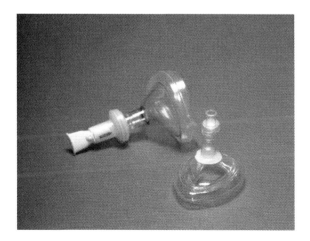

Figure 8-3 Resuscitation mask.

Skill Drill

8-2 Resuscitation Mask Ventilation

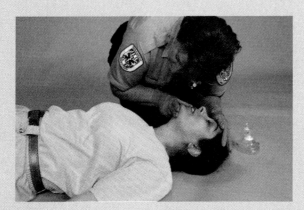

1 Approach the patient from the top of the head, and open the patient's airway with a head tilt-chin lift maneuver.

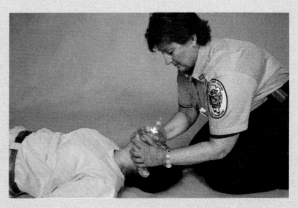

2 Position and seal the mask over the patient's mouth and nose.

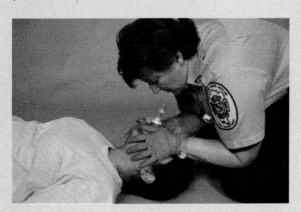

3 Inhale deeply.

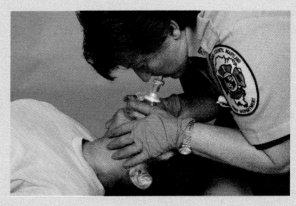

4 Seal your lips to the pocket mask and exhale slowly (1.5 to 2 seconds) until the patient's chest rises.

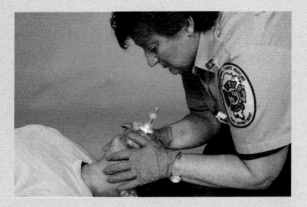

5 Remove your mouth and allow the patient to exhale passively.

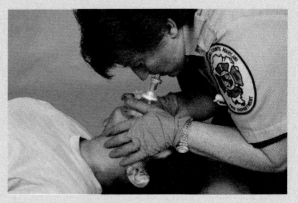

6 Continue ventilation to maintain an acceptable minute volume.

Table 8-3
Resuscitation Mask Ventilation

Indications
- Apnea of any cause

Contraindications
- None in an emergency

Advantages
- Physical barrier between rescuer and patient's blood or body fluids
- One-way valve prevents blood or body fluids from splashing onto the paramedic
- May be easier to obtain face seal

Disadvantages
- Useful only if readily available

Complications
- Hyperinflation of patient's lungs
- Hyperventilation of rescuer
- Gastric distention

Resuscitation mask ventilation allows the rescuer to use both hands to seal the mask, resulting in a mask seal generally superior to that with one-person bag-valve-mask ventilation (◄ **Skill Drill 8-2**). Many resuscitation masks have a one-way valve that diverts the patient's exhaled breath away from the rescuer and/or oxygen ports to increase the percentage of inspired oxygen.

▲ **Table 8-3** lists the indications, contraindications, advantages, disadvantages, and complications of resuscitation mask ventilation.

Bag-Valve-Mask Ventilation

The **bag-valve-mask (BVM)** is the most common device used to ventilate apneic or hypoventilating emergency patients (▼ Figure 8-4). Although a number of manufacturers of bag-valve-mask devices exist, each with its own unique features and characteristics,

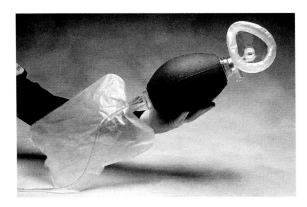

Figure 8-4 Bag-valve-mask device.

Case Study

Case Study, Part 2

Time seems to pass at a crawl as you provide mouth-to-mouth ventilations to the patient. Fortunately you were carrying a barrier device on your key chain, which you are using as you ventilate the patient.

A mall security guard comes up carrying what appears to be a first aid kit.

Inside you see a small cylinder of oxygen and what appears to be an assortment of masks.

Question 2: What would you do next?

CASE STUDY

there are some commonalties. The BVM device consists of a mask that is designed to achieve an airtight seal with the patient's face, usually with a flexible or inflatable silicone gasket. All masks are made in a variety of sizes (pediatric through adult). Some masks are made from hard plastic and are rigid, while others are more pliable (▼ **Box 8-2**). There is less

Box 8-2
Mask Design

Masks are available in several different designs, and some work better than others for emergency ventilation. Ventilation masks vary significantly in material, shape, type of seal, and size. In general, masks used for emergency ventilation (as opposed to those used in operating rooms) should be transparent so you can see any contamination, vomit, or blood in the patient's mouth. All masks have three main parts: the body, seal, and connector. The body is the main structure of the mask, which is made from a variety of materials ranging from rigid hard plastic to flexible transparent rubber or silicone. The body of the mask always increases the amount of dead space, and the more flexible the body the more malleable the mask.

There are two types of seals: inflatable cushion rings and noninflatable flexible gaskets. The pressure in inflatable cushions can usually be adjusted with a syringe. To work properly, they must be neither too full nor too empty. Noninflatable gaskets usually require more effort to obtain a mask seal and have to be sized more carefully. The connector, usually at the top of the body, consists of a 22-mm universal female adapter that connects to all ventilation equipment.

room for error with rigid masks. Pliable masks generally provide a better seal with the face. When selecting a mask, consider also the increase in dead space that the mask creates. Large-volume masks require even more ventilatory volume.

Adult BVM devices include a ventilation bag with a volume of about 1,400 to 1,600 mL. Most manufacturers have other size ventilation bags for infants and children. During ventilation, the bag is squeezed to create the positive pressure necessary to inflate the patient's lungs. The one-way valve between the ventilation bag and the mask prevents the mixing of exhaled breath with fresh gas.

The BVM device can be used with room air, but one of its main advantages is the ability to increase the percentage of inspired oxygen used during ventilation by attaching the device to a constant-flow oxygen supply. If the gas flow needed to fill the ventilation bag exceeds the flow of oxygen from a wall or tank source, a reservoir system is generally necessary. In this case, oxygen flows from the source to the reservoir, into the ventilation bag, and then to the patient (▼ Figure 8-5). When a reservoir bag is used, an oxygen flow rate is needed that prevents complete deflation of the bag. This generally requires a flow of 12 to 15 L/min, which enables you to ventilate the patient with 100% oxygen.

The volume that an operator can deliver depends greatly on the integrity of the seal of the mask and the bag squeezing technique. There is a real skill to squeezing the bag while maintaining a mask seal. Hand size also affects how much volume you can deliver. Small hands cannot expel as much gas as larger hands can. The ventilatory volume also varies slightly from manufacturer to manufacturer. It is important to know how much gas you can expel from the bag using one or two hands with the brand

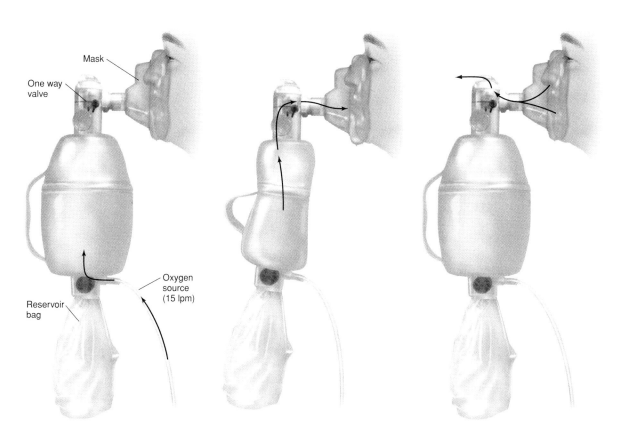

Figure 8-5 A BVM reservoir system. Step 1: Oxygen flows from O$_2$ source into reservoir bag. Inhalation: Oxygen is drawn by the patient from the reservoir bag. The open port provides a safety in the event that the oxygen flow is interrupted, or if the patient "overbreathes" the bag. The presence of the open port prevents 100% oxygen delivery by the device. Exhalation: The patient's exhaled breath is directed from the reservoir by the one way valve, and leaves the mask from the two side ports.

and style of BVM that you generally use. This information enables you to adjust your ventilatory rate if you are unable to ventilate with enough volume for a given patient.

A major advantage of the use of a BVM is the ability to "feel" the ventilation. The pressure needed to cause the lungs to expand, called compliance, is a function of lung stiffness, resistance in the airway (determined by many factors, for example bronchoconstriction or mucous plugging), and chest wall weight. With practice, you will gain a sense of what it feels like to ventilate normal patients. Some patients have poor compliance during resuscitation, and in such cases you should look for a reversible cause (for example bronchoconstriction or tension pneumothorax). In some cases it is difficult to determine whether the patient's lung compliance was poor prior to the current episode of illness, but certainly any changes in compliance during care should alert you to the possibility of rapid deterioration in the patient's condition.

The Importance of Minute Volume

Hypoventilation is defined as an inadequate **minute volume**. Minute volume is the amount of air moved into and out of the lungs in one minute. It is the product of tidal volume and respiratory rate.

Minute volume = respiratory rate (expressed as respirations per minute) × tidal volume

Although you do not often need to calculate the exact minute volume, understanding this concept is critical. Minute volume helps you understand if a patient is ventilating adequately. If a patient is not ventilating adequately, knowing the minute volume will help to determine how much and how often you must breathe for the patient. Neither the rate nor volume alone can tell you if a patient is ventilating adequately. A patient who is breathing slowly but deeply may be breathing adequately. Although there are no absolute numbers, generally tidal volume can compensate only for respiratory rates within the range of 10 to 24 breaths/min (in adults). For that

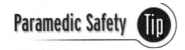

Paramedic Safety Tip

You should use a "test lung" to determine how much volume you can squeeze from a bag-valve-mask using one and two hands. The volume varies with hand size, fatigue, bag design, lung compliance, and technique.

For example, you are treating a 130-kg (280-lb) patient who is breathing slowly and shallowly. Under normal conditions this patient would need a minimum minute volume of 9,360 mL/min (130 kg x 5 cc/kg x 12 breaths/min). To ventilate this patient with positive pressure and room air, you must deliver at least 10 mL/kg (a tidal volume of 1,300 mL/breath) and a minute volume of 15,600 mL/min (1,300 mL/breath x 12 breaths/min). If you have small hands and can only squeeze 650 mL out of the BVM device, you would have to ventilate 24 times a minute just to deliver the minimum minute volume to meet the patient's metabolic needs! Fortunately, once the breathing gas is enriched with oxygen, you can decrease the minute volume to 9,360 mL, or 14 times/min. Although you would rarely make such calculations in emergency situations, keep the fundamental concepts in mind, especially when ventilating large or small patients.

reason, anytime an adult's respiratory rate falls above or below that range, consider the possibility that the patient is hypoventilating.

You can apply the concept of minute volume when ventilating a patient. In particular, you can overcome a small ventilatory volume (caused by your small hands when squeezing a BVM, or your small lungs when giving exhaled breath ventilation) by increasing the rate of ventilations.

One-Person Bag-Valve-Mask Ventilation

The BVM is the most common device used to ventilate emergency patients, and it is most commonly used by only one person. Unfortunately, this is an

Teamwork Tip

It is easy to lose track of ventilation rates during a critical event. It can be helpful for someone to count out loud during ventilations in order to maintain adequate minute volume.

Comprehension Checkpoint

By using a test lung, you know that you are able to deliver 650 mL per ventilation with one hand. You can increase your ventilatory volume to 800 mL by using two hands. How many ventilations per minute do you have to deliver to provide adequate minute volume to a patient weighing 75 kg with room air and 100% oxygen? A 100-kg patient? A 125-kg patient?

inefficient way to ventilate, and significant practice is required to develop and maintain the skill. Because most people do not ventilate patients well using this technique, the one-person technique should not be used, especially if you do not practice it frequently. Anytime that you do ventilate a patient with the one-person technique, it is particularly important to constantly monitor its effectiveness.

The challenge of one-person BVM ventilation involves the need to do three tasks with only two hands (manage the airway, maintain a mask seal, and squeeze the bag) (▼ **Skill Drill 8-3**). Although you may be able to accomplish these three important tasks in some patients, not all patients are the same. Some

patients are more difficult to ventilate than others. Some patients simply cannot be effectively ventilated by one person.

▶ **Table 8-4** lists the indications, contraindications, advantages, disadvantages, and complications of bag-valve-mask ventilation.

▶ **Skill Drill 8-4** describes a technique for effectively obtaining a mask seal.

Most techniques for ventilating patients require an airtight seal between the patient and the delivery device. A good seal is needed between the ventilation mask and patient's face, regardless of the technique used to ventilate. The following two methods can be used to obtain a good seal.

Skill Drill

8-3 One-Person Bag-Valve-Mask Ventilation

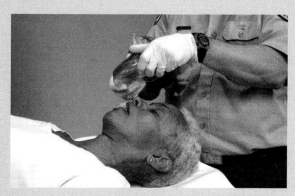

1 Choose the proper mask size to seat the mask from the bridge of the nose to the chin.

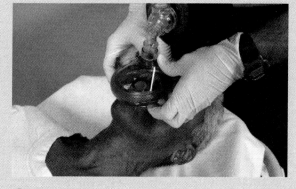

2 Position the mask on the patient's face using the spread/mold/seal technique (Skill Drill 8-4).

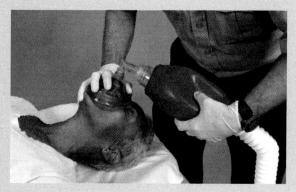

3 Open the patient's airway and hold the mask in place with one hand. Squeeze the bag completely over 1.5 to 2 seconds with the other hand. Allow the bag to reinflate slowly and completely.

Two-Person Bag-Valve-Mask Ventilation

Two-person BVM ventilation is much more efficient than the one-person technique. With two rescuers, one can manage the airway and obtain a mask seal while the other person squeezes the bag (▶ **Skill Drill 8-5**). The major disadvantage is the requirement of an additional person. Two rescuers around the patient's head can make the situation very crowded.

Even though the two-person BVM technique is much more efficient, it is not commonly used. Most often, resuscitation begins with a one-person technique. As long as the patient is being adequately ventilated, the one-person technique can continue. If the patient is not being ventilated properly, however, another person should assist. If you anticipate difficulty in ventilating a patient, begin with the two-person technique. ▶ **Table 8-5** lists the indications, contraindications, advantages, disadvantages, and complications of two-person BVM ventilation.

Three-Person Bag-Valve-Mask Ventilation

A small percentage of unconscious patients have a naturally patent airway and are easily ventilated. On

---

Table 8-4
Bag-Valve-Mask Ventilation

Indications
- Apnea
- Hypoventilation

Contraindications
- None in emergency situations

Advantages
- Minimum requirement of only one person to manage the airway and ventilate the patient
- Excellent blood or body fluid barrier
- Good tidal volume
- Oxygen enrichment possible
- Rescuer can ventilate for extended periods without fatigue

Disadvantages
- Difficult skill to master
- Mask seal may be difficult to obtain and maintain
- Tidal volume delivered depends on mask seal
- One-handed bag squeezing can lead to hypoventilation if the rescuer has small hands or the patient is large

Complications
- Inadequate tidal volume delivery with poor technique or poor mask seal
- Gastric distention

Case Study

Case Study, Part 3

With care and attention, you are ventilating the patient now with a properly fitted mask with supplemental oxygen flowing from the small oxygen cylinder into the mask. As you reassess the patient, you determine the following:

Ongoing Assessment

Recording time
4 minutes after patient contact

Initial assessment
The airway is patent, patient remains apneic, pulse rate appears to be faster and stronger at the carotid.

Intervention reassessment
There are no other changes.

Any other changes
The patient remains unconscious and unresponsive to verbal or physical stimuli.

A member of the local EMS squad arrives, bringing his "first-in" equipment with him. He explains that the ambulance is coming, with a 3-minute ETA. Quickly he assembles the BVM device and hooks it up to his oxygen cylinder.

Question 3: The EMT offers to take over respirations, but instead you suggest that both of you should manage the patient's airway. Why would you suggest this, and how would you execute it?

CASE STUDY

Table 8-7
Using Flow-Restricted, Oxygen-Powered Ventilation for Apneic Patients

Indications
- Apneic patients
- Hypoventilating patients

Contraindications
- Small children

Advantages
- Delivers high-volume/high-concentration O_2
- O_2 volume delivery is restricted to less than 30 cm H_2O, reducing gastric distention

Disadvantages
- Cannot monitor lung compliance
- Requires O_2 source

Complications
- Gastric distention
- Barotrauma
- Hypoventilation in patients with poor lung compliance, increased airway resistance, or airway obstruction

Table 8-8
Flow-Restricted, Oxygen-Powered Ventilation as Supplemental Oxygen to Breathing Patients

Indications
- Self-administration of 100% oxygen to conscious, breathing patients

Contraindications
- Inadequate tidal volume
- Small children
- Unconscious patients or patients with altered sensorium

Advantages
- Can be self-administered
- Delivers high-volume/high-concentration O_2
- O_2 delivered in response to inspiratory effort (no O_2 wasting)

Disadvantages
- Requires the patient's cooperation

Complications
- None

at the midpoint or average for the patient's age. Tidal volume is usually estimated using the formula of 6 to 7 mL/kg because ATVs are oxygen powered and provide oxygen-enriched breathing gas. The tidal volume can be adjusted based on the patient's chest rise and physiologic response. ATVs are considered volume-cycled/rate-controlled ventilators. This means that they deliver a preset volume at a preset respiratory rate, although this does not guarantee that all of the volume is being delivered to the lungs.

Box 8-3
Ventilating a Patient with an Automatic Transport Ventilator (ATV)

1. Attach the ATV to the wall-mounted oxygen source.
2. Set the tidal volumn and ventilatory rate on the ATV as appropriate for the patient's condition.
3. Connect the ATV to the 15/22-mm fitting on the endotracheal tube.
4. Auscultate the patient's breath sounds to ensure adequate ventilation.

Documentation Tip

Record all settings used when an ATV is used, including any changes that were made during transport.

Like the FROPVD, the ATV has a pressure relief valve, which can lead to hypoventilation in cases of poor lung compliance, increased airway resistance, or airway obstruction. ▶ **Table 8-9** lists the indications, contraindications, advantages, disadvantages, and complications of ATVs.

Special Ventilation Situations
Ventilating Trauma Patients

Trauma poses some unique challenges. Three variables with implications for ventilating a patient with traumatic injuries are combativeness, patient positioning (potential for cervical spine injury), and airway obstructions.

Combativeness

For a variety of reasons, many trauma patients are combative. Sudden traumatic injuries create fear and may make a person aggressive. This emotional state may be combined with a preexisting state involving

Paramedic Safety Tip

Consider the cause of combativeness in a trauma patient to be hypoxia and/or head injury until proven otherwise.

Comprehension Checkpoint

List and explain at least five things that you can do to assess the effectiveness of ventilation delivered by an ATV. If you are unable to ventilate a patient with an ATV, what should you do?

alcohol, drug use, or depression/frustration. Combativeness and anxiety are also a result of inadequate cerebral perfusion caused by head injury or shock. This often leads to a diagnostic dilemma in determining whether the patient is combative because of the head injury, shock, or intoxication or is otherwise belligerent. In the first few minutes of care this can lead to a very difficult situation.

If the combativeness is due to head injury or hypoxia, the patient needs to be ventilated with 100% oxygen. If ventilation is successful, combativeness may decrease. Unfortunately, the lack of patient cooperation often makes it extremely difficult to ventilate the patient effectively.

Table 8-9
Automatic Transport Ventilator

Indications
- Extended periods of ventilation

Contraindications
- Poor lung compliance (such as with emphysema or significant pulmonary edema)
- Increased airway resistance (asthma)
- Obstructed airway

Advantages
- Frees personnel to perform other tasks
- Lightweight
- Portable
- Durable
- Mechanically simple
- Adjustable tidal volume
- Adjustable rate
- Adapts to portable O_2 tank

Disadvantages
- Does not detect increasing airway resistance
- Difficult to secure
- Dependent on O_2 tank pressure

Complications
- Unrecognized hypoventilation

If the cause of combativeness is psychological (which is rare), a calm, professional, reassuring approach may be successful. Fully explain what you are doing and why it is important. Realize, however, that some patients are not capable of controlling the stress they are experiencing and will remain combative despite your best efforts to calm them. Getting angry or upset is fruitless and will only worsen the situation.

If help or security personnel are available, it may be necessary to physically restrain the patient. Do not place yourself in danger, and have plenty of assistance to decrease the risk of injury to yourself or the patient. If communication and physical restraint are ineffective and you still have concerns about the patient's cerebral perfusion, a pharmacologic adjunct is typically indicated.

Patient Positioning

You must always assume that a trauma patient has a cervical spine injury. This has two implications. First, all airway procedures must be performed without moving the patient's head. Managing the airway without moving the head is much more difficult, but it can be accomplished effectively. Generally, the head is kept still, and the jaw is thrust forward. This is best accomplished by two people.

The second implication is that all trauma patients are routinely immobilized in the neutral position with a cervical collar and long backboard (▼ Figure 8-8).

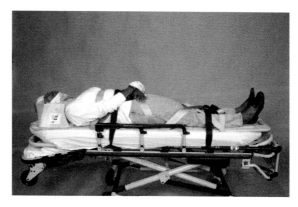

Figure 8-8 Immobilize the patient in the neutral position with a cervical collar and long backboard.

Immobilizing the patient in this position significantly increases the likelihood of an airway obstruction because the patient cannot move or be assisted by gravity to help drain the airway. In fact, gravity works against the patient's own attempts to keep the airway patent. Therefore, you must be vigilant because immobilized patients can quickly succumb to airway problems.

Remember the priorities of patient management. If you absolutely cannot manage a trauma patient's airway without moving the head, you must obtain a patent airway and ventilate the patient. Move the head as little as possible to obtain a patent airway, regardless of the potential compromise to the cervical spine. It is better to risk spinal cord injury than to let a patient die of hypoventilation.

Massive Facial Trauma

Patients with massive facial trauma present a challenge to even the most experienced paramedic. Whether the trauma is blunt or penetrating, considerable risk of airway obstruction and aspiration exists. In addition, traumatic brain injury or cervical spine injury may accompany massive facial trauma, creating a threat to the neuromuscular control of breathing.

Mechanisms of injury for massive facial trauma include gunshot wounds, motor vehicle crashes, falls, battery, and industrial accidents. Airway obstruction may be caused by blood, vomitus, teeth, foreign bodies, edema, the tongue, or structural damage of the face or basilar skull.

The first priority in the care of the patient with massive facial trauma is the assessment and management of the patient's airway and ventilatory status. In addition to evaluation of the mechanism of injury during the scene size-up, the initial assessment may reveal indications of blunt or penetrating trauma to the face. Initial assessment should include consideration of immediate manual stabilization of the cervical spine and the use of the modified jaw-thrust maneuver.

Upon positioning the head, it is important to assess for further indications of airway obstruction.

- Look for obstruction caused by blood, vomit, foreign bodies, edema, or injury of supporting structures. Does movement of the chest indicate respiratory effort?

- Listen for signs of obstruction: gurgling, stridor, or other audible signs of obstruction. Is breathing absent?

- Feel for exhaled air from the patient's mouth and nose.

The next action is to immediately attempt to clear the airway of any obstruction. This is hampered somewhat by the necessity of stabilizing the patient's spine, because turning the head to the side is contraindicated. Suction is vital in removing liquid and smaller particles from the airway. Larger particles must be manually removed using a finger sweep.

Keeping the airway clear is challenging when presented with ongoing bleeding or vomiting. This inability to maintain an airway, regardless of the patient's level of consciousness, is an indication for immediately isolating the trachea with a more advanced airway technique (such as endotracheal intubation). These measures must also be considered immediately when there is edema or structural injury occluding the airway. Ventilation cannot be attempted until the airway is open and clear.

If the airway is cleared by suction and/or manual removal of debris, the patient's ventilatory status must be assessed. In some cases, the patient's breathing may be adequate in both rate and tidal volume upon clearing the airway. In other cases, hypoxia and/or head or spinal injury may create a state of apnea, or of inadequate rate and/or tidal volume. In the event that the airway is cleared and breathing is inadequate, begin BVM ventilations to immediately correct hypoxia and hypercapnia.

In any patient who cannot maintain his or her airway or who does not have adequate respirations, the trachea must be isolated for ventilation. In the presence of massive facial trauma, the first-line mechanisms of intubation, such as direct laryngoscopy, may not be useful. Continued bleeding, vomiting, edema, and/or structural damage may obscure the anatomic landmarks that must be used for direct laryngoscopy. The need for cervical spine immobilization may also limit the usefulness of laryngoscopy. Furthermore, using a BVM device without isolating the trachea in the patient with continued bleeding into the airway or vomiting is contraindicated because it will lead to aspiration, further complicating matters by interfering with the diffusion of gases across the respiratory membrane.

In situations involving massive facial trauma where airway intervention is required but made impossible by direct laryngoscopy, surgical cricothyrotomy, needle cricothyrotomy with jet ventilation, dual lumen airway, or the laryngeal mask airway may be considered, depending on local protocol. These advanced airway techniques will be discussed in detail in subsequent chapters.

The patient with extensive facial trauma often has a difficult airway to manage. The usual techniques of airway management may be contraindicated or impossible due to the nature of the injuries. The techniques above provide some options for both basic and advanced life support providers in managing the patient with massive facial injuries.

Paramedic Safety Tip

Try not to move the head of a trauma patient with a possible cervical spine injury. If the airway or ventilation is threatened and you cannot ventilate effectively, move the head as little as possible to open the airway for ventilation.

Airway Obstruction

Partial and complete airway obstructions are common in trauma patients, especially those who are immobilized. There are numerous causes of airway obstruction in trauma patients, including blood, vomitus, and broken teeth. Managing airway obstruction in trauma patients is the same as in other patients, except that the patient's head should not be moved.

Laryngectomies and Stomas

A **laryngectomy** is a surgical procedure in which all of the larynx (complete or total laryngectomy) or a portion of the larynx (partial laryngectomy) is removed, most commonly as part of the treatment for laryngeal cancer. Patients with laryngectomies have a surgical opening, known as a **stoma**, in the front of their neck, through with they breathe. Stomas affect the delivery of supplemental oxygen and airway management.

Patients with a laryngectomy that require supplemental oxygen therapy must have the breathing gas enriched at the stoma. This enrichment is best accomplished by a tracheostomy collar, which resembles an oxygen mask but is designed to fit the contours of the neck rather than the face. When a tracheostomy collar is not quickly available, a small mask or pediatric mask can be used as a substitute. Patients with laryngectomies are very sensitive to dry and cold air, so you should make every attempt to warm and humidify the gas.

It is actually easier to manage the airway and ventilate laryngectomy patients because the position of the tongue and upper airway soft tissues are irrelevant. Additionally, vomiting generally does not carry a risk of pulmonary aspiration. Finally, the stoma is a relatively direct route to the lungs, and ventilation through the stoma does not usually cause gastric insufflation.

If a patient with a stoma requires artificial ventilation, seal a pediatric mask to the surface of the neck and ventilate. This may seem a bit awkward at first, but it is quite easily accomplished. Some patients with partial laryngectomies or total laryngectomies with a

Case Study

Case Study, Part 4

With the ambulance crew on the scene, transfer of patient care occurs quickly. The crew chief thanks you for your efforts, while the other team members reassess the patient's condition. You observe the following vital signs:

Vital Signs

Recording time
8 minutes after patient contact

Skin signs
Pale, warm

Pulse rate/quality
100 beats/min, strong at the radial

Blood pressure
210/100 mm Hg

Respiratory rate/depth
Assisted at 20 breaths/min

Pupils
Constricted, equal, nonreactive

SpO₂
99% (100% oxygen)

Electrocardiogram
Sinus rhythm

The patient remains unconscious during the entire event. After the crew leaves, you resume your shopping trip, although your mood is a bit more somber.

CASE STUDY

tracheoesophageal puncture (a hole made surgically between the trachea and esophagus that enables air to be forced into the mouth so that modified speech can occur) may have air escape from their mouth and nose during artificial ventilation. If this occurs, simply close the mouth and nose while performing positive pressure ventilation.

Advanced airway management for patients with a stoma is also very straight forward. Simply insert a 5.0 to 6.0 cuffed endotracheal tube into the stoma and advance the tube until the proximal end of the cuff is fully into the trachea. Inflate the cuff and ventilate. The biggest risk of misplacement involves bronchial intubation; so confirm the presence of breath sounds bilaterally.

Ventilation of Stoma Patients

In some respects, ventilating patients with a stoma is easier than ventilating other patients (▶ **Skill Drills 8-9 and 8-10**). First, the airway cannot be occluded by the tongue or any upper airway soft tissue, making the

Skill Drill

8-9 Mouth-to-Stoma Ventilation (Using a Resuscitation Mask)

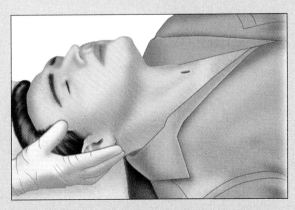

1 Position the patient's head in a neutral position with the shoulders slightly elevated.

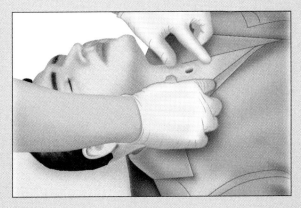

2 Locate and expose the stoma site.

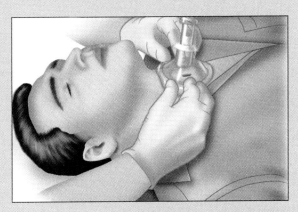

3 Place the resuscitation mask (pediatric mask preferred) over the stoma and ensure an adequate seal.

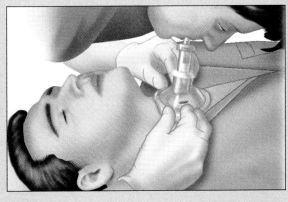

4 Maintain the patient's neutral head position and ventilate the patient by exhaling directly into the resuscitation mask. Assess the patient for adequate ventilation by observing his or her chest rise.

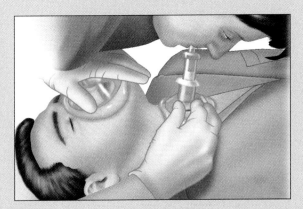

5 If air leakage is evident, seal the patient's mouth and nose and ventilate.

Skill Drill

8-10 Bag-Valve-Mask-to-Stoma Ventilation

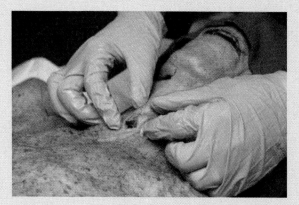

1 With the patient's head in a neutral position locate and expose the stoma.

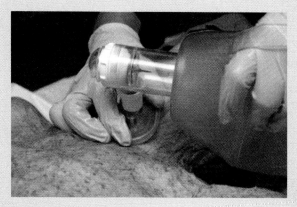

2 Place the bag-valve-mask device over the stoma and ensure an adequate seal.

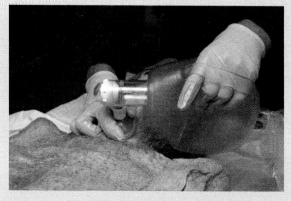

3 Ventilate the patient by squeezing the bag-valve-mask device and assess for adequate ventilation by observing chest rise.

patient's head and jaw position irrelevant to maintaining a patent airway. Second, saliva and vomit do not usually interfere with ventilation because there is no connection between the mouth and the airway. Finally, the air ventilating the patient goes only into the lungs, not the stomach.

The challenge in ventilating patients with a stoma is obtaining an adequate mask seal with the patient's neck. Most ventilation masks, especially pediatric masks, can be made to obtain an airtight seal. Once you have achieved a mask seal, ventilate the patient as usual. If air escapes from the patient's mouth and nose, the patient likely has had an incomplete laryngectomy, leaving a connection between the trachea and the mouth. In this case, simply close the patient's mouth and pinch the nose shut. Then the air will be forced into the patient's lungs. These patients have a risk of gastric distention during positive pressure ventilation.

If you cannot obtain an adequate seal with a ventilation mask, try the two-person technique. If you are alone, you can ventilate the patient using a resuscitation mask, which allows you to use both hands to obtain a seal. If all else fails, or if you are in a nonclinical setting and lack equipment, mouth-to-stoma ventilation is very effective.

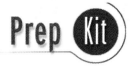

Chapter Summary

Positive pressure ventilation is a lifesaving intervention.

There are a number of techniques for providing ventilation to apneic or hypoventilating patients.

No single technique will work for all patients in all situations.

Paramedics must be skilled in a number of techniques to be able to solve a variety of ventilation challenges.

Vital Vocabulary

<u>automatic transport ventilator (ATV)</u> A fixed flow/rate ventilator that enables the rescuer to set the respiratory rate, the tidal volume, or both.

<u>bag-valve-mask (BVM) device</u> A device with face mask attached to a ventilation bag containing a reservoir and connected to oxygen; delivers more than 90% supplemental oxygen.

<u>flow-restricted, oxygen-powered ventilation device (FROPVD)</u> A fixed flow/rate ventilation device that delivers a breath every time its button is pushed. This device is also referred to as a manually triggered ventilation device, or MTV.

<u>laryngectomy</u> Surgical removal of the larynx.

<u>minute volume</u> The amount of air moved into and out of the lungs in 1 minute, calculated as the product of respiratory rate and tidal volume.

<u>stoma</u> The hole created by a laryngectomy.

Case Study Answers

Question 1: What is the next step in your treatment plan?

Answer: Although the patient has a pulse, it is slow, and she is not breathing. Therefore, you must begin artificial respirations immediately. As a bystander, the mouth-to-mouth ventilation technique is your only option, but risks of infection may be reduced with the use of an inexpensive barrier device.

Question 2: What would you do next?

Answer: Oxygenating the patient now becomes a viable priority. With 100% oxygen delivered to a resuscitation mask, mouth-to-mask ventilations is an effective means of both ventilating and oxygenating a nonbreathing patient effectively.

Question 3: The EMT offers to take over respirations, but instead you suggest that both of you should manage the patient's airway. Why would you suggest this, and how would you execute it?

Answer: With one rescuer securing the mask seal and the other rescuer compressing the bag slowly and effectively, greater ventilation volumes with minimum gastric distention can be achieved over a one-person technique.

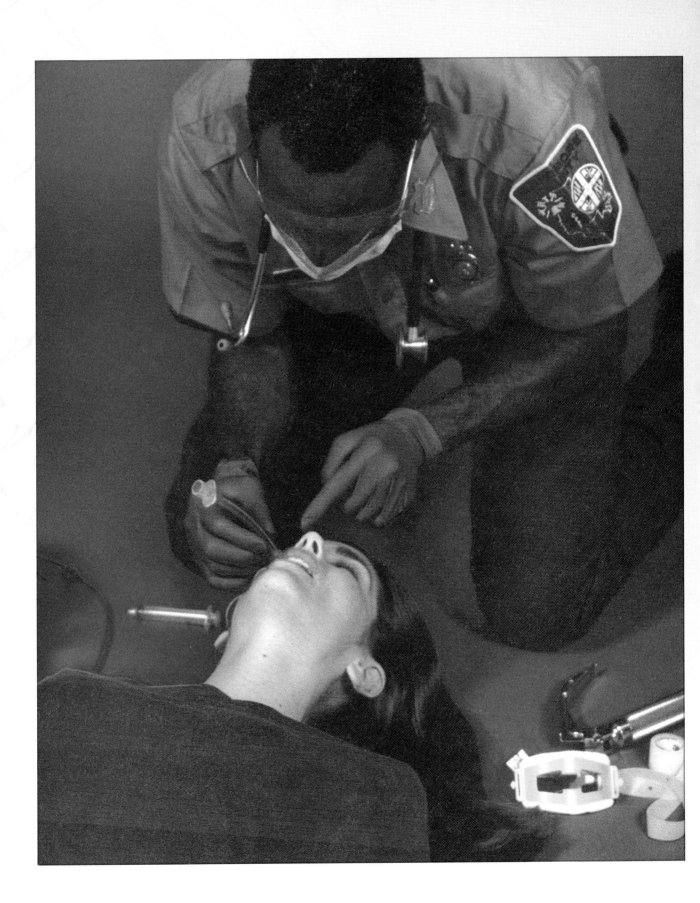

Objectives

Cognitive Objectives

2-1.57 Differentiate endotracheal intubation from other methods of advanced airway management. (p 174)

2-1.58 Describe the indications, contraindications, advantages, disadvantages, and complications of endotracheal intubation. (p 174)

2-1.59 Describe laryngoscopy for the removal of a foreign body airway obstruction. (p 183)

www.Paramedic.EMSzone.com

TECHNOLOGY

Online Chapter Pretest

Vocabulary Explorer

Anatomy Review

Web Links

Chapter FEATURES

Case Studies

Skill Drills

Teamwork Tips

Documentation Tips

Paramedic Safety Tips

Special Needs Tips

Vital Vocabulary

Prep Kit

Endotracheal intubation involves placing a tube through the glottic opening and sealing that tube with a cuff inflated against the wall of the trachea. Endotracheal intubation provides an airtight seal between the patient's lungs and the ventilation device. A sealed cuff placed below the level of the vocal cords is the only form of definitive airway management. All other techniques of airway management are evaluated in comparison to the effectiveness of endotracheal intubation. A solid understanding of the basics of endotracheal intubation is needed when making urgent decisions about when and how to intubate a patient.

Most intubations are performed in the controlled setting of the operating room. Most of what we know about endotracheal intubation comes from the experiences of anesthesiologists managing airways during surgery. This book, however, focuses on the role of endotracheal intubation in the prehospital emergency management of patients. Although there are similarities between intubation in the operating room and intubation during prehospital care, there are also important differences. This chapter will build on what we know about endotracheal intubation in the operating room and apply it to emergency situations.

The Basics

By definition, **endotracheal intubation** means simply placing a tube into the trachea (▼ Figure 9-1). In common usage, however, this term is used in a variety of contexts. For the purposes of this book, the phrase *endotracheal intubation* will be used to mean the process of placing a tube into the trachea.

Many techniques accomplish endotracheal intubation; each has its own advantages and disadvantages. This chapter covers the advantages of having

a tube in the trachea and subsequent chapters will discuss the numerous techniques for putting the tube into the trachea. It is a common error to consider the term endotracheal intubation as synonymous with **direct laryngoscopy**, the most common method of putting a tube in the trachea. Direct laryngoscopy is only one of many techniques used to place a tube into the trachea.

Why Intubate?

Intubating the trachea of critically ill or injured patients has numerous advantages. First, endotracheal intubation provides definitive airway control by providing an unobstructed pathway for airflow into the lungs. Second, endotracheal intubation enables you to finely control the volume, composition, and pressure of the gas being delivered to the lungs. Finally, endotracheal intubation provides a mechanism to deliver liquid or gas medications. Endotracheal intubation is the only airway management technique that enables you to achieve these three objectives. The three major advantages of endotracheal intubation are as follows:

1. to ensure a patent airway
2. to control the ventilation
3. to administer medications

Ensuring a Patent Airway

The **endotracheal tube** is noncollapsible. When it is placed into the trachea, the position of the tongue, epiglottis, and other upper airway soft tissues become irrelevant to maintaining a patent airway. Because the cuff of the endotracheal tube is inflated against the wall of the trachea, secretions from the upper airway and vomitus do not compromise the airway. As long as an endotracheal tube remains properly positioned, unobstructed, and the cuff remains inflated, the patency of the upper airway is virtually assured.

The lumen of the endotracheal tube can become obstructed, however, and the smaller the tube, the

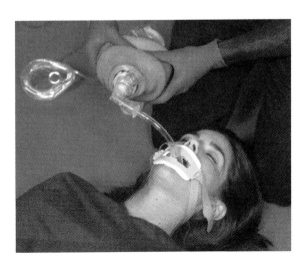

Figure 9-1 Endotracheal intubation.

greater the risk. Additionally, the endotracheal tube does not protect against lower airway obstructions. The most common obstruction within the tube or in the lower airway is mucus secreted from the membranes that line the airway. Thick, sticky mucus can make a plug that is difficult to ventilate around. Depending on where the obstruction is, this plug can become an immediate life threat in intubated patients. Fortunately, most mucous plugs in the endotracheal tube or trachea can be easily removed by suctioning.

Another threat to the patency of the tube in intubated patients is pulmonary fluid. In patients with massive pulmonary edema, pink frothy fluid may bubble up through the endotracheal tube. Trauma patients occasionally are bleeding below the level of the endotracheal tube cuff. Anytime fluid accumulates in the airway, it should be removed by suction. Pulmonary edema may be so copious as to be difficult to suction. Positive pressure ventilations can decrease the volume of pulmonary fluid by forcing it back into the pulmonary circulation.

Controlling Ventilations

When you use a mask to ventilate a patient with an unprotected airway, some of the gas is lost because of mask leakage and some goes into the stomach. When the airway has been secured with an endotracheal tube there is a closed system that enables you to control with precision the pressure, volume, and composition of the gas that reaches the lungs.

Once the patient is intubated, all of the gas coming from the ventilation device goes into the lungs. A closed system distributes pressure evenly and enables you to adjust certain variables to meet the patient's needs. Because no leak in the system exists, all of the air (except for the dead space of the tube, which is much less than the dead space of the anatomic upper airway) reaches the lungs.

Endotracheal intubation enables you to precisely control the breathing gas mixture. In emergency medicine the gas mix is rarely titrated precisely, but the breathing gas is often enriched with oxygen. Supplemental oxygen provided at 15 L/min through a BVM device can provide close to 100% oxygen.

Administering Medications

The alveolar-capillary membrane is thin and therefore offers you the opportunity to administer medications into the central circulation by way of inhalation. Many gases have physiologic effects. Inhalation is the major route of administration for the anesthetic gases and, of course, is the method of delivering oxygen.

Gases are not the only medications administered in the lungs. If medication reaches the alveolar-capillary membrane it quickly diffuses into the blood flowing

Case Study

Case Study, Part 1

"Community ALS 1, respond to a request for ALS backup, 2710 Oak Drive, Ravenswood. Rescue on the scene with a critical medical patient. Time out, 1415."

You head out of the hospital's emergency department ambulance bay in the chase car toward the scene of the call. Although it is the middle of the afternoon on a weekday, traffic is already heavy. Fortunately you are able to make it to the scene with little delay.

As you enter the home you can hear the rescue crew talking to the patient quickly and loudly. You enter the kitchen in time to see the two EMT-Bs moving a heavyset, elderly male from a chair to the floor. The patient appears to be apneic, with agonal efforts to breathe. Quickly, the senior EMT-B reports that they were called to the patient's home for "shortness of breath." On arrival they found him sitting in the kitchen chair, tripoding, in severe respiratory distress. The EMT-B thought he heard audible crackles as he performed an initial assessment. The patient had presented in an agitated state, pulling off the nonrebreathing mask several times and complaining of being "suffocated." The initial vital signs were as follows:

Vital Signs

Recording time
2 minutes prior to your arrival

Skin signs
Cyanotic, diaphoretic, cool

Pulse rate/quality
136 beats/min, irregular

Blood pressure
186/112 mm Hg

Respiratory rate/depth
36 breaths/min, shallow

Pupils
Equal, reactive

SpO₂
N/A

Electrocardiogram
N/A

The patient is becoming lethargic, and his respiratory rate drops dramatically to less than 8 breaths/min. The EMT-B was about to attempt "bagging" the patient while he was still sitting, when the patient began to slump in the chair. The EMT-B decided that he had to move the patient to the floor, where he could better manage the airway.

With the report given, you quickly perform your own initial assessment:

Initial Assessment

Recording time
0 Minutes

Appearance
Cyanotic, diaphoretic, clammy

Level of consciousness
Unresponsive to painful stimulus

Airway
Appears patent with jaw lift

Breathing
Agonal effort, no air exchange felt or heard at the mouth

Circulation
Faint carotid pulse, irregular, slow

Question 1: What are your next steps for the treatment and management of this critical patient?

Question 2: What techniques might you consider in managing this patient's airway?

CASE STUDY

through the pulmonary circulation (▼ Figure 9-2). The administration of medications by the endotracheal route has significant advantages. First, bronchodilators are delivered directly to the site of action and work very quickly. Second, medication is quickly delivered to the central circulation, which is beneficial in cases of cardiac arrest or in other low-flow states.

The key to successfully administering medications by the endotracheal route is to make sure that the active medication reaches the alveolar capillary interface. This is easier said than done. Medications that cause bronchodilation are given to patients with profound bronchoconstriction. The bronchoconstriction itself, however, can prevent the medication from getting deep into the lungs. For these reasons, medications should be nebulized or atomized (aerosolized) to be administered endotracheally.

Nebulization occurs when a high-velocity gas passes through a liquid. This causes the gas to form a mist, which is only slightly heavier than air. The mist is then breathed in or ventilated deep into the lungs. Medications to be administered this way are placed into a plastic nebulization chamber. Some gas, usually oxygen, flows through the medication at high velocity, forming a mist of medication that is instilled into the endotracheal tube.

To administer larger volumes of liquid medication more quickly, it is best to spray the liquid into the stream of air, causing it to be carried as small droplets deep into the airway. If liquid is just squirted down the endotracheal tube of a supine patient, most of it forms a puddle at the end of the tube in the trachea. There are specially designed endotracheal tubes with a medication administration port at the distal tip. If the medication is injected as a breath is being given, it is delivered deeply into the lungs. If you do not have a specially designed endotracheal tube, a similar effect can be accomplished by inserting a straight needle with a medication port adapter into the side of the endotracheal tube. Be careful not to go through both sides of the tube, and use caution not to snag the suction catheter on the needle during endotracheal suctioning.

Not all medications can be given by the endotracheal route. In some cases they simply do not work, and in others they can damage lung tissue. Sometimes damage is caused by the medication itself, the pH of the fluid, or the diluent. The current American Heart Association recommendation is that lidocaine, epinephrine, atropine, and naloxone (Narcan) are safely administered by the endotracheal route.

When you inject a medication directly into a vein, you know that it has been delivered into the bloodstream. When you administer medication into an endotracheal tube, you cannot be as certain. For this reason, the current American Heart Association recommendation for the administration of medication via the endotracheal route is to administer 2 to 2.5 times the dosage and dilute the medication in at least 10 mL of saline or water. Saline is the more common diluent because it causes less cellular damage to lung tissue. Diluting the medication with sterile water facilitates the absorption because an osmotic gradient exists between the drug and the circulation, but water can cause damage to lung tissue.

Indications for Endotracheal Intubation in Emergency Medicine

The general indications for endotracheal intubation are related to the advantages. You should intubate the trachea of any patient when you need to:

- definitively control the patient's airway.
- take control of the patient's ventilations.
- administer endotracheal medications.

Often you will want to accomplish more than one of these objectives.

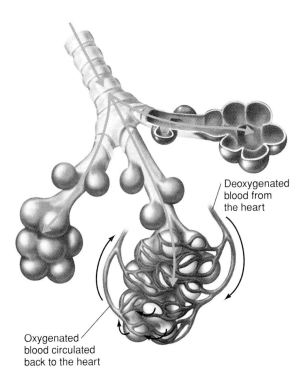

Deoxygenated blood from the heart

Oxygenated blood circulated back to the heart

Figure 9-2 If medication reaches the alveolar-capillary membrane, it quickly diffuses into the blood flowing through the pulmonary circulation.

Intubation to Control the Airway

Patients are at significant risk for losing the patency of their airway if they have any decreased level of consciousness, a suppressed gag reflex, or both. In these patients, their inability to control the soft tissues allows them to partially or completely obstruct the airway. More significantly, these patients cannot clear even small amounts of secretions or vomit from their oropharynx, substantially increasing their risk for aspiration.

Most emergency patients have food in their stomach. A full stomach means there is a high potential for regurgitation and subsequent aspiration. The risk of regurgitation increases as the patient's level of consciousness decreases, the longer they remain unconscious, and the longer they receive positive pressure ventilations. In general, any patient whose level of consciousness is decreased enough that the gag reflex is lost should be intubated to ensure airway patency.

If a patient is able to accept an oral airway without gagging, he or she does not have sufficient protective airway reflexes to prevent aspiration. Also, a noisy airway signifies some type of obstruction. These patients must receive aggressive basic airway management and should be intubated as soon as possible.

Trauma patients are at a particularly high risk for airway obstruction and aspiration. Oral trauma can cause bleeding into the airway, which can be a significant threat to airway patency. Additionally, trauma patients frequently have food or blood in their stomachs and are at a high risk for vomiting and subsequent aspiration.

Intubation to Control Ventilations

A second group of patients who need to be intubated are those requiring respiratory support—specifically, patients in respiratory failure. Many causes of respiratory failure exist, including chronic and acute lung diseases, congestive heart failure, asthma, cardiogenic and noncardiogenic pulmonary edema, and others.

Respiratory failure can be identified if a patient who is having severe difficulty breathing is unable to speak more than a few words at a time. Occasionally such a patient has pale, dusky, or cyanotic skin and begins to experience a decreased level of consciousness (▼ Figure 9-3). These patients are fighting a losing battle to maintain adequate respiration and need aggressive ventilatory support. With experience, you will be able to quickly identify respiratory failure. Patients experiencing respiratory failure are going to need to be intubated eventually, and it is better to intervene early. Because these patients are often conscious, you may need to facilitate the intubation with a pharmacologic agent.

Although subjective assessment data are helpful, objective information makes decision making easier. The following guidelines, taken in the context of a patient's clinical situation, are useful. Anytime a patient's SpO_2 is less than 96%, look for a cause or plausible explanation. An SpO_2 of less than 90% (or a PaO_2 of less than 60 mm Hg) is usually cause for significant concern. Despite aggressive ventilatory support and 100% oxygen administration, intubation is generally indicated. Correspondingly, patients

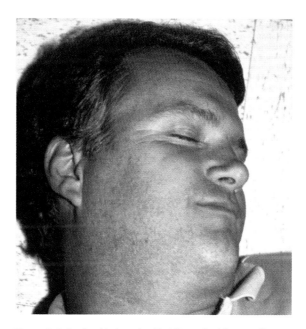

Figure 9-3 Dusky skin is a sign that the patient is cyanotic.

with a $PaCO_2$ greater than 50 mm Hg almost always need to be intubated. ▼ **Box 9-1** lists the objective indicators of respiratory failure.

Complications of Endotracheal Intubation

Endotracheal intubation has great lifesaving potential, but is not risk-free. Always keep in mind the complications of an intubated trachea. For each technique there is a unique set of complications.

Hypoxia

When you intubate a patient, ventilations are interrupted during the procedure. Hypoxia can result from the period of apnea that occurs during the intubation procedure. Therefore, patients should be preoxygenated before an intubation attempt. Preoxygenation enables the patient to better withstand the period of forced apnea.

The question of how much preoxygenation is necessary before intubation is a complex issue and depends significantly on the effectiveness of ventilations. Ideally, the SpO_2 saturation should be above 96% before intubation and not dip below 90% during intubation.

Unfortunately, it is not always possible to achieve a preintubation saturation greater than 96%, so use your judgment. If a patient's oxygen saturation is dropping despite supplemental oxygen therapy and effective ventilation, do not wait to intubate! Intubation is the treatment in these situations. Fortunately, in most cases you can ventilate effectively before intubation and therefore the patient will be adequately preoxygenated.

Patients in cardiac arrest and those in profound shock present a problem because you are unable to obtain a reliable pulse oximetry reading. You will have to make an educated guess regarding the patient's oxygenation status. In general, you should preoxygenate these patients using effective ventilations with 100% oxygen for 2 to 3 minutes prior to attempting intubation. To limit hypoxia during intubation, each attempt should be no longer than 30 seconds. For patients breathing adequately on their own, 2 to 3 minutes of breathing 100% oxygen should be sufficient prior to intubation.

Dysrhythmias

Physical stimulation of the upper airway, either by the tube or the instruments of intubation, can be a powerful vagal stimulus or can cause lethal dysrhythmias. Dysrhythmias occur more commonly when the upper airway is stimulated during a period of hypoxia. Ventricular dysrhythmias, including premature ventricular contractions, ventricular tachycardia, and ventricular fibrillation, can be caused by upper airway instrumentation in adults. Bradycardia is more common in children. The risk of dysrhythmias in adults and pediatric patients is decreased by adequate preoxygenation and by preventing hypoxia during intubation attempts.

Tracheal Trauma

The insertion of a foreign object into the trachea is traumatic. Even when your technique is outstanding, some swelling from tissue trauma should be expected. The amount of swelling significantly decreases with the use of a more gentle technique. Rough technique, poorly lubricated tubes, bleeding disorders, or moving the patient's head excessively may cause significant tracheal trauma and bleeding.

No matter how carefully you intubate, the inflation of the endotracheal tube cuff places pressure on the mucous tissue lining of the trachea. If the cuff is overinflated (greater than 25 to 30 mm Hg) or the tube is in place for a long time without release, the mucous tissue can become ulcerated or necrotic. Mucosal necrosis can be avoided if the cuff is inflated with only enough pressure to prevent leakage. Overinflation of the cuff can also cause pressure on the recurrent laryngeal nerve, causing (usually tempo-

---

Box 9-1

Signs of Respiratory Failure

No one sign indicates respiratory failure. Look at the entire clinical picture and consider combinations of the following signs/symptoms to suggest respiratory failure.

Look of anxiety

Signs of sympathetic overactivity (dilated pupils, sweating)

Acute dyspnea—especially when it results in the inability to talk

Use of accessory muscles

Self-PEEP (breathing against pursed lips, expiratory grunting, groaning)

Cyanosis

Restlessness and fidgeting, progressing to apathy or coma

SpO_2 < 90% despite ventilatory support with 100% oxygen

PaO_2 < 60 mm Hg despite ventilatory support with 100% oxygen

$PaCO_2$ > 60 mm Hg despite ventilatory support with 100% oxygen

Uncompensated respiratory acidosis

rary) vocal cord paralysis. The tube passing through the glottic opening can damage the vocal cords. Almost everyone who has been intubated experiences some hoarseness after the tube has been removed. In a small percentage of patients this hoarseness does not go away. Direct vocal cord damage and vocal cord paralysis are also potential complications of endotracheal intubation.

Laryngospasm

The vocal cords are not only important organs of speech, they also play an important role in protecting the lungs from aspiration. When contracted, the vocal cords create an airtight and watertight seal that protects the lungs from objects entering the upper airway. The spasmodic contraction of the vocal cords, accompanied by an infolding of the arytenoid and aryepiglottic folds, is called **laryngospasm**, and can be lifesaving. Fortunately, laryngospasm usually lasts only a minute or two. Unfortunately, persistent laryngospasm can also be life threatening if no air can pass into the lungs.

Persistent laryngospasm may be managed with an aggressive jaw thrust, which elevates the hyoid and stretches the epiglottis, forcing the aryepiglottic folds to open. This procedure accompanied by positive pressure ventilation stops most laryngospasm. Persistent laryngospasm may need to be treated with succinylcholine.

Barotrauma

The closed pressure system created by the insertion of a cuffed endotracheal tube makes it possible to generate high intrapulmonary pressures. Pressure is evenly distributed throughout the closed system. If the lung tissue has a weakness, or the ventilatory pressures are too high, the lungs can become overpressurized. Pulmonary overpressurization can cause a pneumothorax, pneumomediastinum, subcutaneous emphysema, or tension pneumothorax.

Bronchial Intubation

If the tube is inserted too deeply into the patient or migrates inferiorly, it can come to rest in one of the mainstem bronchi, resulting in complete absence of ventilation in the opposite lung. Because the right bronchus is straighter and larger than the left, this is the typical location for mainstem bronchial intubation (▸ Figure 9-4); however, left mainstem intubation may also occur. The proper position of the endotracheal tube tip is halfway between the vocal cords and the carina, which places the tip of the tube just inferior to the sternal notch. Keep in mind that the patient's head movements can cause

the tip of the endotracheal tube to move as much as 5 cm. Head movement can cause the tube to move deeper into, or, out of, the trachea.

Mainstem intubation can be avoided by using any number of techniques. The most common technique involves inserting the tube under direct visualization until the proximal end of the cuff just past the cords. It is important to be able to estimate the correct depth of insertion (▸ Table 9-1). For blind techniques or reconfirmation of tube placement, bilateral breath sounds are an important finding during reassessment. Another strategy that helps you avoid mainstem intubation is deliberately inserting the tube too far and then withdrawing the tube until breath sounds return on the silent side. The last strategy involves palpation of the cuff at the sternal notch.

Esophageal Intubation

As previously mentioned, even an endotracheal tube that is properly positioned in the trachea can become displaced by either the patient's head movement or an

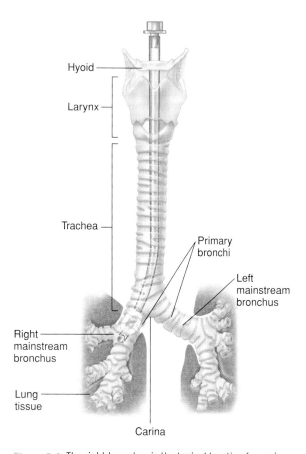

Hyoid

Larynx

Trachea

Primary bronchi

Left mainstream bronchus

Right mainstream bronchus

Lung tissue

Carina

Figure 9-4 The right bronchus is the typical location for mainstem bronchial intubation.

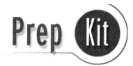

Chapter Summary

Endotracheal intubation can greatly decrease the morbidity and mortality in any situation in which patients cannot maintain their own airway or are in need of respiratory support. The decision to intubate should not be taken lightly. In some cases, it is clear that the patient needs aggressive airway management. Other situations require clinical judgment and experience to make the right decision. In emergency situations there are no absolute contraindications to endotracheal intubation, but the risks must always be weighed against the benefits. The art of medicine involves thoughtful consideration of alternatives and intelligent decision-making, not a programmed response.

Reasons to intubate the trachea include the assurance of a patent airway, the control of ventilation, and the ability to administer certain medications.

As with any invasive procedure, there are significant complications from endotracheal intubation, including hypoxia, dysrhythmias, trauma, laryngospasm, barotrauma, esophageal intubation, and bronchial intubation.

An endotracheal tube does not replace the physiologic functions of upper airway structures. However, in critical situations an artificial airway is better than none at all.

Vital Vocabulary

<u>direct laryngoscopy</u> A technique to accomplish endotracheal intubation by visualizing the glottic opening with the aid of a laryngoscope.

<u>endotracheal intubation</u> Placement of a tube into the trachea.

<u>endotracheal tube</u> A tube designed to be placed into the trachea for the purpose of airway management, ventilatory control, and/or medication delivery.

<u>esophageal intubation</u> The placement of a tube into the esophagus. When discussed in the context of airway management, esophageal intubation usually refers to the misplacement of a tube intended for the trachea, into the esophagus.

<u>laryngospasm</u> The spasmodic contraction of the vocal cords, accompanied by an infolding of the arytenoid and aryepiglottic folds.

<u>Mallampati airway classification</u> A classification system designed to predict the difficulty of intubation/laryngoscopy based on the view of the faucial pillars and the uvula.

<u>nebulization</u> The process of creating a fine mist by passing high-velocity gas through a liquid.

Case Study Answers

Question 1: What are your next steps for the treatment and management of this critical airway?

Answer: The patient needs to be quickly ventilated manually. There has been a marked change for the worse in terms of his ability to maintain a patent airway, as evidenced by the report of the EMT-B. Basic airway maneuvers should continue, with a BVM device or positive pressure ventilation device used to provide artificial ventilations; 100% oxygen should be provided as soon as possible. A basic airway adjunct, such as a nasal airway or oropharyngeal airway, should be used to help control the tongue if tolerated by the patient.

Question 2: What techniques might you consider in managing this patient's airway?

Answer: The answer to question 1 includes a few techniques to manage the patient at the basic level. With the decreasing level of consciousness, however, it is becoming clear that an advanced airway management technique such as endotracheal intubation will be needed to provide a patent airway and avoid aspiration secondary to potential vomiting.

Question 3: You have decided to intubate the patient in order to protect his airway and deliver positive pressure ventilations into the lungs. What size intubation tube would you select?

Answer: For a heavy-set male, a size 8.5 intubation tube would be a smart initial choice. It is sometimes a good idea to have a tube one size smaller and one size larger available to you, just in case.

Question 4: What other adjunct equipment would you want to have immediately available to you during the procedure?

Answer: Because vomiting may occur during an invasive airway maneuver, some type of suction equipment needs to be immediately available to you during any intubation procedure.

Question 5: What concerns might you have about this particular intubation attempt?

Answer: The patient's short, thick neck and recessed jaw may be indicators that a more difficult intubation than typical can be expected. In addition, there may still be some form of intact gag reflex to overcome during the intubation procedure.

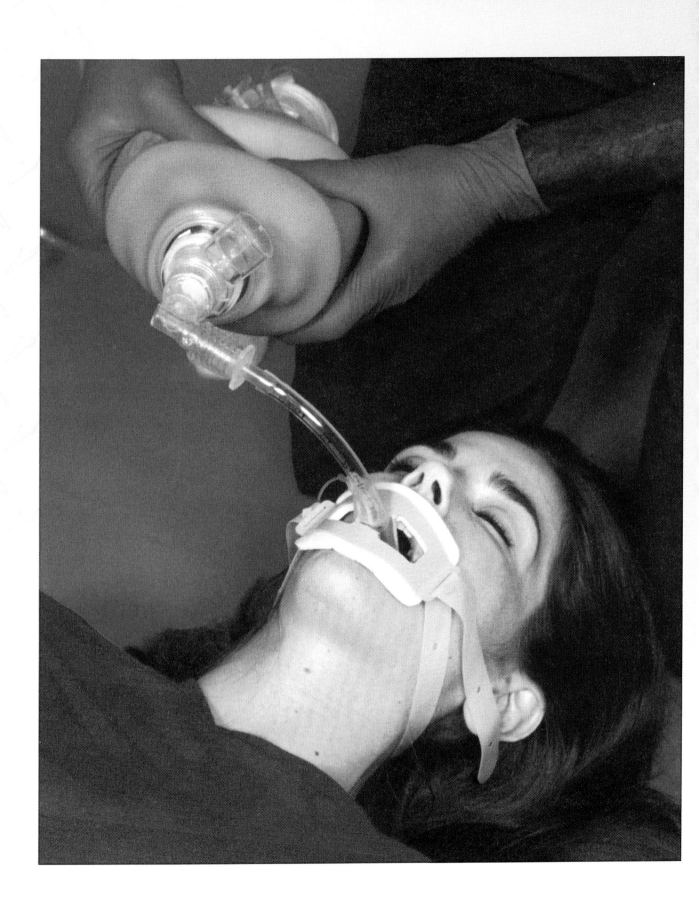

Objectives

Cognitive Objectives

2-1.60 Describe the indications, contraindications, advantages, disadvantages, complications, equipment, and technique for direct laryngoscopy. (p 192)

2-1.61 Describe visual landmarks for direct laryngoscopy. (p 193)

2-1.62 Describe use of cricoid pressure during intubation. (p 205)

2-1.63 Describe indications, contraindications, advantages, disadvantages, complications, equipment, and technique for digital endotracheal intubation. (p 216)

2-1.69 Describe the indications, contraindications, advantages, disadvantages, complications, equipment, and technique for nasotracheal intubation. (p 206)

2-1.73 Describe methods of assessment for confirming correct placement of an endotracheal tube. (p 206)

2-1.74 Describe methods for securing an endotracheal tube. (p 206)

Psychomotor Objectives

2-1.80 Perform body substance isolation (BSI) procedures during basic airway management, advanced airway management, and ventilation. (p 201)

2-1.104 Intubate the trachea by the following methods:

- Orotracheal intubation (p 194) (Skill Drill 10-1)
- Nasotracheal intubation (p 210) (Skill Drill 10-4)
- Digital intubation (p 220) (Skill Drill 10-5)
- Transillumination (p 222) (Skill Drill 10-6)

2-1.105 Adequately secure an endotracheal tube. (pp 208 and 209) (Skill Drills 10-2 and 10-3)

www.Paramedic.EMSzone.com

TECHNOLOGY

- Online Chapter Pretest
- Vocabulary Explorer
- Anatomy Review
- Web Links

Chapter FEATURES

- Case Studies
- Skill Drills
- Teamwork Tips
- Documentation Tips
- Paramedic Safety Tips
- Special Needs Tips
- Vital Vocabulary
- Prep Kit

Skill Drill

10-1 Intubation of the Trachea Using Direct Laryngoscopy

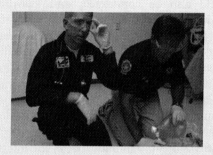

1 Use body substance isolation precautions (gloves and face shield).

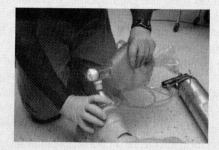

2 Preoxygenate the patient whenever possible with a bag-valve-mask device and 100% oxygen.

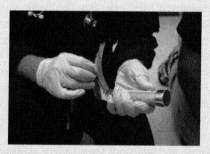

3 Check, prepare, and assemble your equipment.

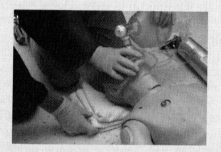

4 Place the patient's head in the sniffing position.

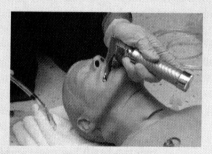

5 Insert the blade into the right side of the patient's mouth and displace the tongue to the left.

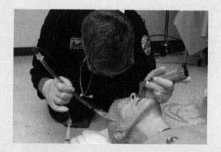

6 Gently lift the long axis of the laryngoscope handle until you can visualize the glottic opening and the vocal cords.

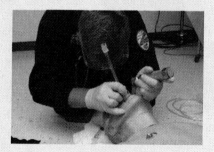

7 Insert the endotracheal tube through the right corner of the mouth and place it between the vocal cords.

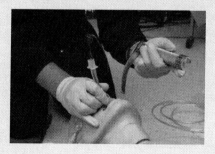

8 Remove the laryngoscope from the patient's mouth.

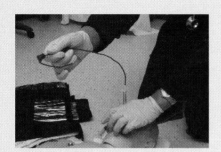

9 Remove the stylet from the endotracheal tube.

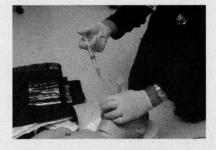

10 Inflate the distal cuff of the endotracheal tube with 5 to 10 mL of air and detach the syringe.

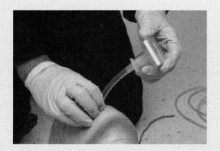

11 Attach the end-tidal carbon dioxide detector to the endotracheal tube.

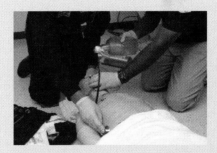

12 Attach the bag-valve device, ventilate, and auscultate over the apices and bases of both lungs and over the epigastrium.

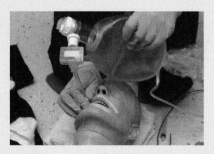

13 Secure the endotracheal tube.

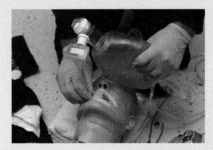

14 Place a bite block in the patient's mouth.

Trauma patients can be challenging to intubate using direct laryngoscopy because one component of obtaining a good laryngoscopic view is proper positioning of the head. All patients with significant traumatic injures should be treated as if they have a cervical spine injury until they have been examined clinically and radiographically. Keeping the head in the neutral position significantly decreases the likelihood of successful laryngoscopy. Also, a cervical collar often makes it difficult to adequately open the patient's mouth.

Nonetheless, in practice, direct laryngoscopy is often performed on trauma patients. If you choose to intubate a trauma patient, you must keep the patient's head in a neutral position. This is best accomplished with an assistant maintaining manual in-line stabilization. While trauma is not a contraindication to direct laryngoscopy (and may in some cases represent an absolute emergent indication), the inability to move the patient's head makes it much more difficult to visualize the glottic opening.

Complications of Direct Laryngoscopy

Many types of complications can occur as a result of direct laryngoscopy. The risk of complications can be dramatically decreased with strict attention to proper technique, but it cannot be eliminated. Even the most experienced paramedics occasionally encounter complications. The most significant complication of direct laryngoscopy is hypoxia. Hypoxia can result from a prolonged attempt at intubation or from misplacement of the tube. To decrease the incidence of hypoxia during the intubation attempt, certain guidelines should be followed.

Did You Know ?

An absolute contraindication to direct laryngoscopy is epiglottitis. The insertion of a laryngoscope blade can cause an increase in soft tissue swelling and/or induce laryngospasm, which may totally occlude an already compromised airway. Even a little air exchange is better than nothing. Patients with epiglottitis are usually taken to the operating room for intubation. If attempts to intubate are unsuccessful and upper airway swelling worsens, the airway is accessed surgically.

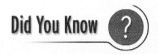

Did You Know ?

It is difficult to perform direct laryngoscopy with a cervical collar in place. A properly fitting collar not only limits head movement (its desired effect), it makes it difficult to open a patient's mouth. When you are intubating a trauma patient, have an assistant provide manual in-line stabilization and release the collar.

A **pulse oximeter** is an invaluable tool to help you decide when to start and stop intubation attempts in patients with a pulse. You should hyperoxygenate patients prior to intubation attempts. A properly hyperoxygenated patient will have 100% oxygen saturation for at least 2 minutes, assuming that the patient is normovolemic and hemodynamically stable. Of course, the patient should be continuously monitored during the intubation attempt. If the level of oxygen saturation falls below 96%, the attempt should be terminated and the patient reoxygenated.

In cardiac arrest, it is often more difficult to determine the patient's oxygenation status because the pulse oximeter usually cannot find a pulse. The amount of time that it takes to hyperoxygenate a patient depends on how long the patient has been hypoventilating or apneic and the effectiveness of the artificial ventilation. If you are unable to quantify oxygenation, a general guideline is to ventilate the patient approximately 24 times/min for at least 2 minutes before the intubation attempt. This should enable the patient to maintain reasonable oxygenation for about 30 seconds. If you are not able to intubate the patient in 30 seconds, halt the attempt and hyperventilate the patient again. There is *no* problem with attempting intubation multiple times as long as the patient is adequately oxygenated before and after each attempt.

Remember that these are guidelines only and that your decisions about whether to intubate should also be based on physiologic monitoring. If the patient's oxygen saturation decreases (especially if it is below 96%) or if the patient experiences a dysrhythmia, *stop the attempt at intubation and ventilate the patient.* Pulse oximetry is unreliable in patients who are hypovolemic, anemic, hypothermic, or in cardiac arrest. If a patient's oxygen saturation is falling despite every attempt to improve ventilatory efficiency, it is probably best to immediately intubate the patient.

Hypoxia can also result from improper placement of an endotracheal tube. If the tube is placed in

Paramedic Safety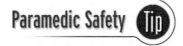

You should preoxygenate all patients to reduce the possibility of hypoxia during an intubation attempt. It is not always easy to determine when a patient has been adequately preoxygenated. Ideally, the patient should have a SpO$_2$ of 100% prior to the intubation attempt, and it should never fall below 96% during intubation. Unfortunately, the pulse oximeter is not reliable in cardiac arrest. If you are unable to obtain a SpO$_2$ reading, you should moderately hyperventilate (24 breath/min) the patient for at least 2 minutes before attempting to intubate. If you are attempting to preoxygenate the patient, and the SpO$_2$ continues to drop despite your best efforts at manual airway management and ventilation, it is best to intubate immediately.

Paramedic Safety

Do not let patients become hypoxic during intubation attempts. Monitor the pulse oximeter and halt your attempts if the SpO$_2$ level falls below 96%. In cardiac arrest patients, limit intubation attempts to 30 seconds. If you are not able to intubate the patient in 30 seconds, halt the attempt and hyperventilate the patient.

the esophagus, no pulmonary ventilation will occur for an apneic patient. **Gastric insufflation** will severely limit the ability of the diaphragm to move. Esophageal intubation that is undetected is a lethal situation. Mainstem intubation is usually not an immediate life threat but significantly decreases oxygenation. Unilateral ventilation is poorly tolerated in patients who are already compromised and should be corrected quickly.

A common and almost always avoidable complication of direct laryngoscopy is **iatrogenic trauma**. Oral, dental, and laryngeal trauma usually occur from poor technique. Most laryngoscope blades are metal and can easily cause hard-tissue and soft-tissue damage. Dental trauma and lip lacerations occur when the paramedic levers back on the teeth or uses the teeth as a fulcrum. The metal blade can injure the epiglottis, vocal cords, larynx, lips, and oral mucosa. Forcing the tube against resistance can also cause serious damage, especially when a stylet is used. Gentle technique and using equipment free of rough edges minimizes soft-tissue damage.

During proper intubation technique, your left forearm is against the patient's face. If you wear a watch, be careful not to scratch the patient's face and eyes.

While aspiration is a complication of all intubation techniques, it is relatively common for patients to retch and vomit when the laryngoscope blade is placed into the posterior pharynx. Because of the possibility of vomiting, suction should be available before beginning an intubation attempt. If the patient is not a trauma patient, turn his or her head to the side and suction the airway. *Do not* ventilate

the patient at this time unless it is necessary, because ventilation may force vomitus that is in the posterior pharynx into the trachea. Quickly clear the airway and then ventilate the patient. Check for the presence of a gag reflex before attempting intubation or inserting an oral airway. The risk of aspiration decreases if you ensure that the patient has no gag reflex before making an intubation attempt. Although not always true, patients without an eyelash reflex usually do not have a gag reflex.

Laryngoscopy and endotracheal intubation may produce a strong sympathetic response characterized by tachycardia, hypertension, and increased intracranial pressure. The physical stimulation caused by the laryngoscope can cause supraventricular and ventricular dysrhythmias. The combination of physical stimulation and preexisting hypoxia (which may be the reason for intubation or result from prolonged attempts) is particularly dangerous. Bradyarrhythmias may also occur in adults, but are common in pediatric patients and require continuous monitoring. Lethal ventricular dysrhythmias are more common in patients with high myocardial irritability, such as those having an acute myocardial infarction or those experiencing hypothermia.

Laryngoscopy causes a dramatic transient increase in intracranial pressure. This increased intracranial pressure is usually well tolerated in patients with normal intracranial pressure, but can be neurologically disastrous in patients with elevated intracranial pressure. When intubation is necessary in patients with brain injury, intracranial bleeding, or neoplasms, steps should be taken to keep the increase in intracranial

Paramedic Safety Tip

The tip of the straight blade is designed to lift the epiglottis, whereas the tip of the curved blade should be placed in the vallecula. Neither should be used like the other. In particular, using a curved blade to lift the epiglottis can cause damage (such as laceration or contusion of the epiglottis).

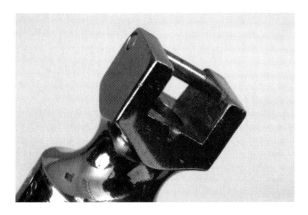

Figure 10-7 The laryngoscope's handle has a bar designed to mate with a notch on the blade.

pressure to a minimum. The first strategy is to ensure that the patient is adequately ventilated. Specifically, be sure that the $PaCO_2$ is not elevated before intubation. Patients with a preintubation increase in intracranial pressure may benefit from premedication with lidocaine.

The role of lidocaine in intubation is controversial, but most of the literature suggests that an intravenous dose of 1.5 mg/kg of lidocaine 3 minutes before intubation will reduce the intracranial pressure spike. Lidocaine may also decrease gagging, coughing, laryngospasm, and (possibly) bronchospasm. The best way to decrease the increased intracranial pressure associated with intubation is to aggressively manage hypoxia, hypercarbia, hypotension, and acidosis *and* then pretreat the patient with lidocaine.

Equipment for Direct Laryngoscopy

The main piece of equipment used in direct laryngoscopy is the <u>laryngoscope</u> (▼ Figure 10-6). The laryngoscope consists of a handle and interchangeable blades. Laryngoscopes come in different varieties (eg,

fiberoptic, disposable) and are made by many manufacturers, but there are more similarities than differences among them.

The handle contains the power source for the light. Most laryngoscopes run on batteries, but some are rechargeable. In either case, make sure there is adequate energy to provide a bright, steady light. The handle has a bar designed to mate with a notch on the blade (▲ Figure 10-7). When the blade is moved into the perpendicular position, the bright light shines near the tip of the blade.

There are many types of laryngoscope blades, each with its own advantages and disadvantages, depending on personal preferences. The two most common blades are the straight (Miller) and the curved (Macintosh) blades. Many other blade designs are manufactured for specialty purposes, with the Wisconsin blade having gained much popularity, especially for use in intubating children. Various blade designs have been shown to be effective, although the curved and straight blades are the most commonly used and readily available. In most emergency situations it is unlikely that you will have

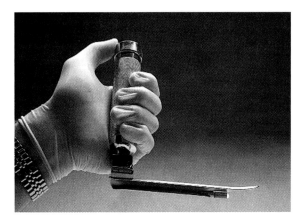

Figure 10-6 Laryngoscope.

Did You Know ?

Blade choice is mainly a matter of personal preference and is more related to experience than to functional differences. Nevertheless, the two blades are used differently. The straight blade is narrow and has a curved channel. Its tip is rounded and is designed to lift the epiglottis to provide the laryngoscopic view. The curved blade has a broad flange that is used to move the tongue out of the way. The tip of the curved blade is flat and broader and is designed to fit into the vallecula. Because of the hyoepiglottic ligament, upward pressure in the vallecula moves the epiglottis, providing the laryngoscopic view.

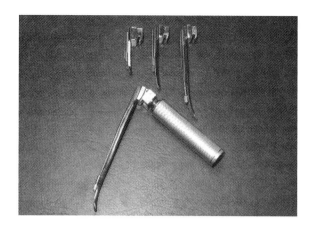

Figure 10-8 A straight blade.

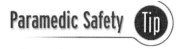

Before you consider intubation, ensure that the patient is being adequately ventilated if possible. Intubation can be painful, so ensure that the patient is receiving adequate ventilation first, if possible.

immediate access to other blades unless you bring them yourself.

Blade choice is mainly a matter of personal preference and is more related to experience than to functional differences. Nevertheless, the two blades are used differently. The straight blade is narrow and has a curved channel. Its tip is rounded and is designed to lift the epiglottis to provide the laryngoscopic view (▲ Figure 10-8). The curved blade has a broad flange that is used to move the tongue out of the way. The tip of the curved blade is flat and broader and is designed to fit into the vallecula (▼ Figure 10-9). Because of the hyoepiglottic ligament, upward pressure in the vallecula moves the epiglottis, providing the laryngoscopic view.

Two other pieces of equipment have specific uses in direct laryngoscopy. The first is the stylet. In the controlled setting of the operating room, many intubators choose not to use a stylet, but it is strongly recommended that you always use a stylet for prehospital emergency intubations. It is common, especially in emergency situations, to be unable to obtain a full view of the glottic opening. The stylet enables you to guide the tip of the tube over the arytenoid

cartilages, even if you cannot see the entire glottic opening. Unlike in the operating room, you may not get a second chance, and it is better to have the stylet and not need it than to need it and not have it.

Blade sizes range from 0 to 4. Infants and children use sizes 0, 1, and 2, while 3 and 4 are considered adult sizes. Most adults of average size can be best visualized with a size 3 straight or curved blade. For pediatric patients, blade sizes are often recommended based on patient age or height. Most practitioners choose the blade for adults based on experience and the size of the patient (3 for average-sized adults and 4 for larger persons).

Another piece of equipment used during direct laryngoscopy is the Magill forceps. Magill forceps have two uses in the emergency setting. First, they are used to remove obstructions from the airway under direct visualization. If you see a solid obstruction in the airway, hold the Magill forceps in your right hand and remove the obstruction (▼ Figure 10-10). The Magill forceps can also be used to guide the tip of the endotracheal tube through the glottic opening if you are unable to get the proper angle with simple manipulation of the tube.

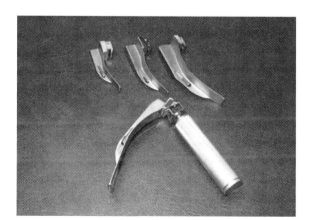

Figure 10-9 A curved blade.

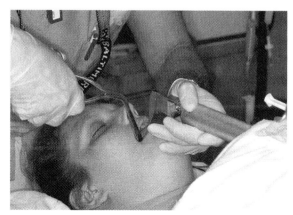

Figure 10-10 Remove obstructions with the Magill forceps.

Technique for Direct Laryngoscopy

Intubation skill involves paying strict attention to the details of technique. Direct laryngoscopy is a psychomotor skill that can be developed and maintained only through practice. Success in intubation results from always following the same sequence of steps. Approaching each intubation in the same way provides a structure and format that is helpful in stressful times. The intubation process can be divided into preintubation, intubation, and post-intubation procedures.

The first procedure described here is for the uncomplicated intubation of a patient in respiratory arrest. Procedurally, this represents the simplest situation, although it may be very challenging technically, depending on the anatomy of the patient. When you understand the sequence of events for a patient in respiratory arrest, you can apply the same principles and steps in other situations. It is assumed here that the decision has already been made to intubate the patient. If possible, you have already evaluated the patient and predicted how difficult intubation will be. Finally, a patient about to be intubated should always be placed on a cardiac monitor and pulse oximeter.

In general, emergency airway management should be considered a two-person procedure. Although situations will occur when you have to manage a patient's airway alone (especially if you practice in the out-of-hospital setting), it is better to have an assistant. The assistant ventilates the patient while you assemble, prepare, and check your equipment; provides cricoid pressure by performing the Sellick maneuver; and hands you equipment. The following procedure description assumes that an assistant is ventilating the patient while you perform the intubation.

The first step in intubation is to ensure that adequate ventilation is being accomplished using basic techniques, including proper airway positioning, use of an oral or nasal airway, and use of positive pressure ventilation techniques, as described in earlier chapters. A later section here discusses what to do in the rare situation where you cannot adequately ventilate the patient first.

Table 10-1
Preparing Equipment for Intubation

Piece of equipment	What to check/prepare/assemble
Ventilation equipment	Have an assistant ventilate the patient while you are assembling, checking, and preparing your equipment. Check to make sure that the patient is being ventilated with 100% oxygen and that the pulse oximeter is reading 96% to 100%.
Endotracheal tube, stylet, 10-cc syringe, water-soluble lubricant	Select the proper size endotracheal tube (7.0 to 7.5 female; 8.0 to 8.5 male). Insert 10 cc of air in the cuff and check that it holds air. Check to make sure that the 15/22-mm adapter is firmly inserted into the tube. Insert the stylet and be sure that the tip is proximal to Murphy's eye. Bend it to be sure that the stylet does not protrude. Bend the tube/stylet into a hockey stick configuration. Increase the angle of the bend if you anticipate a difficult intubation.
Laryngoscope handle and blades	It is best to have an assortment of blades available, since some patients are easier to intubate with one than another. Check the blade that you are going to use. Be sure that it is free from any nicks in the metal (which could easily cause a laceration). Check the bulb to be sure that the light is "bright, white, steady, and tight." The light should be bright enough that it is uncomfortable to look directly at it. It should be white, not yellow or dim. The light should not flicker, especially as the blade is moved on the handle. Most importantly, the bulb *must* be tightly screwed into the handle to prevent its loss in the airway.
Magill forceps	Have available to guide the tip of the tube into the trachea, or to remove foreign body airway obstructions.
Tape or commercial tube securing device	Have tape torn or the device ready before you start.
Suction	You will not need it 9 times out of 10, but when you need it, you need it fast!
Towels	Needed to position the patient's head.

Check/Prepare/Assemble Your Equipment

It is important to prepare and check the equipment before beginning the intubation attempt (▼ **Table 10-1**). It is easy to become complacent with this step. With practice, you will find that most intubations are relatively easy and uncomplicated. In most cases you do not use some of the extra equipment that you assemble for an intubation attempt. Unfortunately, this usual experience may lull you into a false sense of security. When you do encounter a difficult airway, you need to have the necessary extra equipment immediately available. Remember that you are preparing for difficulty, even though you hope that you have none. Even though you may use extra equipment only in a small percentage of cases, you will be glad to have it when you need it.

BSI

Intubation is a procedure that may expose you to body fluids and therefore proper precautions should be taken. In addition to gloves, your face will be relatively close to the patient's mouth and nose. You should always wear a mask and eye shield to protect you in the event of vomiting. Masks with eye protection included are inexpensive, easy to put on, and unobtrusive. They should be considered mandatory parts of your airway kit.

Preoxygenate

The importance of preoxygenation cannot be overstated. During an intubation attempt, the patient will undergo a period of forced apnea. The goal is to prevent hypoxia from occurring during this period in which the patient is not breathing or being ventilated. In general, stable patients can undergo 2 to 3 minutes of apnea provided that they are adequately preoxygenated. In the operating room, patients commonly go a few minutes between ventilations, although these patients are hemodynamically and cardiovascularly stable. Their hemoglobin and hematocrit levels are known, and the patient is being closely monitored.

Unfortunately, this is not the case in the prehospital setting or even in the emergency department, where there is seldom the opportunity to do an extensive preintubation evaluation of the patient. Many patients to be intubated are physiologically compromised. To prepare them for the apnea during intubation, they must be preoxygenated, and the amount of time between breaths significantly limited.

Pulse oximetry has dramatically changed how patients are monitored before and during intubation. Ideally, the patient should have an oxygen saturation of 100% for 2 minutes before intubation, and it should never fall below 96% during an intubation attempt. Since we do not know the patient's baseline level before the crisis, we cannot rely entirely on the pulse oximeter reading, but it nevertheless provides us with important trending information.

For patients who are breathing, it is first important to have them breathe 100% oxygen. Even if they are 100% saturated, more oxygen can be forced into the blood. Hyperoxygenation delays desaturation and the resulting hypoxia. If a patient is apneic or hypoventilating, you should mildly hyperventilate (approximately 24 breaths/min) him or her for 2 to 3 minutes prior to intubation.

The consequences of brief periods of hypoxia can be disastrous. Do not rely too heavily on the pulse oximeter reading because it may be falsely high even if the patient is profoundly hypoxic. Although some of the sequelae of hypoxia are dramatic and immediate, most are subtle and occur gradually. Clearly some of the poor neurologic outcomes following aggressive airway management result from intubation-induced hypoxia. These incidents can be avoided by adequate preintubation hyperoxygenation.

Position the Patient

Proper positioning of the patient is one of the main keys to successful laryngoscopy. An understanding of the proper positioning for intubation by direct laryngoscopy depends on knowledge of basic airway anatomy. There are three axes of the airway: the mouth, pharynx, and larynx. Ordinarily these axes are at sharp angles, facilitating the entry of food into the esophagus and reducing the likelihood of food entering the airway. Although this is an obvious advantage for everyday life, the angles between these three axes make intubation difficult (▶ Figure 10-11).

To facilitate visualization of the airway, you want to align these axes to the extent possible. This is

Did You Know ?

Intubation is a procedure that may expose you to body fluids and therefore proper precautions should be taken. In addition to gloves, your face will be relatively close to the patient's mouth and nose. You should always wear a mask and eye shield to protect you in the event of vomiting. Masks with eye protection included are inexpensive, easy to pout on, and unobtrusive. They should be considered mandatory parts of your airway kit.

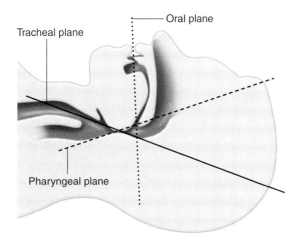

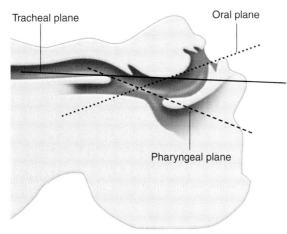

Figure 10-11 Three axes of the airway: oral, tracheal, and pharyngeal.

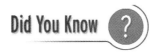

In most supine patients, the sniffing position is achieved by extension of the head and elevation of the occiput. The most practical guide to the amount of elevation necessary in a given patient is to elevate the head until the ear is at the level of the sternum. Elevation of the head is best achieved with folded towels positioned under the head and/or neck. In obese patients, however, padding under the head alone my not result in the sniffing position. You may need to pad also under the shoulders, neck, and head.

achieved by placing the patient in the "sniffing" position. The sniffing position is so-named because this is the position of the head when intentionally sniffing. The position involves approximately a 20° extension of the **atlanto-occipital joint** and 30° flexion of the neck at C6 and C7.

In most supine patients, the sniffing position is achieved by extension of the head and elevation of the occiput 2.5 to 5 cm. The most practical guide to the amount of occipital elevation necessary in a given patient is to elevate the head until the ear is at the level of the sternum. Elevation of the head is best achieved with folded towels positioned under the head and/or neck (▶ Figure 10-12). The advantage of using towels is that the thickness can easily be adjusted by changing the number of folds (▶ Figure 10-13). In obese patients, however, padding under the head alone may not result in the sniffing position. You may need to pad also under the shoulders, neck, and head. When in doubt as to whether the patient is in

a true sniffing position, looking at the person from the side usually provides the best view for evaluating the adequacy of the head tilt.

After the patient is in the sniffing position, have the assistant stop ventilating. The intubation attempt should take no more than 30 seconds, or the amount of time that it takes for the SpO_2 level to fall below 96%, whichever comes first. The attempt should be stopped at 30 seconds, if the oxygen saturation falls significantly, or if the patient's heart rate or rhythm changes dramatically.

If you stop an intubation attempt, simply reoxygenate the patient (generally for 2 to 3 minutes of ventilation at 24 breaths/min with 100% oxygen) and try again. Repeated attempts do not harm the patient, but prolonged attempts do.

Insert the Blade

The tongue is a sticky, amorphous structure that is a major hindrance to visualizing the airway. The

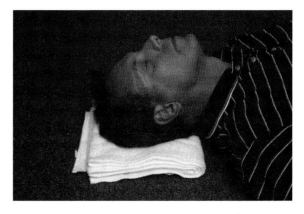

Figure 10-12 Head elevation is best achieved with folded towels positioned under the head and/or neck.

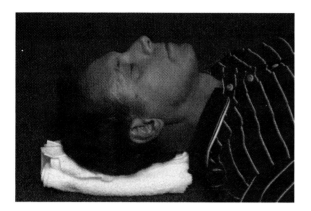

Figure 10-13 The advantage of using towels is that the thickness can easily be adjusted by changing the number of folds.

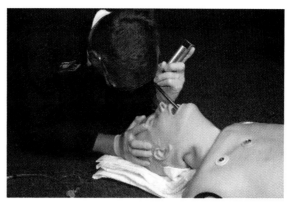

Figure 10-14 If the patient is on the floor or ground, you may need to kneel down and lean forward, or lie down on the floor, to get into the proper position.

proper use of the laryngoscope blade is critical to controlling the tongue; this is difficult to simulate in practice with manikins. Nonetheless, you need to develop excellent technique in manikins to help avoid difficulties in patients.

Position yourself at the top of the patient's head. If the patient is on a gurney, you can squat down to put your head at the level of the patient's face. If the patient is on the floor or ground, you may need to kneel down and lean forward, or lie down on the floor, to get into the proper position (▶ Figure 10-14).

All laryngoscope handles and blades are held in the left hand. Some custom-made or specialty blades can be held in the right hand, but these are rare in traditional emergency settings. Hold the laryngoscope in your left hand and the prepared, lubricated tube like a pencil in your right hand.

Be sure the patient's mouth is open. Most patients' mouths naturally fall open when the head is placed in the sniffing position. If the patient's mouth is not open, the easiest technique is to place the side of your right-hand thumb just below the bottom lip and push the mouth open or scissor your thumb and forefinger between the molars (▼ Figure 10-15).

Regardless of the blade being used, it should be inserted into the right side of the patient's mouth. Use the flange of the blade to sweep the tongue to the left side of the mouth while the blade is moved into the midline. Moving the tongue from right to left is a critical step. If you simply insert the blade in the midline, the tongue will hang over both sides of the blade and you will see only the tongue (▶ Figure 10-16).

If you are using a straight blade, insert the tip of the blade all the way to the posterior pharyngeal wall and then lift the jaw. If you are using a curved blade, insert the tip into the vallecula. With both, the goal is to *lift* the jaw. The most common beginning error is to pull the jaw back using the patient's teeth as a leverage point (▶ Figure 10-17). This can break the teeth and does not provide a view of the glottis.

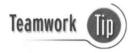

In emergency intubations, the standard of care is to stop an intubation attempt if the patient's oxygen saturation falls below 96%, a significant dysrhythmia develops, or when 30 seconds has elapsed—*whichever comes first*. It is helpful to have a second team member time the intubation effort in order to ensure an adequate safety margin.

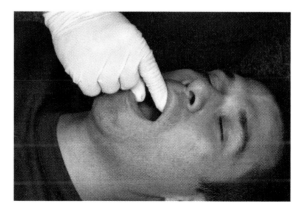

Figure 10-15 Place the side of your right-hand thumb just below the bottom lip and push the mouth open, or scissor your thumb and forefinger between the molars.

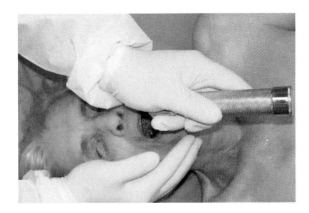

Figure 10-16 If you simply insert the blade in the midline, the tongue will hang over both sides of the blade and you will see only the tongue.

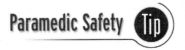

Paramedic Safety Tip

Think right, midline, and lift. Insert the blade in the right side of the mouth, sweep the tongue to the midline, and lift the jaw. *Do not pull the jaw back* or use the teeth as a fulcrum. When proper technique is used, the blade moves away from the teeth.

Lifting the patient's jaw is accomplished by keeping your left wrist straight, elbow bent, and back straight (▶ Figure 10-18). The correct motion is similar to holding a wine glass and offering a toast.

Visualize the Glottic Opening

Now is the stressful part. As you look down the blade you should start to see some familiar airway landmarks. Identifying either the epiglottis or arytenoids is very important at this point. Identifying these structures enables you to make small adjustments in the position of the blade to aid in visualization of the glottic opening. If you are not able to identify any familiar structures it is generally fruitless to continue and it may be better to start over. With the curved blade, it is best to walk the blade down the tongue because you know that the vallecula and the epiglottis lie at the base of the tongue. With the straight blade, insert the blade straight back until the tip touches the posterior pharyngeal wall. This is the proper depth of insertion.

As you continue to work the tip of the blade into the proper position (lifting the epiglottis or in the vallecula) the glottic opening should come into view as you *lift*. Do not be concerned if you do not have a full view of the glottic opening. ▶ **Box 10-1** describes two techniques for improving your laryngoscopic view.

The **gum bougie** is an ingenious device that can make intubation possible in some difficult situations, especially when you have limited glottic visualization. The gum bougie is a flexible device that is roughly a centimeter in diameter. It is rigid enough to be able to be easily directed through the glottic opening, but flexible enough so that it does not cause damage to the tracheal walls. There is a slight angle at its distal tip.

The gum bougie is inserted through the glottic opening under direct visualization. Because it is much smaller than an endotracheal tube, it is useful if you cannot obtain a full glottic view. The angle at its distal tip facilitates entry into the airway and

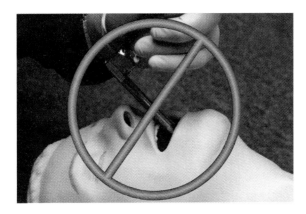

Figure 10-17 The most common beginning error is to pull the jaw back using the patient's teeth as a leverage point.

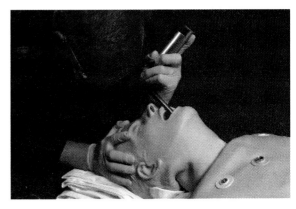

Figure 10-18 Lifting the patient's jaw is accomplished by keeping your left wrist straight, elbow bent, and back straight.

Improving Your Laryngoscopic View: The Sellick Maneuver and the BURP Maneuver

When the angle of the pharynx and the larynx is particularly acute, it is often difficult to see the entire glottic opening. You can do two things to increase the percentage of the glottic opening that you can see. You can employ either the Sellick maneuver or the BURP maneuver.

The Sellick maneuver, which reduces the incidence of gastric distention during positive pressure ventilation, also moves the airway structures more posteriorly. If applied by an assistant during direct laryngoscopy, it reduces the acuity of the angle between the pharynx and larynx and can improve the laryngoscopic view (▼ Fig 10-19).

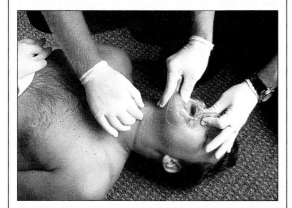

Figure 10-19 The Sellick maneuver.

The **BURP maneuver** is an acronym for **B**ackward, **U**pward, **R**ightward **P**ressure. If you are having difficulty seeing the glottic opening, take your right hand and locate the lower third of the thyroid cartilage. By applying backward, upward, and rightward pressure, you can often move the larynx into view (▼ Figure 10-20). Unfortunately, sometimes when you let go to pass the tube with your right hand, you will lose the view. If possible, once you have visualized the glottic opening, have an assistant hold the larynx in position as you pass the tube. The BURP maneuver can also be applied to the cricoid ring or the hyoid bone.

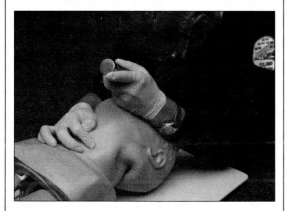

Figure 10-20 BURP maneuver.

enables you to "feel" the ridges of the tracheal wall. Once the gum bougie is placed deeply into the trachea, it becomes a guide for the endotracheal tube. Simply slide the tube over the device and into the trachea. Remove the gum bougie, ventilate, and confirm placement.

Pass the Tube

Once you have visualized the glottic opening, the next step is to insert the tube. When you find the glottic opening, *do not take your eye off it.* Losing sight of the glottic opening is a major cause of failed intubation. Have the tube ready in your right hand so that you can advance it immediately upon identification of the vocal cords.

A major mistake of beginners is to try to pass the tube down the barrel of the blade. The laryngoscope is not designed as a guide for the tube; it is a tool used only to visualize the glottic opening. Placing the tube down the blade would obscure your view of the glottic opening (▼ Figure 10-21). Pass the tube as far to the right as possible and at an angle that lets you watch the tip as you insert it through the vocal cords. Continue to insert the tube until the proximal end of the cuff is 1 to 2 cm past the cords. If you take your eye off the tip of the tube, even for a second, you significantly increase the likelihood of allowing the tube to slip into the esophagus.

Ventilate

After watching the tube pass between the patient's vocal cords, gently remove the blade and begin to ventilate the patient. Hold the tube with your right hand and carefully remove the stylet. Have your assistant attach the ventilation device to the tube with an end tidal carbon dioxide detector (note, if you are using an esophageal detection device, it is important to use it before the first breath is taken).

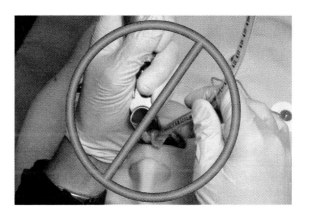

Figure 10-21 Placing the tube down the blade would obscure your view of the glottic opening.

Did You Know ?

A word of caution. Posterior pressure on the superior third of the thyroid cartilage causes the top of the larynx to tip downward, obscuring your view. A common error when using either of these techniques is to simply push posteriorly on the laryngeal prominence. In the case of the Sellick maneuver, it is important to apply posterior pressure to the cricoid ring (not the thyroid cartilage). For the BURP maneuver, be sure to apply backward, upward, and rightward pressure on the inferior third of the thyroid cartilage to avoid tilting the larynx forward.

As the first breaths are delivered, watch the patient's chest rise.

You should now listen to breath sounds as another tube location confirmation technique. You should listen to both lungs at both the apices and bases and to the stomach over the epigastrium. If you are properly positioned in the trachea, you will hear bilaterally equal breath sounds and a quiet epigastrium. Gurgling over the stomach suggests esophageal placement, and the tube should be immediately removed and the patient ventilated. Unilateral breath sounds generally indicate a mainstem intubation. Place your stethoscope over the quiet side of the chest and slowly withdraw the tube until you hear breath sounds return.

Fill the tube cuff with just enough air to stop the leaking sound around the tube. If the tube is properly sized, it will take 4 to 6 mL of air to achieve an airtight seal. Be careful to avoid cuff pressures in excess of 25 mm Hg because they can cause mucosal tissue necrosis.

Ventilation should continue as indicated according to the patient's size and clinical condition. It is prudent to slightly hyperventilate the patient for 30 seconds to 1 minute immediately after intubation to blow off any accumulated carbon dioxide.

Confirm Placement

Watching the tube pass between the vocal cords is your first method of confirming tube placement, but this alone is not completely reliable. You must continue the process of gathering information to assess the location of the tube. Remember that a misplaced tube that goes undetected is a fatal error. You *must* incorporate multiple assessment findings into the determination of where the tube is located. If the tube must be repositioned or removed, be sure to remove the air from the cuff first.

Secure the Tube

The last, and very important step, is to secure the tube (▶ Skill Drills 10-2 and 10-3). Inadvertent extubation caused by either the patient or someone else is *common* and very traumatic to the patient. A second intubation would not be as easy as the first due to swelling and possible bleeding. It is very disheartening to accomplish a difficult intubation and then find that the tube has been accidentally dislodged. Be sure to secure the tube well to prevent this from happening.

Many commercial tube holders are available that have varying degrees of efficiency. If one is available in your facility, become familiar with its use. Every paramedic should know how to secure a tube using tape, because it is almost always available (▼ Figure 10-22).

After the tube is secured, be sure that a bite block or oral airway is inserted into the patient's mouth. If the patient bites the tube or has a seizure, there is a risk of occluding the only airway. A rigid device that will not damage the teeth but that is hard enough to prevent biting the tube should be placed in the mouth. Finally, it is important to limit head movement in the intubated patient. With a firmly secured tube, the tip can move as much as 5 cm during head flexion and extension. If you are going to move the patient, consider placing the patient on a rigid board and using a cervical collar and/or head immobilization device to reduce the likelihood of tube dislodgement during head movement.

Nasotracheal Intubation

Nasotracheal intubation is the process of passing an endotracheal tube into the nostril, past the nasopharynx, and then through the glottic opening (▶ Skill Drill 10-4). Functionally, the tube works exactly the same as a tube passed through the

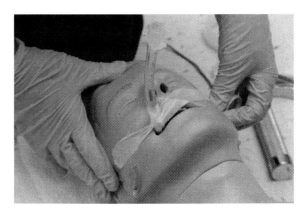

Figure 10-22 Every paramedic should know how to secure a tube using tape, because it is almost always available.

Documentation (Tip)

On the patient care record, be sure to document the means of assessing placement of the endotracheal tube, such as breath sounds, visualization, and capnometry readings.

mouth. In the operating room, nasotracheal intubation is done primarily to avoid having a tube in the way when the surgeon is working in or near the mouth. When nasotracheal intubation is performed on anesthetized patients in the operating room, the tube is often advanced into the nasopharynx and then placed through the glottic opening with Magill forceps under direct visualization. This procedure is rarely performed in the prehospital setting.

The procedure described here is occasionally referred to as "blind nasotracheal intubation." This technique has some advantages over the orotracheal route in emergency situations. Blind nasotracheal intubation uses the patient's own breathing to guide the tube into the trachea and confirm proper tube placement.

Advantages and Disadvantages of Nasotracheal Intubation

The main advantage of blind nasotracheal intubation is that it can be used to intubate a patient who is awake and breathing. Nasotracheal intubation does not require that you place anything into the mouth. Since the strongest gag reflex is stimulated by a foreign object deep in the throat, the nasotracheal route causes much less retching and a smaller risk of vomiting in patients with an intact gag reflex.

Another major advantage of nasotracheal intubation is that there is no need for a laryngoscope. Nasotracheal intubation may be an option if there is an equipment failure. Because no laryngoscope is used, the risk of dental or oral trauma is virtually eliminated, which may be a consideration when intubating a patient with loose or unstable teeth. The mouth need not be opened for nasotracheal intubation to be accomplished, and this can be a significant advantage for patients with limited temporomandibular joint mobility (patients with wired jaws,

Case Study

Case Study, Part 2

With one EMT immobilizing the cervical spine manually, you quickly release the cervical collar. To your relief there appears to be no injury to the patient's jaw; you are able to suction the airway quickly. Meanwhile your partner has been preparing your intubation equipment, and hands over a laryngoscope handle with a number 3 straight blade attached. With your left hand guiding the suction catheter, you insert the tip of the blade into the mouth, trying to visualize the glottic opening. However, the amount of blood filling the posterior oropharynx is greater than the motorized suction unit can handle, thereby blocking your field of view.

Meanwhile another EMT has completed her rapid trauma exam and vital signs. She reports the following:

Physical Examination

Recording time
2 minutes after patient contact

Level of orientation
Deeply unconscious

Head
Abrasions, lacerations to scalp, face

Neck
Abrasions

Chest
Abrasions, contusions, minor lacerations to anterior and posterior chest wall

Lung sounds
Equal, crackles

Abdomen
Soft, nontender, flat

Pelvis
Appears intact

Upper extremities
Angulated fracture right forearm, abrasions to both arms

Lower extremities
Lacerations, abrasions

Back
Abrasions and bruising to lower lumbar region

Vital Signs

Skin signs
Pale, cool

Pulse rate/quality
126 beats/min, regular, weak at radius

Blood pressure
100/70 mm Hg

Respiratory rate/depth
12 breaths/min, irregular; assisted with a BVM device

Pupils
Midpoint, sluggish to react, equal

SpO$_2$
85% (100% oxygen)

Electrocardiogram
Sinus tachycardia

Your suction machine is nearly full, and you are no closer to visualizing the glottic opening. You are starting to get a little anxious.

Question 3: What are some of your options in managing this patient's airway? What are some of the drawbacks to each procedure?

CASE STUDY

Skill Drill

10-2 Securing an Endotracheal Tube with Tape

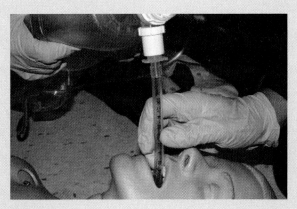

1 Note the cm marking on the tube at the level of the patient's teeth.

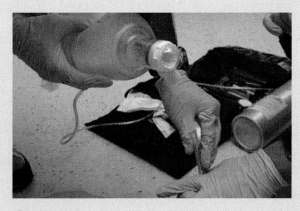

2 Remove the bag-valve device from the endotracheal (ET) tube.

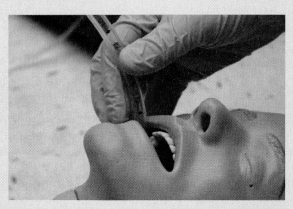

3 Move the ET tube to the corner of the patient's mouth.

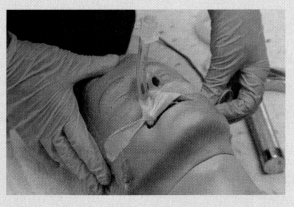

4 Encircle the ET tube with tape and secure the tape to the patient's maxilla (using tincture of benzoin to facilitate tape adhesion).

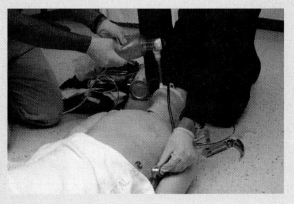

5 Reattach bag-valve device and auscultate again over the apices and bases of the lungs and over the epigastrium.

Skill Drill

10-3 Securing an Endotracheal Tube with a Commercial Device

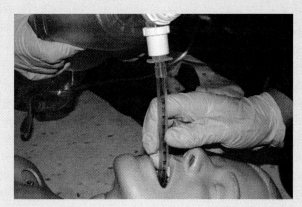

1 Note the cm marking on the tube at the level of the patient's teeth.

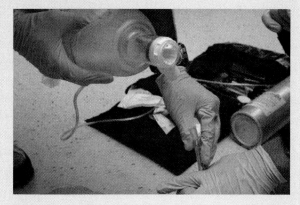

2 Remove the bag-valve device from the endotracheal tube.

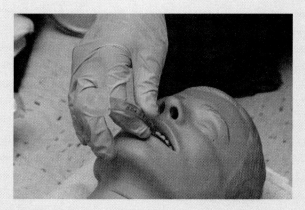

3 Position the endotracheal tube in the center of the patient's mouth.

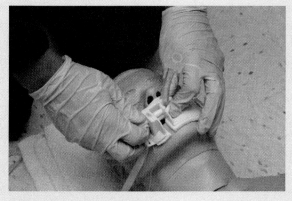

4 Place the commercial device over the endotracheal tube and secure.

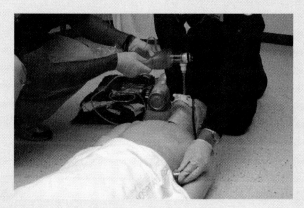

5 Reattach the bag-valve device and auscultate again over the apices and bases of the lungs and over the epigastrium.

Skill Drill

10-4 Blind Nasotracheal Intubation

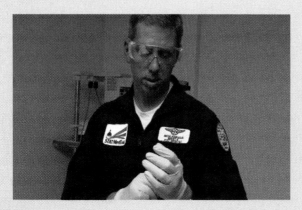

1 Take body substance isolation precautions (gloves and face shield).

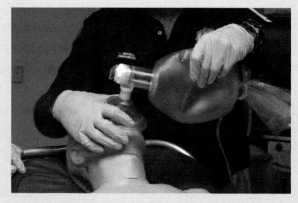

2 Preoxygenate the patient whenever possible with a bag-valve-mask device and 100% oxygen.

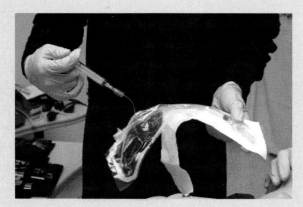

3 Check, prepare, and assemble your equipment.

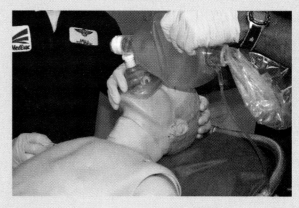

4 Place the patient's head in a neutral position.

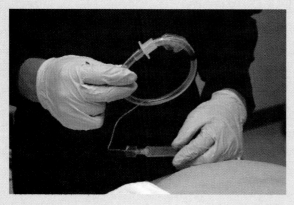

5 Pre-form the endotracheal (ET) tube by bending it into a circle.

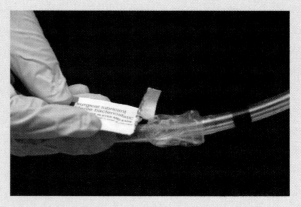

6 Lubricate the tip of the ET tube with a water-soluble gel.

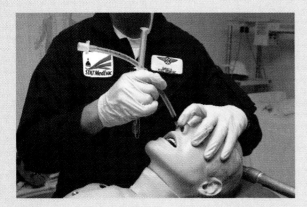

7 Gently insert the ET tube into the most compliant nostril with the bevel facing toward the nasal septum and advance the tube along the nasal floor.

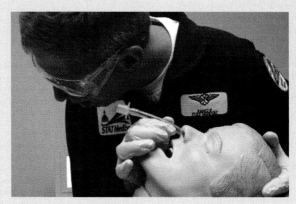

8 Advance the ET tube through the vocal cords when the patient inspires.

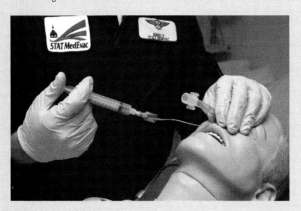

9 Inflate the distal cuff of the ET tube with 5 to 10 mL of air and detach the syringe.

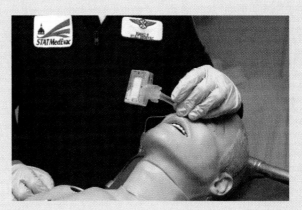

10 Attach the end-tidal carbon dioxide detector to the ET tube.

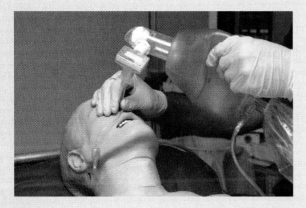

11 Attach a bag-valve device, ventilate, and auscultate over the apices and bases of both lungs and over the epigastrium.

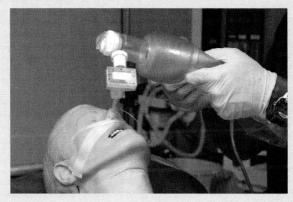

12 Secure the ET tube.

mandibular fractures, active seizures, fractured mandible). Nasotracheal intubation does not require the patient to be placed in the sniffing position, which is not possible in trauma situations. Finally, because the tube is placed through the nose, the patient cannot bite the tube; it is furthermore easier to secure.

Blind nasotracheal intubation requires the patient to be breathing to guide placement and to pull the tube into the trachea. Blind nasotracheal intubation should not be performed in apneic patients in emergency settings. Some anesthesiologists have developed modifications to the blind nasotracheal procedure and use it in nonbreathing patients in the operating room, but these techniques have not been studied in emergency settings and offer few advantages over other intubation techniques.

Unfortunately, emergency nasotracheal intubation is a blind technique. This means that you lack the advantage of one of the main tube confirmation steps (ie, watching the tube pass through the cords). Of course, confirming the location of the tube is always important, but you must be even more diligent when utilizing a blind technique. Since this technique is often used in breathing patients, the presence of breath sounds alone does not indicate that the tube is in the trachea. Most research indicates that nasotracheal intubation takes longer than orotracheal intubation. Because the patient is breathing, however, it is not critical to accomplish the intubation in 30 seconds or less.

Indications and Contraindications for Nasotracheal Intubation

The most common use of the technique is for patients who need to be intubated but who are awake and breathing. This is a common situation as patient's progress into respiratory failure from chronic obstructive pulmonary disease, asthma, or pulmonary edema. Early intubation in these patients can be a lifesaving intervention, and waiting until they become unresponsive would deprive them of the oxygen they desperately need.

The second most common use for blind nasotracheal intubation is for unresponsive breathing patients with a gag reflex. Direct laryngoscopy in these patients can lead to retching and/or vomiting upon insertion of the blade or repeated gagging on the tube. The nasotracheal route causes much less upper airway stimulation. While it is mildly uncomfortable for the patient, it is much more comfortable than an oral endotracheal tube, and it rarely causes gagging or vomiting. Blind nasotracheal intubation is also indicated when a patient needs to be intubated who is breathing but

cannot open his or her mouth adequately for direct laryngoscopy. Occasionally, nasotracheal intubation is useful in patients who cannot be placed into the sniffing position. Blind nasotracheal intubation is contraindicated in apneic or near-apneic patients. While some combination of techniques may be useful (nasotracheal intubation combined with lighted stylet, fiberoptics, etc), these procedures have not been evaluated in emergency settings. An inability to pass the tube through the nostril is another absolute contraindication to nasotracheal intubation. Obstruction can be caused by a foreign object, an anatomic abnormality (eg, deviated septum), or pathologic condition (eg, masses, trauma).

Blood clotting abnormalities and anticoagulation therapy are considered to be relative contraindications because they increase the likelihood and severity of epistaxis. Nasal bleeding following nasotracheal intubation attempts in these patients can be severe, and if you are unable to secure the airway, this bleeding can cause substantial additional airway problems.

The role of nasotracheal intubation in patients with severe nasal and/or facial fractures is highly debated. There have been a few reported cases of endotracheal tubes inserted into the cranial vault. Although this is highly unlikely, the catastrophic nature of this risk must be considered. Most paramedics avoid nasotracheal intubation in cases of severe midface fractures.

Complications of Nasotracheal Intubation

Of course, patients undergoing nasotracheal intubation can experience any of the general complications of intubation. As mentioned previously, bleeding is by far the most common complication specific to nasotracheal intubation. Usually, however, the bleeding is minor. If the intubation is successful, the airway is protected and bleeding is just an annoyance. Unfortunately, severe bleeding can occur and can pose an additional threat to an already compromised airway. Two guidelines can reduce the incidence of bleeding. First, be very gentle when inserting the tube into the nostril. The angle of insertion should be straight back (towards the ear) and *not* up (towards the eye). Using a tube 1.0- to 0.5-mm smaller than you would use for the oral route can also reduce bleeding. Using an anesthetic lubricant containing a vasoconstricting agent increases the patient's comfort and decreases the likelihood and severity of nasal bleeding. Finally, avoiding nasotracheal techniques in patients who are taking anticoagulants will reduce the risk of severe bleeding episodes.

Perforation of the nasal or nasopharyngeal mucosa is possible if excessive force is used but can be avoided with gentle technique, adequate lubrication, and avoiding the use of rigid stylets. A long-term complication of nasotracheal intubation is paranasal sinusitis.

Equipment for Nasotracheal Intubation

Nasotracheal intubation requires no special equipment, although some equipment has been developed specifically to make blind nasotracheal intubation easier. Standard endotracheal tubes can be used for both orotracheal and nasotracheal intubation. In general, select tubes 1.0- to 0.5-mm smaller when intubating via the nasotracheal route. Although you can use a standard endotracheal tube for nasotracheal intubation, the Endotrol tube was designed specifically for nasotracheal intubation and can be very useful. The Endotrol tube is slightly more flexible than standard endotracheal tubes and contains a trigger, which is attached to a piece of line attached to the tip of the tube. Pulling the trigger moves the tip of the tube anteriorly and increases the overall curvature (▶ Figure 10-23). The Endotrol tube is not required for successful nasotracheal intubation, but it makes the procedure much easier, more efficient, and safer.

During nasotracheal intubation, the movement of air though the tube helps to determine the proper position of the tube. One option is for the paramedic to place his or her ear or cheek next to the tube and listen and feel for air movement. Unfortunately, body fluids often accompany the exhaled breath from the tube, presenting a risk for transmission of infectious

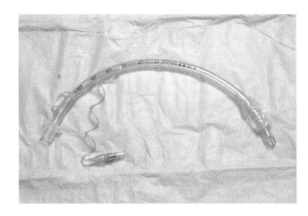

Figure 10-23 Endotrol tube.

disease. A number of devices have been developed to potentially avoid the necessity of placing your face so close to the end of the tube. None of these devices has yet been shown to be effective (▼ Table 10-2).

Technique for Nasotracheal Intubation

There is a pattern in all the techniques described in this chapter. Each technique has nine steps. In each case the three preintubation steps (check/prepare/assemble equipment, preoxygenate, and position the patient) and the three postintubation steps (ventilate, confirm placement, and secure the tube) are the same. Although these general steps are the same, the specifics of each step vary depending on the procedure. The

Table 10-2
Devices Used to Determine Maximum Airflow Through the Tube During Nasotracheal Intubation

Humid-Vent 1	Device that attaches to the 15/22-mm adapter at the end of the endotracheal tube to prevent secretions from being expelled from the tube.
BAAM	A small whistle that attaches to the 15/22-mm adapter and emits a high-pitched sound as air moves in and out of the tube. The BAAM enables the paramedic to keep his or her face away from the end of the tube.
Stethoscope with head removed	Stethoscope tubing placed in the proximal 2 to 3 cm of the endotracheal tube enables the paramedic to hear air movement without placing the face next to the tube.
IV tubing attached to an earpiece	The tubing placed in the proximal 2 to 3 cm of the endotracheal tube enables the intubator to hear air movement without placing the face next to the tube.

Table 10-3
Preparing Equipment for Nasotracheal Intubation

Piece of equipment	What to check/prepare/assemble
Ventilation equipment	Because the patient is breathing, you may only need to supplement the breathing gas with 100% oxygen, but more often than not, the reason for intubation is that the patient cannot maintain adequate oxygen saturation on his or her own. In this case, have an assistant ventilate the patient while you are assembling, checking, and preparing your equipment. Check to make sure that the patient is being ventilated with 100% oxygen and that the pulse oximeter reading is 96% to 100%.
Endotracheal tube, 10-cc syringe, lubricant	Select the proper size endotracheal tube, which will be a half to a full size smaller than you would use for oral intubation (6.0 to 6.5 for a female; 7.0 to 7.5 for a male). Inject 10-cc of air in the cuff and make sure that it holds air. You do not use a stylet for nasotracheal intubation. If possible, use a lubricant that has anesthetic and a vasoconstrictor agent.
Laryngoscope handle and blades, and Magill forceps, towels	While blind nasotracheal intubation does not use the laryngoscope, it is best to have it available in case something goes wrong. The Magill forceps can be used to guide the tip of the tube into the glottic opening if direct laryngoscopy becomes necessary.
Tape or commercial tube securing device	Have tape torn or the device ready before you start.
Suction	Although vomiting is less likely than with direct laryngoscopy, it is possible.

only steps that change completely are the middle three steps, which describe the actual intubation procedure.

Check/Prepare/Assemble Equipment

Less equipment is needed for nasotracheal intubation than for direct laryngoscopy, but you should still assemble the direct laryngoscopy equipment so that it is immediately available if something goes wrong and you need it quickly (▲ **Table 10-3**).

Preoxygenate

As with all intubation techniques, it is imperative that the patient be adequately oxygenated before the intubation attempt. Patients undergoing blind nasotracheal intubation are breathing but doing so inadequately (that is why you are intubating them). In some cases, having the patient breathe 100% oxygen will bring the oxygen saturation level above 96%. If that fails to provide adequate preoxygenation, you should assist the patient's ventilations with a bag-valve-mask device. Ideally, you should have the patient's oxygen saturation level at 100% for 2 minutes or more before you begin.

While you are preoxygenating the patient, if time permits, insert a nasopharyngeal airway that has been well lubricated with an anesthetic and vasocon-

strictor. The nasopharyngeal airway should be the same size as the endotracheal tube and left in place for 3 to 5 minutes. This will significantly increase patient comfort, decrease the probability of bleeding, and prelubricate the passageway for the tube.

Position the Patient

For nasotracheal intubation the patient can be either in the supine or semi-Fowler's position. A major advantage of nasotracheal intubation is that the patient does not have to be in the sniffing position. In fact, nasotracheal intubation can be easily performed while the patient is in a semi-Fowler's position, which is a particular benefit when intubating patients in respiratory failure because they often refuse to lie down flat and may experience decompensation if forced to do so.

With the patient in either the supine or semi-Fowler's position, the natural curvature of the endotracheal tube directs the tip of the tube toward the glottic opening, if the head is slightly extended.

Insert the Tube

After the patient has been prepared and the tube properly lubricated, the tube should be inserted into the nostril with the bevel facing toward the nasal

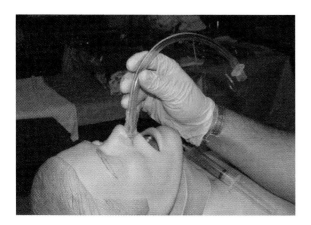

Figure 10-24 Be sure to aim the tip of the tube straight back toward the ear.

septum. Usually the right nostril is used because the curvature of the tube is in the correct orientation in relation to the bevel. If the left nostril is used (due to an obstruction or difficulty in passing the tube on the right), the tube should be rotated 180° as the tip enters the nasopharynx.

The angle of insertion is critical. Be sure to aim the tip of the tube straight back toward the ear (▲ Figure 10-24). The goal is to follow the floor of the nasal cavity until the tube is into the nasopharynx. *Do not* insert the tube with the tip aimed upward toward the eye. This can damage the turbinates and cause significant bleeding.

It is common to meet slight resistance as the tip of the tube has to make the bend in the posterior pharynx. Be gentle. If you are using an Endotrol tube, pull the trigger to increase the curvature of the tube and slowly advance it. If you are using a standard endotracheal tube, tilt the patient's head back slightly to decrease the angle that the tube has to make in negotiating the turn.

Position the Tip at the Glottic Opening

As you advance the tube into the oropharynx, you will begin to hear air rushing in and out of the tube as the patient breathes. Your goal is to position the tube right at the glottic opening so that the patient will literally suck the tube into the airway with a deep inspiration. Moving the patient's head controls the position of the tip of the tube. Cup your left hand (if you have inserted the tube in the right nostril) under the occiput of the patient's head. Move the patient's head until you have found the position that offers the maximum amount of air moving through the tube. You are now positioned just above the glottic opening.

Advance the Tube

If you have properly positioned the tube at the glottic opening, the patient ends up doing most of the

work of inserting the tube into the trachea. As the patient takes a deep breath, the negative pressure created by the inspiration facilitates the movement of the tube through the glottic opening. Instruct the patient to take a deep breath, and gently advance the tube with the inspiration. You will know if you are in the trachea because the air movement through the tube will increase.

If you advance the tube and the airflow decreases or stops, there are three places the tube may have gone: the vallecula, pyriform fossa, or the esophagus. If the tube has been advanced into the vallecula, in most patients you will see a soft-tissue bulge anteriorly, just above the thyroid cartilage. Slightly withdraw the tube and flex the head slightly forward and advance the tube again. If you are using an Endotrol tube, release the trigger to decrease the curvature of the tube.

If you see a soft-tissue bulge on either side of the airway, you probably have inserted the tube into the pyriform fossa. Hold the head still and withdraw the tube slightly. If the bulge is on the left, rotate the tube clockwise; if the bulge is on the right, rotate the tube counterclockwise. Once you detect maximum airflow, advance the tube on inspiration. If you see no soft-tissue bulges and there is no airflow through the tube, the tube has entered the esophagus. Withdraw it until you detect airflow, and then extend the head. If you are using an Endotrol tube, pull the trigger to increase the curvature of the tube (▼ Figure 10-25). With a little practice, these corrective measures will become second nature. ▶ **Box 10-2** describes a procedure for inserting a nasotracheal tube under direct laryngoscopy if the patient stops breathing during intubation.

Ventilate

Once you have achieved maximum airflow through the positioned tube, inflate the cuff with the minimum amount of air necessary to achieve an airtight seal.

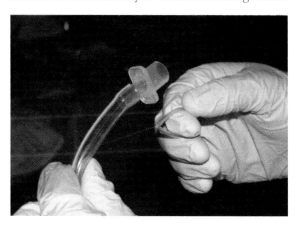

Figure 10-25 Pull the trigger to increase the curvature of the tube if you are using an Endotrol tube.

Attach a ventilation device to the endotracheal tube, and ventilate the patient as needed according to the patient's clinical condition.

Confirm Placement

Tube confirmation is more important following blind nasotracheal intubation than with other intubation techniques. With blind nasotracheal intubation you do not have the benefit of having watched the tube pass through the vocal cords. Air coming through the tube is a good indication that the tube is in the trachea, but this is not a foolproof indicator. The most common situation is that only the tip

has passed through the glottic opening and the tube is precariously positioned. Even a small movement by the patient may dislodge the tube and cause it to slip, potentially unrecognized, into the esophagus. Movement of the tube can also cause mainstem intubations. Be sure to employ numerous tube confirmation techniques and continuously monitor the tube's placement.

Secure the Tube

Securing a tube after nasotracheal intubation is generally easier than securing a tube that has been inserted orally because there are generally fewer secretions and the patient cannot bite the tube. Clean up any secretions or excess lubricant and secure the tube with tape (▼ Figure 10-27). Record the depth of insertion at the nostril to help monitor for any tube migration.

Digital Intubation

<u>Digital intubation</u> is one of the oldest techniques for intubating the trachea. Digital intubation involves palpating and elevating the epiglottis with your middle finger while guiding the endotracheal tube into position by feel. Since the development of the laryngoscope, digital intubation is not routinely used but still has significant utility in a number of situations in emergency medicine. Although digital intubation is rarely your first choice, being adept at the skill gives you an option in some extreme situations.

Advantages and Disadvantages of Digital Intubation

Digital intubation has a number of advantages over more traditional techniques of intubation. First, it does not require a laryngoscope. Digital intubation is an option in the event of an equipment failure if a working laryngoscope is not available. Digital intubation may also be a viable option in such extreme situations as an entrapment, building collapse, disaster

---

Box 10-2

Inserting a Nasotracheal Tube under Direct Laryngoscopy

If you are attempting nasotracheal intubation and the patient stops breathing, do not remove the tube from the nostril. You can ventilate the patient through the tube even if it is not in the trachea. Simply pinch the nostrils and close the mouth. Open the airway with a head tilt-chin lift maneuver and ventilate through the tube.

Next, perform laryngoscopy as you would normally. Once you identify the glottic opening, grasp the endotracheal tube just proximal to the cuff with the tip of the Magill forceps. Guide the tip of the endotracheal tube through the glottic opening by rotating your right hand using the same motion used to hit a ping-pong ball (▼ Figure 10-26).

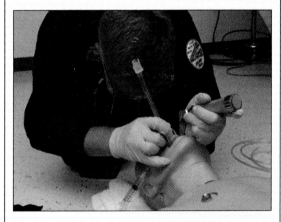

Figure 10-26 Guide the tip of the endotracheal tube through the glottic opening by rotating your right hand.

The same technique is used for nasotracheal intubation of nonbreathing patients. This procedure is not usually done in emergency situations because it offers few advantages and has some disadvantages (bleeding) over conventional direct laryngoscopy.

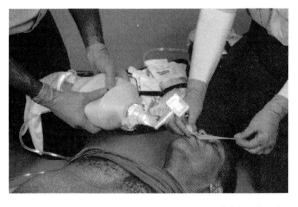

Figure 10-27 Clean up any secretions or excess lubricant and secure the tube with tape.

situation, or wilderness environment, when an endotracheal tube is available but you either cannot use or do not have a laryngoscope. Digital intubation may also be useful in cases of massive tissue damage where the visual identification of intubation landmarks is impossible (such as gunshot wounds or blast injuries to the face).

The technique is tactilely (rather than visually) guided. This fact makes it ideal in situations in which the glottic view is hopelessly obliterated because of large quantities of uncontrollable secretions. Having the patient in the sniffing position makes placement easier, although it is not required for digital intubation. Therefore, digital intubation can be valuable for trauma patients and for obese and/or short-necked patients.

Digital intubation has some significant limitations, however. First, the safety of the paramedic must be ensured. Significant risks are associated with insertion of your fingers into a patient's mouth. The most obvious risk is the possibility that you can be bitten. Digital intubation should therefore be performed only in patients who are deeply unconscious *and* who have had something placed in their mouth to prevent closure. A dental prod or an oropharyngeal airway *must* be inserted into the mouth to reduce the chances of significant injury to you. Even if the patient is deeply unconscious, a seizure or sudden or transient increase in consciousness could result in the patient biting you.

Another less obvious risk is exposure to infectious disease. Gloves must be worn during the procedure, but the patient's teeth (especially if they are broken) can *easily* rip gloves and cut the paramedic. Ideally, you should avoid contact with the teeth and wear two pair of good-quality gloves while performing digital intubation.

Digital intubation is a blind procedure, and misplacement of the tube is common. The success of the procedure depends on the experience, manual dexterity, and anatomic characteristics of the paramedic's hand and fingers. People with short fingers or fingers that are large in diameter have great difficulty performing the skill. Finally, most people understandably are reluctant to insert their fingers so deeply into a patient's mouth. This very real consideration means that part of the decision to perform digital intubation is a matter of personal choice that should be respected.

Indications and Contraindications for Digital Intubation

Digital intubation is indicated only for patients who are deeply unconscious, apneic, and who have no gag reflex. It should be performed only if some device can be placed in the mouth to prevent injury to the

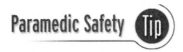

paramedic. If these conditions are met, digital intubation may be a valuable adjunct to traditional airway management techniques when:

- other techniques have failed.
- the patient is obese or has a short neck.
- a laryngoscope is not available.
- the patient is in a confined space.
- secretions are obscuring the view.
- the head cannot be moved due to trauma, or immobilization equipment is complicating direct laryngoscopy.
- massive trauma has made the visual identification of intubation landmarks impossible.

In theory, digital intubation can be performed in pediatric patients, but the size of the paramedic is a factor. The patient's mouth has to be big enough to accommodate two of the paramedic's fingers.

Digital intubation is absolutely contraindicated in patients who have a gag reflex. It should never be performed without a bite block, and therefore it is contraindicated if no suitable device is available or can be inserted.

Complications of Digital Intubation

The major complication of the procedure is a misplaced endotracheal tube. Even though the intubation is tactilely guided, it is easy to misdirect the tip of the tube during insertion. Careful attention to tube confirmation is absolutely essential following digital intubation. Although dental trauma does not result as it may from a laryngoscope, a dental prod or other bite block can cause lip trauma, tooth damage, or both. Obviously, prolonged intubation attempts can result in hypoxia. Vigorous attempts at insertion or careless insertion technique can cause airway trauma and swelling.

Technique for Digital Intubation

Continual practice at digital intubation is needed to develop and maintain the skill. Like many alternative airway techniques, digital intubation is often not attempted until other techniques have failed. Cases in which digital intubation must be employed are therefore almost always particularly challenging. You should work to become just as skilled and competent with alternative techniques as you are with more common airway management techniques.

Check/Prepare/Assemble Equipment

Less equipment is needed for digital intubation, and, in fact, you may be attempting the digital technique because you have limited equipment available. Proper preparation of the equipment is necessary before starting the procedure.

As with all intubation techniques, prepare the equipment you will need. Select, check, and lubricate the endotracheal tube as you would for any intubation. You may find it slightly easier to intubate digitally with a tube a half to a full size smaller than that used for direct laryngoscopy. A stylet is very important for digital intubation. The technique calls for the tip of the tube to be guided into the trachea while using your index finger as a leverage point. Therefore, a stylet is used to provide the tube with the rigidity necessary to make the bend. Two configurations are recommended, and you should practice with both to determine which you prefer.

1. In an "Open J" configuration, the stylet is inserted and a large J shape is made in the distal tip of the tube.
2. In the "U-Handle" configuration, the tube is bent into a U and the proximal half of the tube is bent into a 90° handle toward your dominant hand (▼ Figure 10-28).

Preoxygenate

Make every attempt to preoxygenate the patient so that a period of apnea does not result in hypoxia. Patients who need emergency intubation obviously have a problem significant enough to require the procedure in the first place. Unnecessarily prolonged periods of hypoxia would clearly be detrimental to the patient's outcome.

Position the patient

For digital intubation, the patient does not need to be placed in the sniffing position. Unlike with other intubation procedures, the paramedic is positioned at the patient's left side facing toward the head. If the patient is trapped in a seated or standing position, digital intubation can be accomplished from a position facing the patient (▼ Figure 10-29).

Insert a Bite Block

The first step of the intubation procedure is to protect your fingers by inserting a bite block into the patient's mouth. A commercially available device known as a dental prod, which is used commonly for oral surgery, is inserted at the level of the first molar (▼ Figure 10-30). It is generally desirable to insert the dental prod on the patient's right side. Alternatively, the flange of an oral airway can be inserted into the mouth and turned sideways (▶ Figure 10-31). Although less effective than the dental prod, this flange prevents complete mouth closure and affords

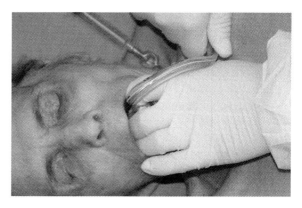

Figure 10-29 If the patient is trapped in a seated or standing position, digital intubation can be accomplished from a position facing the patient.

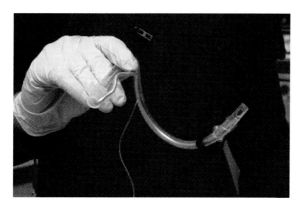

Figure 10-28 U-handle configuration.

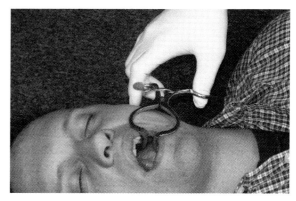

Figure 10-30 Dental prod.

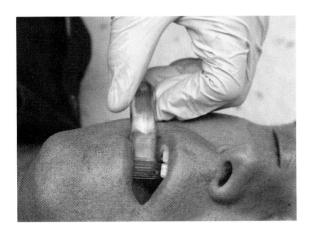

Figure 10-31 The flange of an oral airway can be inserted into the mouth and turned sideways to act as a dental block.

significantly more protection in the event of a sudden change in consciousness or seizure.

Palpate the Epiglottis

After the dental prod has been inserted, "walk" the index and middle finger of your left hand down the tongue until you feel the epiglottis deep in the oral cavity at the base of the tongue. It is a common mistake to simply insert your fingers and feel nothing but "mush." By following the tongue, however, you stay oriented and increase the likelihood of successfully identifying the epiglottis. The epiglottis feels like a slimy earlobe. The middle finger then lifts the epiglottis.

Insert the Tube

As you hold the epiglottis with your middle finger, insert the tube. There are two commonly used techniques for insertion of the tube. Insert the tube between the patient's mandible and the palmar surface of your index finger. Insert the tube over your middle finger and across onto the tip of your index finger

With both insertion techniques, the tip of the index finger guides the tip of the tube into the glottic opening, which lies just below the middle finger. The curvature of the tube is leveraged against the tip of the index finger to provide the proper angle for insertion. As the tube is passed into the airway, remove the stylet.

Postintubation Procedures

After insertion of the tube, standard postintubation procedures are followed. Ventilate the patient according to the clinical presentation. Because this is truly a blind technique, rigorous tube confirmation protocol must be followed. After subjective and objective confirmation of proper tube placement, secure the tube in place.

Transillumination Techniques

Like digital intubation, <u>transilluminated intubation</u> (▶ Skill Drill 10-6) is rarely considered a first-line technique but may prove valuable in some situations. The concept of transillumination is simple, based on the fact that the tissues that overlie the trachea are relatively thin. A bright light source placed inside the trachea emits a bright, tightly circumscribed light visible on the outside of the trachea.

A number of devices can be used to intubate the trachea that use transillumination. Some are pieces of equipment designed for other purposes and adapted for airway management, whereas others are specifically designed for intubation. It is the intent of this text not to explain the use of any specific devices but to describe the general principles of the technique. Consult the manufacturer's instructions for device-specific directions. We use the term "lighted stylet" as a generic term for any malleable stylet with a bright light source at its distal end that can be used to guide intubation.

Advantages and Disadvantages of Transillumination Techniques

Transillumination has some significant advantages for intubation. Since a laryngoscope is not used, the problems of laryngoscopy (eg, dental trauma, soft-tissue trauma) are minimized or eliminated. Transillumination does not require glottic visualization, so it can be used when secretions are copious and obstruct the laryngoscopic view. In addition, because the patient's head does not need to be in the sniffing position, the technique has great potential for use in trauma patients.

The most significant disadvantage of transillumination involves not the procedure but the fact that special equipment is required. Without a bright light source at the tip of a malleable wire stylet, the procedure cannot be performed. In addition, transillumination may be difficult in obese patients or those with short, muscular necks because more soft tissue overlies the trachea. Finally, transillumination can be difficult or impossible in well-lit environments. Inside, you may be able to dim the lights, but outside in direct sunlight it is extremely difficult to discern the transilluminated light. Although it may be possible to shield the patient with a blanket, this would add more steps to the procedure and decrease its utility.

Indications and Contraindications for Transillumination Techniques

There are no specific indications for transillumination as a technique for intubation. It can be used anytime

Skill Drill

10-5 Digital Intubation

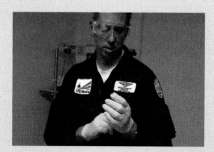

1 Take body substance isolation precautions (gloves and face shield).

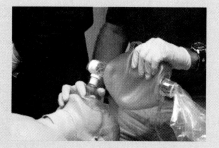

2 Preoxygenate the patient for at least 2 minutes with a bag-valve-mask device and 100% oxygen.

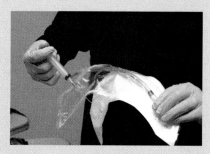

3 Check, prepare, and assemble your equipment.

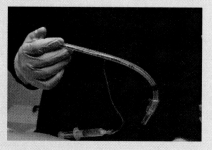

4 Bend the endotracheal (ET) tube by placing a slight curve at its distal end (like a hockey stick).

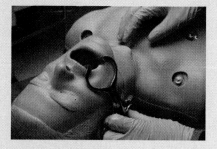

5 Place the patient's head in a neutral position.

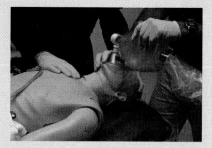

6 Place a bite block in-between the patient's molars to prevent the patient from biting your fingers.

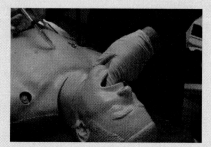

7 Insert your left middle and index fingers into the patient's mouth and shift the patient's tongue forward as you advance your fingers toward the patient's larynx.

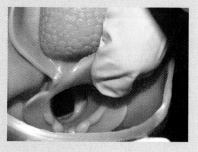

8 Palpate and lift the epiglottis with your left middle finger.

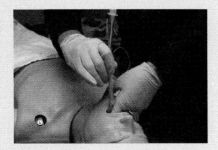

9 Advance the tube with your right hand and guide it in-between the vocal cords with your left index finger.

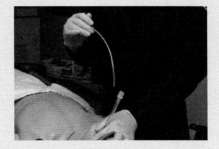

10 Remove the stylet from the ET tube.

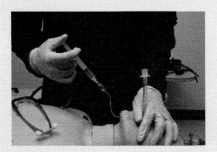

11 Inflate the distal cuff of the ET tube with 5 to 10 mL of air and detach the syringe.

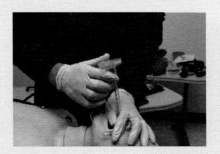

12 Attach the end-tidal carbon dioxide detector to the ET tube.

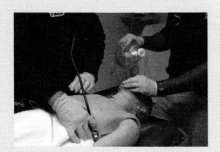

13 Attach the bag-valve-mask device, ventilate, and auscultate over the apices and bases of both lungs and over the epigastrium.

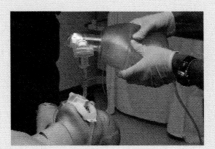

14 Secure the ET tube.

Skill Drill

10-6 Transillumination Intubation

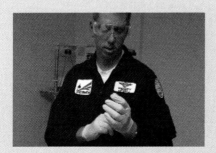

1 Take body substance isolation precautions (gloves and face shield).

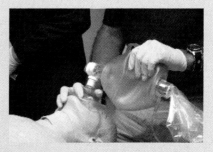

2 Preoxygenate the patient for at least 2 minutes with a bag-valve-mask device and 100% oxygen.

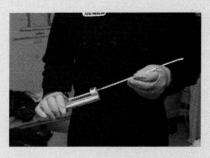

3 Check, prepare, and assemble your equipment.

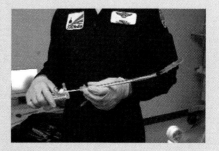

4 Insert lighted stylet into endotracheal (ET) tube.

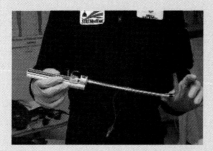

5 Bend the ET tube by placing a slight curve at its distal end (like a hockey stick) and turn on the lighted stylet.

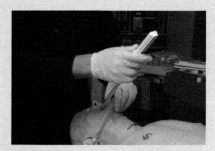

6 Lift the patient's tongue and mandible anteriorly.

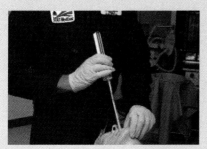

7 Insert the ET tube into the midline of the patient's mouth and slowly advance toward the larynx.

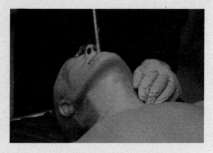

8 Observe for illumination of the thyroid and cricoid cartilages and advance the ET tube 1 to 2 cm further.

Skill Drill

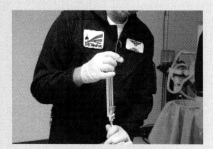

9 Remove the stylet from the ET tube.

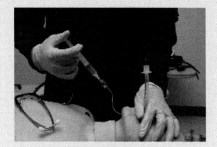

10 Inflate the distal cuff of the ET tube with 5 to 10 mL of air and detach the syringe.

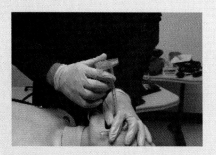

11 Attach the end-tidal carbon dioxide detector to the ET tube.

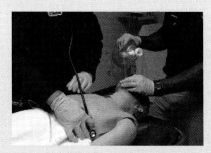

12 Attach the bag-valve-mask device, ventilate, and auscultate over the apices and bases of both lungs and over the epigastrium.

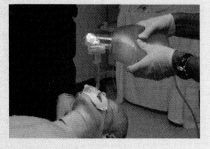

13 Secure the ET tube.

a patient needs to be intubated. Although it does not need to be saved for a final effort, transillumination is usually employed after other techniques have failed.

Transillumination is absolutely contraindicated in cases of airway obstruction. Consider the amount of soft tissue overlying the trachea when determining whether transillumination should be attempted. Obese patients and persons with short, muscular necks may be difficult to transilluminate. Although theoretically it is possible to perform transillumination with pediatric patients, the stylet must fit into the tube. Most lighted stylets do not fit in tubes smaller than 6 mm.

Complications of Transillumination Techniques

While transillumination is not an entirely blind technique, this technique lacks the advantage of direct observation of the tube passing through the vocal cords. Therefore, passage of the tube into the esophagus is the main complication. Pay strict attention to tube confirmation procedures following transilluminated intubations.

Equipment for Transillumination Techniques

The most significant piece of equipment necessary for transillumination guided intubation is a device with a rigid stylet and a bright light source at the end. At the time of this writing, a number of devices have been specifically designed for, or can be easily modified for, intubation.

The ideal transillumination device should have a bright light source at the end of a rigid stylet. The light source should shine laterally as well as forward, because the light source may not always be aiming directly at the skin surface. The light source must be securely held in place; with early equipment adapted for intubation, there were some cases of the bulb becoming dislodged as the tube was advanced over the stylet. The stylet should be long enough to accommodate a standard-length endotracheal tube. There should be some method of securing the tube to the stylet.

Technique for Intubation Utilizing Transillumination

As mentioned earlier, this technique has some significant variations based on manufacturers' differences. A general description of the technique for transillumination-guided intubation follows. For use of a specific device, refer to the specific instructions from the manufacturer.

Check/Prepare/Assemble Equipment

First, check the tube to ensure that the cuff holds air. Lubricate and insert the lighted stylet so that the light is positioned immediately at (but not beyond) the tip of the tube and be sure that the tube is firmly seated into the handle. The crucial step in preparation is bending the tube in the proper shape to facilitate entry of the tube into the trachea and orientation of the light so that it will be visible at the anterior neck.

The stylet should be straight. Place a sharp 90° angle in the tube/stylet just proximal to the cuff. It is important that this bend be sharp because this will be the pivot point as you direct the stylet into the trachea. The proper bend not only facilitates entry of tube into the trachea but also places the light in the proper orientation to illuminate the anterior neck.

Preoxygenate

As with all intubation techniques, remember to preoxygenate the patient.

Position the Patient

The patient should be placed in the neutral or slightly extended position. This position moves the epiglottis off the posterior pharyngeal wall and facilitates entrance of the endotracheal tube into the glottic opening. The extension also provides maximum exposure of the anterior neck. Although other positions are possible, the intubator most commonly assumes a traditional position at the head of the patient.

Scoop the Epiglottis

Hold the lighted stylet in your dominant hand. As the procedure begins, forwardly displace the jaw of the patient by grasping the jaw with your thumb and forefinger. This is an important step to further ensure that the epiglottis is not covering the glottic opening. With your dominant hand, turn on the stylet light and insert the device deep into the mouth, all the way to the posterior pharyngeal wall. The goal is to lift the epiglottis with the tip of the tube/stylet combination. This is accomplished by moving your hand in an imaginary arc back towards you. Place the tube in the midline of the patient's body, with the tip directed toward the laryngeal prominence.

Identify the Light

As you draw your wrist back toward you, the light should become visible at the midline of the neck. If the light is tightly circumscribed and slightly below the thyroid cartilage, the tip of the tube has been inserted into the trachea. If a faint glow and a soft tissue bulge is identified above the thyroid cartilage, the tip has been placed into the vallecula. Withdraw the tube slightly, forwardly displace the jaw and/or slightly flex the head, and re-advance the tube/stylet assembly. A dim glow on either side of the larynx indicates placement in the pyriform fossa. Slightly withdraw the tube/stylet and rotate the assembly accordingly to position the tip at the glottic opening.

A dim, diffuse light generally indicates esophageal placement. If time and patient conditions permit, slightly withdraw the tube/stylet and extend the head slightly. You may also increase the angle of the bend in the tube. This should reposition the tube/stylet at the glottic opening.

Advance the Tube into the Trachea

Once a bright, tightly circumscribed glow of light is visible in the midline and just below the thyroid cartilage, hold the stylet in place and advance the tube approximately 2 to 4 cm into the trachea. When the tube is securely in the trachea, hold it in place with your nondominant hand and carefully withdraw the lighted stylet.

Postintubation Procedures

Following insertion of the tube, follow standard postintubation procedures for confirming the location of the tube. After confirmation of the location of the tube, ventilate the patient according to the clinical presentation. Transillumination must always be followed with rigorous attention to tube confirmation protocol. Following subjective and objective confirmation of proper tube placement, secure the tube in place. ▼ **Box 10-3** lists other uses for transillumination and the lighted stylet.

Box 10-3

Other Uses for Transillumination and Lighted Stylet

While useful in its own right as an intubation technique, transillumination of the soft tissues of the neck has also been advocated for other purposes.

Tube confirmation: Placing a flexible lighted stylet into a tube that has already been inserted is another method of verifying tube placement. If a bright, tightly circumscribed light appears in the trachea, suspect tracheal placement. A diffuse light usually indicates esophageal placement.

Nasal intubation: A flexible lighted stylet inserted into a tube before nasotracheal intubation is another method of guiding and verifying tube placement.

Tube positioning: The proper depth of insertion of the endotracheal tube places the tip midway between the carina and the vocal cords. The proper external landmark is the sternal notch. A bright light source placed immediately at the tip of an endotracheal tube can be used to adjust the depth of insertion of a tube. Insert the tube until the glow of light begins to disappear at the sternal notch.

Direct laryngoscopy: Some cases of difficult intubation are due to inadequate light from the laryngoscope. A lighted stylet increases the light available during direct laryngoscopy and may increase success in some cases.

Digital intubation: Using a lighted stylet during digital intubation is another potential method for guiding and verifying tube placement during digital intubation.

Case Study

Case Study, Part 3

With your gloved hand you reach into the patient's mouth, "walking down" the tongue into the posterior pharynx with your index and middle fingers. You reach the tip of the epiglottis, flipping it up and holding it with your fingers. With the other hand you snake down the endotracheal tube, maneuvering the distal tip so that it travels between your fingers that will guide it into the glottic opening. A few seconds later, the tube is in, with confirmation of accurate tube placement obtained with capnometer readings, fogging of the proximal tube, and equal breath sounds auscultated bilaterally.

After securing the tube, the patient is quickly moved to the ambulance, and rapid transport to the trauma center begins. An IV of normal saline is initiated, using a large-bore angiocatheter. Bloods are carefully drawn for type and crossmatch. A detailed secondary exam does not reveal any further injuries. A repeat set of vital signs is obtained as follows:

Vital Signs

Recording time
12 minutes after patient contact

Skin signs
Pale, cool

Pulse rate/quality
120 beats/min, regular, remains weak at the radial

Blood pressure
102/82 mm Hg

Respiratory rate/depth
Assisted at 20 breaths/min

Pupils
Midpoint, equal, reactive

SpO_2
92% (100% oxygen)

Electrocardiogram
Sinus tachycardia

The patient is transferred to the emergency department, but is quickly moved to surgery to determine the cause of his bleeding at the oropharynx. You find out later that the patient did well after exploratory surgery, where an esophageal tear was repaired. He remained in the hospital for several weeks, where he had additional surgery for his fractured arm and recovered from a concussive type of brain injury. A police report later indicated that the patient had not been wearing a seatbelt at the time of the accident.

CASE STUDY

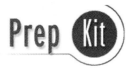

Chapter Summary

Endotracheal tubes come in a variety of sizes and styles to accommodate varying airway presentations. Select a tube of the appropriate size to minimize chances of both mechanical trauma and barotrauma.

There are many techniques used to get a tube into the trachea. By far the most common in both emergency and elective situations is direct laryngoscopy. While this is the mainstay of advanced airway management by most paramedics, there are other techniques of intubation. Skilled paramedics are familiar with a number of alternative techniques that can provide advantages over direct laryngoscopy in some situations and with some patients.

The steps to oral intubation using direct laryngoscopy are as follows:

1. Check/prepare/assemble your equipment
2. Body substance isolation
3. Preoxygenate your patient
4. Position the patient
5. Insert the laryngoscope blade
6. Visualize the glottic opening
7. Pass the tube
8. Ventilate the patient
9. Confirm tube placement
10. Secure the tube

Each step is critical to the success of any intubation attempt.

The steps to a nasotracheal intubation attempt are similar to an oral intubation using direct laryngoscopy:

1. Check/prepare/assemble your equipment
2. Body substance isolation
3. Preoxygenate your patient
4. Position the patient in a supine, or semi-Fowler's position
5. Advance the tube to the glottic opening
6. Time insertion of the tube with the inspiratory effort of the patient
7. Ventilate the patient
8. Confirm tube placement
9. Secure the tube

Digital intubation can be used as an effective alternative to direct laryngoscopy. However, there is potential of being inadvertently bitten by the patient, so use this technique carefully!

As is the case with any alternative technique, transillumination of the upper airway during intubation can be effective under certain conditions. Practice with your equipment often in order to be comfortable with this (and any other) airway technique.

Vital Vocabulary

anode (armored) endotracheal tube A special type of endotracheal tube that has wire reinforcements built into the wall of the tube itself that prevents kinking of the tube. The tube is rarely used in the prehospital setting.

atlanto-occipital joint Joint formed at the articulation of the atlas of the vertebral column and the occipital bone of the skull.

BURP maneuver Acronym for **B**ackward, **U**pward, and **R**ightward **P**ressure.

digital intubation A blind technique of intubation in which you palpate and elevate the epiglottis with your middle finger while guiding the endotracheal tube into position by feel.

double-lumen endobronchial tube A specialty tube that is used when one lung must be isolated from the other. This tube is rarely used in the prehospital setting.

endotracheal intubation The technique of inserting an endotracheal tube through the vocal cords and into the trachea in order to maintain a patent airway.

endotracheal (ET) tube Tube that is placed into the trachea during intubation. The ET tube has a standard 15/22-mm fitting on its proximal end, which makes it compatible with any type of ventilatory device (such as a bag-valve-mask device or mechanical ventilator).

endotrol tube Tube made from a material that is more flexible than that of standard endotracheal tubes.

epiglottitis A bacterial infection of the epiglottis that results in laryngeal swelling and airway closure.

gastric insufflation Instillation of air into the stomach when the endotracheal tube is inadvertently placed into the esophagus instead of the trachea.

gum bougie A device that is placed in-between the vocal cords under direct laryngoscopy. The endotracheal tube is then advanced over the gum bougie and into the trachea. This device is useful when you are unable to obtain a full view of the glottic opening.

iatrogenic trauma Injury caused to the patient by the rescuer. In the case of intubation, this would include damaging the soft tissues of the mouth or breaking the patient's teeth.

laryngoscope An instrument used in conjunction with a straight or curved blade to give a direct view of the patient's vocal cords during endotracheal intubation.

malleable stylet Flexible wire that is placed into the endotracheal tube and makes the tube formfitting. This device facilitates maneuvering of the ET tube during intubation.

<u>Murphy's eye</u> The hole at the distal end of the endotracheal tube that enables ventilations to occur even if the tip becomes occluded by blood, mucus, or the tracheal wall.

<u>nasotracheal intubation</u> Intubation of the trachea via the nasopharynx.

<u>pilot balloon</u> Small pouch at the end of the inflation port on the endotracheal tube that indicates if the cuff is inflated or deflated once the distal end of the tube is inserted into the patient.

<u>pulse oximeter</u> Assessment tool that measures oxygen saturation of the blood through the capillary bed. The pulse oximeter reading is expressed as either the SpO_2 or SaO_2.

<u>temporomandibular joint</u> Joint that connects the mandible (lower jaw bone) to the temporal bone of the skull.

<u>transilluminated intubation</u> Technique in which a lighted stylet is used to illuminate the trachea and facilitate intubation.

Case Study Answers

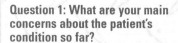

Question 1: What are your main concerns about the patient's condition so far?

Answer: Managing this patient's airway quickly and decisively is critical. Besides the obvious signs of trauma and significant mechanism of injury, the blood coming out of the patient's mouth is of significant concern. Where is it coming from? Is the blood being aspirated by the patient? He clearly needs a definitive airway.

Question 2: What are your next immediate series of actions in the management of the patient's airway?

Answer: While maintaining manual cervical spine precautions, suctioning the airway is a critical first action step. If the airway can be cleared with suction, then basic ventilation procedures, followed by endotracheal intubation, can proceed. However, if the potential aspirate cannot be cleared adequately, intubation may have to occur much earlier, using techniques not involving direct laryngoscopy.

Question 3: What are some of your options in managing this patient's airway using endotracheal intubation? What are some of the drawbacks to each procedure?

Answer: Inserting an endotracheal tube in this particular patient with an unstable airway will require some quick decision making on your part.

Your options include:

A. Direct laryngoscopy–With the view of the glottic opening obscured by frank blood, it will be difficult to pass the tube through the vocal cords successfully. Additionally, as the patient exhales, blood may become aerosolized, splattering your face and eyes.

B. Nasal intubation–Although the patient is breathing, the presence of facial injuries and mechanism of injury may indicate the presence of a fractured cribriform plate, increasing the danger of brain injury if a nasal intubation procedure is selected.

C. Digital intubation–This may be a good option, although being bit by the patient is a potential drawback. However, in this case, the patient's level of consciousness appears to be appropriate for the use of the digital technique.

D. Transillumination–The potential drawback to this device is the level of ambient light that might obscure the view of the lighted stylet as it passes through the trachea.

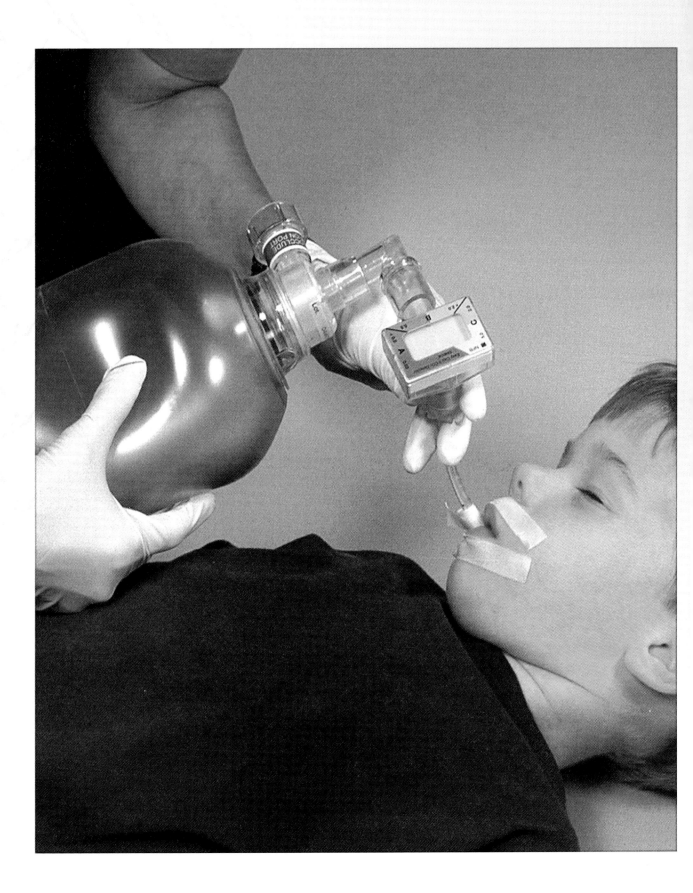

Objectives

Cognitive Objectives

2-1.36 Describe the indications, contraindications, advantages, disadvantages, complications, equipment, and technique of tracheobronchial suctioning in the intubated patient. (p 230)

2-1.38 Identify special considerations of tracheobronchial suctioning in the intubated patient. (p 231)

2-1.73 Describe methods of assessment for confirming correct placement of an endotracheal tube. (p 232)

2-1.75 Describe the indications, contraindications, advantages, disadvantages, complications, equipment, and technique for extubation. (p 241)

Psychomotor Objectives

2-1.82 Perform end-tidal CO_2 detection. (p 236) (Skill Drill 11-2)

2-1.89 Perform tracheobronchial suctioning in the intubated patient by selecting a suction device, catheter, and technique. (p 232) (Skill Drill 11-1)

2-1.108 Perform extubation. (p 242) (Skill Drill 11-3)

www.Paramedic.EMSzone.com

TECHNOLOGY

Online Chapter Pretest

Vocabulary Explorer

Anatomy Review

Web Links

FEATURES

Case Studies

Skill Drills

Teamwork Tips

Documentation Tips

Paramedic Safety Tips

Special Needs Tips

Vital Vocabulary

Prep Kit

Chapter

eople often relax once they have intubated a patient, but this is not the time to become complacent! Remember, the goal is oxygenation and ventilation! First, you must ensure that the tube is in the right place, and then you should ensure that it stays there by securing it properly. Of course, the patient must be ventilated effectively. Finally, you must ensure that the tube and airways remain free from solid or liquid obstructions. The order and priorities of these postintubation procedures will be dictated by the situation, and require judgment and experience.

Tracheobronchial Suctioning

After a patient has been intubated, it is important to ensure that you are able to provide adequate ventilation and oxygenation. Copious secretions in the trachea and upper airway that are not removed will be forced into the lungs during ventilation, thus impairing adequate ventilation and oxygenation. As a result, hypoxia will develop and the patient's condition could potentially worsen. This is a situation that can easily be avoided by suctioning the trachea via the endotracheal tube (▶ Skill Drill 11-1).

Suction Apparatus

Either a fixed or portable mechanical suction device can be used when performing tracheobronchial suctioning. Fixed suction devices are permanently mounted on the wall of the ambulance and operate off of the vacuum generated by the vehicle engine's manifold (▼ Figure 11-1). Fixed suction devices should be capable of furnishing an air intake of at least 40

L/min and a vacuum of at least 300 mm Hg when the suction tubing is occluded or clamped.

The fixed suction device should be mounted in a location where it is easily accessible should tracheobronchial suctioning need to be performed during transport of the patient. In most ambulances, the device is mounted to the immediate right of the patient's head.

The portable mechanical suction device, whether it is powered by oxygen, air, or electricity, should be able to furnish an air intake of at least 20 L/min in order to be effective (▼ Figure 11-2).

Suction Catheters

For tracheobronchial suctioning, the soft, flexible suction catheter, also called a "whistle-tip" catheter, should be used (▶ Figure 11-3). The **whistle-tip catheter** is designed to slide down the endotracheal tube easily. It has holes on the side and molded ends that will minimize trauma of the tracheal and

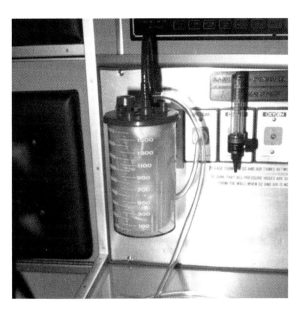

Figure 11-1 Fixed suction device.

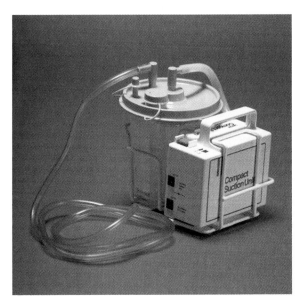

Figure 11-2 Portable mechanical suction device.

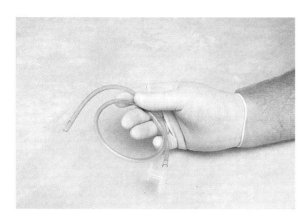

Figure 11-3 Whistle-tip suction catheter.

bronchial walls. A port on the proximal end of the catheter is occluded with the thumb to generate suction. Prior to performing tracheobronchial suctioning, the whistle-tip catheter should be prelubricated with a water-soluble gel.

Special Considerations

It is important to realize that any time suctioning is performed, especially via the endotracheal tube, ventilations must be interrupted; therefore, it is imperative to limit tracheobronchial suctioning to a maximum of 15 seconds. Additionally, if the patient is not already on a cardiac monitor, one should be applied in order to monitor the patient for hypoxia-related cardiac arrhythmias, which can occur during the suctioning procedure. The patient's oxygen saturation level should also be monitored with a pulse oximeter. If arrhythmias develop or the level of oxygen saturation begins to drop, suctioning must be discontinued immediately and ventilations resumed, even if you have not cleared all secretions.

Preoxygenation

Prior to performing **tracheobronchial suctioning**, the patient must be preoxygenated for at least 5 minutes (▶ Figure 11-4). Preoxygenation of the patient with 100% oxygen will minimize the risk of significant hypoxia during the procedure.

Suctioning Technique

Prior to performing tracheobronchial suctioning, it may be necessary to inject 3 to 5 mL of sterile water or saline down the endotracheal tube in order to loosen any thick secretions. After preoxygenating the patient as previously described, the suction catheter is gently inserted into the endotracheal tube using sterile technique, until resistance is felt. Resistance indicates that the tip of the catheter is

Case Study

Case Study, Part 1

You and your paramedic partner are dispatched to a residence for a 50-year-old man in acute respiratory distress. When you enter the residence, you find the patient in obvious distress, sitting upright on the corner of his bed. Cyanosis is noted around the patient's lips as are traces of dried blood. He tells you that he was suddenly awakened by the feeling that he was "suffocating." The fire department, with first responders, arrives at the scene a short time later.

You make the following determinations on your initial assessment:

Initial Assessment

Recording time
0 minutes

Appearance
Leaning forward, struggling to breathe

Level of consciousness
Appears alert

Airway
Coarse rhonchi are audible without a stethoscope.

Breathing
His ventilations are rapid and labored.

Circulation
A weak, rapid radial pulse is detected.

Question 1: On the basis of your initial assessment findings, what is your immediate management for this patient?

CASE STUDY

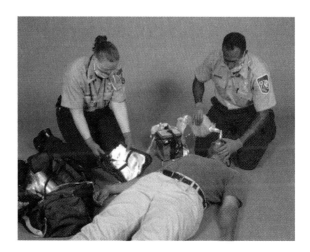

Figure 11-4 Preoxygenate the patient.

Skill Drill

11-1 Performing Tracheobronchial Suctioning

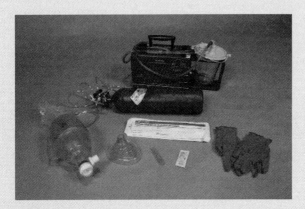

1 Check, prepare, and assemble your equipment.

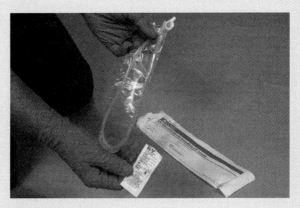

2 Lubricate the suction catheter.

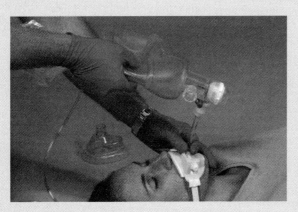

3 Preoxygenate the patient.

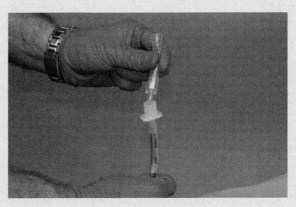

4 Detach the ventilation device and inject 3 to 5 mL of sterile water down the endotracheal tube.

about at the level of the carina. Suction is then applied while removing the catheter by occluding the proximal port. You should rotate the catheter as suction is being applied. *Remember to suction only while you are withdrawing the catheter and for no longer than 15 seconds.*

After suctioning has been completed, immediately reconnect the ventilation device to the endotracheal tube and resume ventilation and oxygenation. Should you need to resuction the patient, preoxygenation should occur for at least 30 seconds.

Determining Tube Placement

The most difficult part of intubating is the decision-making processes surrounding the procedure, not the procedure itself. The first challenge is to determine when to intubate. In some cases the answer is obvious, whereas in others it may be difficult to weigh the relative benefits and risks. The next challenge, which is even more important, is to determine exactly where the tube is. In some cases its location is obvious, but in other cases the findings can be

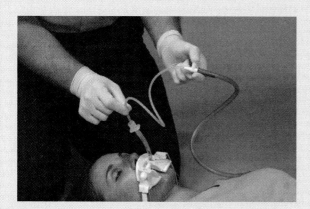

5 Gently insert the catheter into the endotracheal tube until resistance is felt.

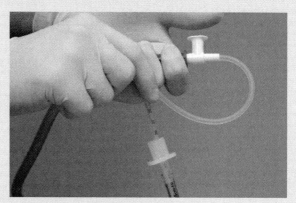

6 Suction in a rotating motion while withdrawing the catheter. Monitor the patient's cardiac rhythm and oxygen saturation during the procedure.

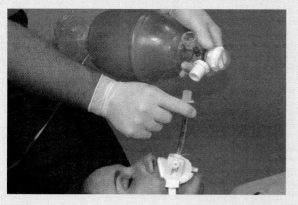

7 Reattach the ventilation device and resume ventilation and oxygenation.

conflicting or confusing. Incorrectly interpreting assessment findings about a tube's position can place the patient in tremendous jeopardy.

In this age of high technology, it is unfortunate that a method of rapidly confirming an endotracheal tube's placement with absolute certainty has not yet been developed. **No single test for endotracheal tube placement is 100% accurate.** A lot of new "gadgets" have been invented, but they all have limitations. Each test has to be evaluated on its sensitivity and specificity. Sensitivity is the probability

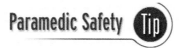

Paramedic Safety **Tip**

Unrecognized esophageal intubation is lethal. Failure to recognize that the endotracheal tube was either placed into or has moved into the esophagus is inexcusable and indefensible. When you take the responsibility of intubating a patient, you also assume responsibility for ensuring that the tube is properly placed and that it remains in the trachea.

Paramedic Safety Tip

Even if you put the tube in the trachea initially, it can become dislodged. Tubes (especially uncuffed pediatric tubes) *commonly* slip out of the trachea when you are removing the laryngoscope blade or securing the tube, or during ventilation or moving the patient. Simply flexing or extending the patient's head can move the tube tip as much as 5 cm, and rotation causes tube movement also. Many people advocate the immobilization of intubated patients with a cervical collar and head immobilization device to limit movement of the head, and thereby decrease the likelihood of the tube slipping out of the trachea while the patient is being moved.

that the test will correctly identify when the tube is in the trachea (the number of true positive results). Specificity is the probability that the test will correctly identify when the tube is not in the trachea (the number of true negative results).

The best way to be confident about the tube's location is to use a combination of different assessments to increase the accuracy of your interpretation. Do not be lulled into a false sense of security by relying on only one test to make a decision that is so important to the patient's survival.

Visualization

When you are performing endotracheal intubation by **direct laryngoscopy**, watching the tube pass through the cords is an important part of verifying that the tube is placed into the trachea. Unfortunately, you cannot always get a clear view of the glottic opening, and in some cases you cannot watch the tube actually pass through the cords. The tube may also become dislodged by removal of the laryngoscope. The fact that a tube was initially placed properly does not mean that it will stay in place.

Repeat visualization is an excellent way to reconfirm tube placement, but it is not as simple as some people think. If visualization was difficult in the first place, it will likely be difficult on subsequent attempts to confirm placement, when visualization is really useful. A technique to improve visualization of the glottic opening in intubated patients is to gently displace the tube posteriorly toward the palate. This action alters the direction of the tube and provides a better view of the passage of the tube through the vocal cords.

Another visualization technique uses a **bronchoscope**. The bronchoscope is inserted through the lumen of the endotracheal tube to identify the tracheal rings. The bronchoscope can also be used as an intubation guide for patients with an anticipated difficult airway. The use of fiberoptic bronchoscopes is effective for intubation confirmation, but this equipment is expensive and quite delicate, making it impractical in most prehospital settings.

Auscultation

Auscultation is an important part of confirming proper tube placement but can be difficult. Unfortunately, underlying pathologic conditions and large patient size can yield confusing or misleading findings. Because breath sounds are transmitted throughout the thoracic cage, they are more clearly transmitted through smaller patients with thinner chest walls. In obese patients, the large amount of chest wall tissue represents a significant barrier for the sound to traverse. Traumatic injuries (such as pneumothorax or obstructions), medical conditions (such as chronic obstructive pulmonary disease, bronchospasm, or pulmonary edema), or surgical interventions (such as pneumonectomy) can all make auscultation more difficult.

The movement of air through the esophagus may sound like adventitious breath sounds. The presence of gastric sounds does not always indicate esophageal intubation. Gastric distention that is present may have occurred prior to intubation.

To be effective, listen to the chest in at least *six* places: the right and left apices in the midclavicular line, the right and left bases in the midaxillary line, over the epigastrium, and at the sternal notch. You should hear bilaterally equal sounds in all lung fields, a quiet stomach, and a rush of air with ventilation at the sternal notch. More than any single auscultatory finding, gurgling in the stomach most likely indicates esophageal intubation. If you suspect esophageal intubation, immediately stop ventilating the patient and remove the tube.

There are two possible ways to auscultate to confirm tube placement:

1. If you are auscultating after direct laryngoscopy and you had good visualization of the tube passing through the cords, you are fairly confident that the tube is properly placed. In this case, listen to the left base first. If you hear breath sounds there, check the right base, left apex, right apex, stomach, and sternal notch. If you hear no breath sounds at the left base, check the stomach next. If you hear gurgling, remove the tube.

If the stomach is quiet, but you have breath sounds on the right side and not the left side, the right mainstem has been intubated. Place the stethoscope over the left apex, and auscultate as you ventilate while slowly withdrawing the tube. As breath sounds return to the left side, secure the tube.

2. If you are auscultating after direct laryngoscopy and had poor visualization or are using a blind technique (nasal or digital), check the epigastrium first. If it is quiet, check the four lung fields and the sternal notch.

Observation and Palpation of the Chest

Observing the rise and fall of the chest provides some indication of tube placement. If the chest moves symmetrically during each ventilation, this suggests proper tube placement. Placing your hands on the thoracic cage provides additional tactile information: both sides of the patient's chest should expand equally with ventilation. You should palpate the thoracic cage to feel the separation of the ribs with chest expansion.

Chest wall movement can be very difficult to detect in obese patients, women with large breasts, patients with rigid chest walls, and patients with poorly compliant lungs. Endotracheal tubes that have been placed in the esophagus can result in the inflation and deflation of the stomach and/or esophagus, which can cause the chest wall to move in a way that mimics the movements associated with lung ventilation.

End-Tidal Carbon Dioxide

The continual presence of carbon dioxide in the patient's exhaled breath is the established standard for confirming endotracheal tube placement. End-tidal carbon dioxide (CO_2) has become the standard for determining placement in the operating room (▼ Figure 11-5). Because no respiration occurs in

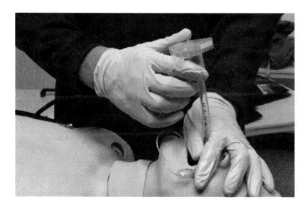

Figure 11-5 End-tidal CO_2.

Case Study

Case Study, Part 2

You place the patient on a non-rebreathing mask set at 15 L/min. As your partner is applying a cardiac monitor, you complete a focused history, physical examination, and baseline vital signs. Your findings are recorded as follows:

Physical Examination

Recording time
2 minutes after patient contact

Level of orientation
Alert

Head
Cyanosis around the lips, coughing up blood-tinged sputum

Neck
Accessory muscle use

Chest
Unremarkable

Lung sounds
Coarse rhonchi in both bases with scattered rales and rhonchi to both apices

Abdomen
Soft and nontender

Pelvis
Unremarkable

Extremities
Moves all extremities

Back
Unremarkable

History

Age, sex, weight
50-year-old man, 75 kg

Signs and symptoms
Patient complains of acute onset of shortness of breath that woke him from sleep.

Allergies to medications
Codeine, aspirin

Medications taken
Vasotec (Enalapril maleate)
Digoxin (Lanoxin)
Furosemide (Lasix)

Past pertinent medical history
Hypertension, acute myocardial infarction, congestive heart failure

Last food/fluid intake
Ate supper approximately 8 hours earlier

Events prior to onset
No sentinel events reported

Onset of symptoms
Sudden, while sleeping

Provoking/palliative factors
The patient reports a 2-day history of exertional intolerance and generalized weakness.

Quality of discomfort
The patient is clearly in distress. He denies having pain.

Radiating/related signs/symptoms
Patient is coughing up secretions that are tinged with blood.

Severity of complaint
The respiratory distress is worse, even more so than when he called EMS.

Time
The episode began 20 minutes ago.

Vital Signs

Skin signs
Pale, cool, dry

Pulse rate/quality
120 beats/min, regular

Blood pressure
160/94 mm Hg

Respiratory rate/depth
28 breaths/min, significantly labored

Pupils
Equal, reactive

SpO$_2$
83% (100% oxygen)

Electrocardiogram
Sinus tachycardia

Question 2: Is the management that you are providing for this patient producing a noted improvement in his condition?

Question 3: Should you consider a more aggressive management approach? Why?

CASE STUDY

Skill Drill

11-2 Performing End-Tidal CO₂ Detection

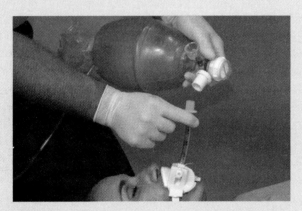

1 Detach ventilation device from the endotracheal tube.

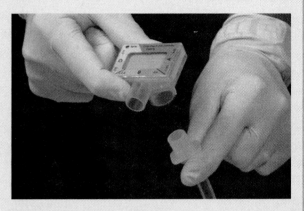

2 Attach in-line capnograph or capnometer to proximal adaptor of the endotracheal tube.

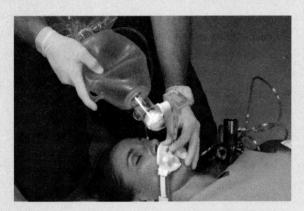

3 Reattach the ventilation device to the endotracheal tube and resume ventilations.

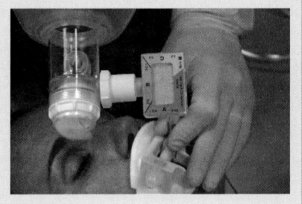

4 Monitor the capnograph or capnometer for appropriate reading (appropriate color change or digital reading).

the stomach, the presence of carbon dioxide indicates that the tube is in the trachea. The continual presence of more than 2% carbon dioxide (corresponding to approximately 15 mm Hg) in the exhaled breath is considered a positive finding.

In theory, carbonated beverages or antacids in the stomach could produce false-positive results. Although this does occur, the carbon dioxide from these sources is quickly vented from the stomach and is not replaced. Therefore, it is generally considered that carbon dioxide in exhaled breath after six breaths strongly suggests tracheal tube placement. The most likely cause of a false-positive result is from the tube not being inserted far enough into

the trachea. In the case of a supraglottic placement of the tube, there will still be carbon dioxide in the exhaled breath yet positive control of the airway does not exist. The risk of tube dislodgement is great, and the risk of aspiration remains.

The most common cause of a false-negative result is a significant disruption in pulmonary blood flow. It takes a severe interruption in pulmonary blood flow to drop the concentration of carbon dioxide in the exhaled breath below 2%, but the concentration in many emergency patients falls into this category. The most common situation occurs in cardiac arrest. In this state of very low blood flow, pulmonary perfusion is often insufficient to increase carbon dioxide levels above 2%. In fact, it has been suggested that end-tidal CO_2 indicates the amount of cardiac output generated by compressions during cardiopulmonary resuscitation. The amount of end-tidal CO_2 has even been correlated with the likelihood of successful resuscitation.

Other causes of interrupted pulmonary blood flow that are sufficient enough to cause false-negative results are low cardiac output, hypotension, pulmonary embolism, and severe bronchospasm. Therefore, the continual presence of end-tidal CO_2 (greater than 15 mm Hg, or 2%) almost guarantees that the tube is not in the esophagus, but the absence of end-tidal CO_2, however, does not mean that the tube is in the esophagus. The patient may not be generating enough carbon dioxide to register a positive result, as is often the case during cardiac arrest. Two devices are generally used to measure end-tidal CO_2—the capnometer and the capnographer.

Capnometer

A **capnometer** simply measures the amount of carbon dioxide in expired gas. Capnometers are either colorimetric or electronic.

Colorimetric Capnometers

The colorimetric capnometer, also known as an end-tidal CO_2 detector, is a simple and ingenious device that uses a chemical reaction of carbon dioxide to detect its presence in the exhaled gas. In the presence of carbon dioxide, metacresol purple changes color to yellow. If a piece of filter paper containing metacresol purple is placed in-between the endotracheal tube and the ventilation device, the paper will turn from purple to yellow if the carbon dioxide concentration is greater than 2% in the exhaled breath (◄ Skill Drill 11-2). This chemical reaction is very rapid and should occur with each breath.

Unfortunately, colorimetric capnometers do not make quantitative measurements. With more than 2% carbon dioxide in the gas sample, the color change is dramatic and usually obvious in well-lit environments (some adjustment may be needed for incandescent lights by using an alternative color chart). The filter will not change at all when exposed to a concentration of carbon dioxide of less than 0.05%. In carbon dioxide concentrations between 0.05% and 2%, the chemical reaction is incomplete and may indicate poor pulmonary perfusion or improper tube placement. It is generally recommended that such an intermediate color change after 6 breaths requires confirmation of tube placement using other techniques.

The colorimetric capnometer has some limitations. The end-tidal CO_2 detector is not affected by temperature but is affected by humidity. The device becomes ineffective when exposed to room air for more than a few hours and after about 15 minutes of

continual ventilation. It should not be used with humidified breathing gas. The color change is apparent in fluorescent light but has to be adjusted for incandescent light. The color change can be difficult for colorblind individuals to detect.

Electronic Capnometers

Electronic capnometers detect and calculate the amount of carbon dioxide in the exhaled breath. These devices calculate this information very quickly and accurately, providing a real-time indication of the patient's carbon dioxide levels. With modern electronics these devices are now smaller,

Case Study

Case Study, Part 3

Noting that oxygen by nonrebreathing mask is not producing a notable improvement in the patient's condition, you begin assisting ventilations with a BVM device attached to 100% oxygen. The patient does not resist. Your partner and a first responder load the patient into the ambulance and begin transport to the hospital, which is approximately 20 minutes away. You request that the first responder accompany and assist you in the back of the ambulance. You reassess the patient's condition and vital signs:

Ongoing Assessment

Recording time
7 minutes after patient contact

Initial assessment
You note decreased compliance with bag-valve-mask ventilations. The patient continues to produce blood-tinged secretions.

Intervention reassessment
Diffuse coarse rhonchi are now audible in all lung fields.

Any other changes
The patient's level of conscious has markedly decreased.

Vital Signs

Skin signs
Remains pale, cool, and dry

Pulse rate/quality
132 beats/min, regular

Blood pressure
156/88 mm Hg

Respiratory rate/depth
30 breaths/min, assisted with BVM device

Pupils
Dilated, but reactive

SpO_2
86% (with BVM ventilation and 100% oxygen)

Electrocardiogram
Sinus tachycardia

Question 4: On the basis of your ongoing assessment findings, what intervention should you consider at this point?

Question 5: Are there additional interventions that might improve this patient's condition?

more reliable, cheaper, and lighter than they have been in the past.

Electronic capnometers usually have an adapter that fits between the endotracheal tube and the ventilation device. The amount of carbon dioxide is displayed quantitatively or with a bar graph of LED lights.

The major advantage of electric capnometers is that they quantify the carbon dioxide. This is not only valuable for the verification of endotracheal tube placement but also provides an approximation of $PaCO_2$. In most cases, end-tidal CO_2 is about 5 to 6 mm Hg below $PaCO_2$. This information makes it possible and practical to adjust minute volume (by altering ventilatory rate and/or volume) to maintain normal $PaCO_2$ during ventilation. End-tidal CO_2 becomes an unreliable approximation of $PaCO_2$ in cases of significant ventilation-perfusion mismatch (V-Q mismatch).

Capnograph

A **capnograph** instantly plots the level of carbon dioxide in a gas sample on a printout known as a capnogram. The information from the capnogram allows you to track trends in the end-tidal CO_2 and quickly identify problems that would not be obvious in a simple quantitative reading. Any pattern on the capnogram that is irregular and oscillating, always returning to baseline between breaths, should alert you to a potential problem.

Some capnographs are bulky, requiring calibration, a warm-up period, paper, and AC power. These types are obviously not practical for prehospital use. Newer models are now small, light, and battery operated. Some manufacturers are even incorporating capnography into other monitors (such as an electrocardiogram monitor). The capnograph has great potential for use not only in verifying tube placement, but in guiding ventilation rate and depth.

The Esophageal Detection Device

The trachea is a rigid structure that is essentially noncollapsible. In contrast, the esophagus is a flaccid tube that expands only when something is placed into it. Because of this anatomic distinction, you cannot draw air when negative pressure is applied to the tip of an endotracheal tube placed in the esophagus because the walls of the esophagus will occlude the tip of the tube. In contrast, the trachea, being rigid, will not form an airtight seal with the tip of an endotracheal tube subjected to negative pressure. You can draw air from the lungs by applying negative pressure.

The simple anatomic distinction is the basis for the **esophageal detection device (EDD)**. The EDD is a bulb or syringe with a 15/22-mm adapter. The syringe is attached to the end of the endotracheal tube. The plunger is withdrawn, creating negative pressure. If the tube is in the trachea, air is easily drawn into the syringe and the plunger does not move when released. If the tube is in the esophagus, a vacuum is created as you withdraw the plunger, and the plunger moves back toward zero when released.

With the bulb model, the bulb is collapsed and then attached to the end of the endotracheal tube. If it remains collapsed, the tube is in the esophagus. If the bulb briskly expands, the tube is properly positioned in the trachea.

The main limitation of the EDD is that gastric or esophageal air may fill the bulb or syringe. It is important therefore to apply the device before ventilation has begun. The bulb must be collapsed before being connected to the tube as well, because squeezing it while it is attached to the tube would instill a small amount of air that could theoretically cause a false-positive result. There is a low incidence of false-negative results in very obese patients. The EDD cannot detect mainstem intubation or oropharyngeal placement.

Transillumination

In most patients the tissue overlying the trachea is relatively thin. If a bright bulb is positioned at the tip of a properly placed endotracheal tube, a point of light should be visible in the midline of the neck, at the level of the sternal notch. A number of commercially available devices use **transillumination** for confirmation of tube placement and for intubating. When used as a tube confirmation technique, a bright light is positioned at the tip of the inserted endotracheal tube. A tightly circumscribed light visible through the tissue of the neck at the midline strongly suggests proper tube placement.

A main advantage of transillumination is the ability to judge the depth of insertion. The proper location for the tip of the tube is halfway between the glottic opening and the carina. The sternal notch is the external landmark for this location. When you are placing an endotracheal tube under direct visualization, the proper depth of insertion is estimated by advancing the proximal end of the cuff 1 to 2 cm beyond the glottic opening, typically to a depth of 21 to 23 cm in an adult of average height. With transillumination, you can adjust the depth of the endotracheal tube until the light is right at the sternal notch. The main disadvantage of transillumination is the fact that it can be difficult to see the light in obese, bullnecked patients or in situations where ambient light is particularly bright.

Miscellaneous Techniques for Determining Tube Placement

The best assurance that a patient is properly intubated is to use a combination of verification techniques. Although the following techniques are generally not reliable enough to be used individually, they provide important confirmatory information. When those techniques are combined with other verification techniques, the confidence that you have in the interpretation of the results will be increased.

As a patient passively exhales, the gas from the lungs is warm and moist. If the tube is properly positioned in the trachea, mist will form on the inside of the tube. Unfortunately, misting can also sometimes occur in a patient who has a significant amount of gastric air who has been esophageally intubated. Even when the tube is correctly positioned, mist may not form in a hot, humid environment.

When the tube is in the trachea, there will be a small "puff" of exhaled air as the patient's sternum is depressed. This can be heard or felt at the proximal end of the tube during external chest compressions.

If the tube is properly placed, a pressure wave in the pilot balloon can be felt when a gentle force is applied to the trachea just above the sternal notch. An assistant who is providing the Sellick maneuver often can feel the tube pass through the cricoid ring into the trachea. Because of the ridges in the wall of the trachea, this sensation has been described as "washboardlike."

If the patient's SpO_2 improves, the tube is likely in the trachea. The SpO_2 can improve, however, in a spontaneously breathing patient who is esophageally intubated. Furthermore, it is hard to obtain saturation in pulseless patients, and readings below 80% can be inaccurate.

Regurgitation of stomach contents through the endotracheal tube indicates that the tube is in the esophagus. Some patients have copious tracheal secretions, but these should be easily distinguished from vomitus.

If the patient is able to make any noise (such as talk, grunt, or moan) by moving air past the vocal cords, the tube is in the wrong place and should be immediately removed. This rule does not apply to pediatric patients intubated with uncuffed tubes. ▼ **Table 11-1** summarizes these techniques and their false-positive and false-negative findings.

Table 11-1
Errors of Tests Used to Determine Endotracheal Tube Placement

	False-Positive Findings	**False-Negative Findings**
Visualization	Tube may slip out after visualization	Misinterpretation of anatomic landmarks
	Poor visualization	
	Misinterpretation of anatomic landmarks	
Observation/palpation of the chest	Gastric ventilation causing chest wall movement	Limited chest wall mobility in poorly compliant lungs
		Difficult to detect chest wall movement in obese, barrel-chested, or large-breasted patients
Breath sounds	Gastric sounds can mimic breath sounds	Difficult to hear in obese patients, traumatic injuries, pneumothorax, obstructions, COPD, bronchospasm, pulmonary edema, pneumonectomy
	Transmitted breath sounds	
	Transmitted bronchial sounds	

Ventilating the Intubated Patient

Effective ventilation is a real art. It requires experience, attention to detail, and a certain touch. Once a patient is intubated, ventilation becomes much easier. In fact, increased efficiency of ventilation is one of the main reasons to intubate. Nonetheless, ventilation technique is still important after the patient has been intubated.

When the patient has been endotracheally intubated, none of the air forced into the mouth goes to the stomach, but it is still necessary to deliver the ventilatory volume slowly, over 1 to 2 seconds. A slow inspiratory time reduces the airflow and hemodynamic complications of positive pressure ventilation and keeps intrapulmonary pressure low, reducing the chances of barotrauma.

Another advantage of ventilating the intubated patient is that you no longer have to worry about the mask seal. The cuff on the endotracheal tube provides a virtually airtight seal. With an intubated patient the dead space of the mask is eliminated, and you can usually decrease the ventilation volume to 5 to 7 cc/kg.

The 15/22-mm adapter on the end of the endotracheal tube is a universal connector to all ventilation equipment. In emergency medicine, there are a number of options for ventilating the intubated patient, as described in the following sections.

Bag-Valve-Mask Device

Bag-valve-mask ventilation is the most common method of ventilating intubated patients in emergency care. You will often use the **bag-valve-mask (BVM) device** while moving patients and while awaiting a ventilator. In addition to being fast, ventilation with a BVM device provides a "feel" for the breathing. You can judge the **compliance** of the lungs, possibly becoming alert to significant bronchospasm or an evolving pneumothorax. You can feel the rattling and gurgling of fluid or mucous obstructions and the need for tracheobronchial suctioning.

One of the biggest advantages of the BVM device lies in the ventilation of breathing patients. You can time your ventilations to the patient's own breathing pattern. If the minute volume is inadequate, you can increase the patient's tidal volume by gently squeezing the bag during inhalation and/or interspersing breaths between the patient's own breaths, thereby increasing the respiratory rate.

The main disadvantage of BVM ventilation is that it requires one person to be constantly vigilant about ventilation. The ventilator cannot be distracted by other tasks and interrupt ventilations.

The BVM device is also a bit awkward. If the ventilator is not paying close attention, the tube can inadvertently be moved.

The Flow-Restricted, Oxygen-Powered Ventilation Device

The **flow-restricted, oxygen-powered ventilation device (FROPVD)**, also referred to as a **manually triggered automatic ventilator (MTV)**, can be used to ventilate an intubated patient. The FROPVD is a valve that attaches to an oxygen regulator and provides 100% oxygen at constant flow rate of 60 L/min when a button is depressed. The constant flow keeps intrapulmonary pressure reasonably constant throughout the ventilation. The FROPVD has a pressure valve that prevents ventilation pressures in excess of 40 cm of water, which may decrease the incidence of **barotrauma**. The controlled flow rate and pressure relief are particularly important in cases of chest trauma. Any form of positive pressure ventilation will likely increase the size of a preexisting pneumothorax, but the flow restriction afforded by the FROPVD may keep the increase in intrapleural air minimal.

The FROPVD can be triggered in two ways. For nonbreathing patients, a button on the device is depressed, opening the valve, and starting the flow of oxygen. For breathing patients, the device is triggered by intrinsically generated negative pressure. It can therefore be attached to the endotracheal tube of a breathing patient to provide 100% oxygen. As with the BVM device, the minute volume can be increased if the patient is hypoventilating by increasing the rate and/or volume of the breaths.

One disadvantage of ventilating intubated patients with the FROPVD is the loss of the "feel" for the ventilations. The FROPVD also requires one person to be dedicated to ventilating the patient. Finally, the flow restriction and pressure pop-off may make it impossible to ventilate a patient with poor lung compliance, increased airway resistance, or a heavy chest wall. The FROPVD is not recommended for the ventilation of children.

Automatic Transport Ventilator

The **automatic transport ventilator (ATV)** has a number of advantages over the FROPVD and the BVM device. After you set the tidal volume and respiratory rate of the ATV, it will ventilate the patient automatically. With the ATV, one person need not be dedicated to ventilation. Most ATVs do not allow patients to control their own breathing, however, which can be very upsetting to conscious patients able to breathe on their own.

Paramedic Safety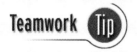

Accidental extubation can occur if the BVM device pulls on the tube. It is strongly recommended that the BVM device be disconnected when it is not being used (such as during patient movement or defibrillation).

Ventilator

A ventilator is frequently used to ventilate patients after the emergency phase of care. Ventilators allow precise control of all the variables of ventilation. Ventilators are used on both breathing and apneic patients. Some ventilator settings require that the patient do some of the work of breathing. These settings can be used to help "wean" patients off ventilatory dependence. The proper setup and use of ventilators is beyond the scope of this book, but you should know the basic functions of ventilators used in your facility.

Extubation in Emergency Medicine

Extubation is the process of removing the tube from an intubated patient (▶ **Skill Drill 11-3**). In the critical care environment, the decision to extubate a patient is very complicated and depends on many factors. It may take days or weeks to wean a patient off of a ventilator and be confident that the person will be able to ventilate and maintain his or her own airway. The decision to extubate the critical care patient is beyond the scope of this book.

In emergency medicine we rarely extubate patients. The major indication for extubation is when the patient's level of consciousness improves and he or she begins gagging on the tube. In general,

Teamwork

It takes considerable effort to coordinate the efforts of the rescuers managing an advanced airway such as an endotracheal intubation. Determining roles of various team members prior to the actual call is useful in minimizing confusion at the scene.

Case Study

Case Study, Part 4

You perform endotracheal intubation on this patient as his condition is clearly not improving with basic airway management. The ambulance is briefly stopped and your partner assists you in the back. After sedating the patient, you successfully place the endotracheal tube. Correct placement is confirmed by auscultation of the lungs and an end-tidal CO_2 detector. Because of the obvious fluid in the lungs and the secretions evident in the endotracheal tube, you decide to perform tracheobronchial suctioning. The patient's condition is improved following intubation and suctioning. You arrive at the hospital approximately 5 minutes later and give your report to the charge nurse. His last set of vital signs are noted below:

Vital Signs

Recording time
35 minutes after patient contact

Skin signs
Pink, cool, and dry

Pulse rate/quality
94 beats/min, regular

Blood pressure
128/66 mm Hg

Respiratory rate/depth
24 breaths/min, intubated

Pupils
Equal and reactive

SpO_2
94% (intubated with ventilatory assistance)

Electrocardiogram
Normal sinus rhythm

The patient is later admitted to the hospital, with a diagnosis of acute exacerbation of his congestive heart failure.

CASE STUDY

it is better to sedate the patient than to remove the tube, but this may not be an option in some systems or in patients who are hemodynamically unstable.

There are a number of risks in extubating emergency patients. The most obvious is overestimating the ability of the patient to protect his or her own airway. Once you remove the tube, there is no guarantee that you will be able to replace it. Patients who are awake are at a high risk for laryngospasm upon removal of an endotracheal tube, and most patients experience some degree of upper airway swelling because of the trauma of having a tube in their throat. These two facts, complicated by the

Skill Drill

11-3 Performing Extubation

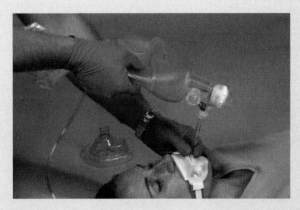

1 Hyperoxygenate the patient.

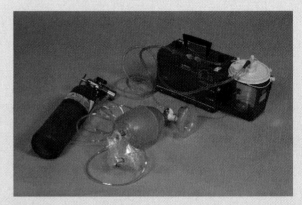

2 Ensure that ventilation and suction equipment are immediately available.

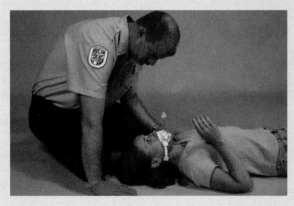

3 Confirm patient responsiveness.

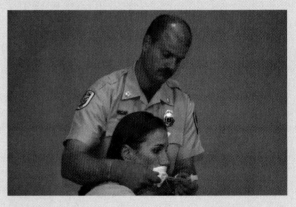

4 Lean the patient forward.

ever-present possibility of vomiting, make reintubation challenging, and maybe impossible. These risks must be factored against the benefit of removing the tube.

Field extubation is indicated when the patient is able to protect and maintain the airway, the patient is not sedated, and you are confident that you will be able to ventilate and reintubate if necessary. Field extubation should never be performed if there is a risk of continued or recurrent respiratory failure.

Keep in mind that postextubation vomiting and/or laryngospasm is possible.

Field extubation is accomplished by first hyperoxygenating the patient. Discuss the procedure with the patient, and explain what you are going to do. If possible, it is best to have the patient sit up, or lean slightly forward. Be sure to assemble and have available all equipment to suction, ventilate, and reintubate, if necessary. After you have confirmed that the patient remains responsive enough to protect his or

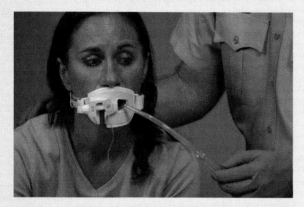

5 Suction the oropharynx.

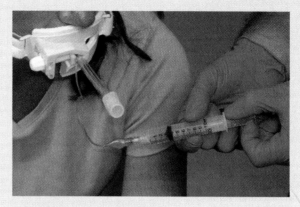

6 Deflate the distal cuff of the endotracheal tube.

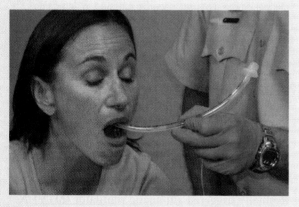

7 Remove the endotracheal tube upon cough or when the patient exhales.

her own airway, suction the oropharynx to remove any debris or secretions that may threaten the airway. Deflate the cuff on the endotracheal tube at the beginning of an exhalation so that any accumulated secretions just above the cuff are not aspirated into the lungs. On the next exhalation, remove the tube in one steady motion, following the curvature of the airway. You may find it useful to hold a towel or emesis basin in front of the patient's mouth, in case the patient gags or vomits.

Paramedic Safety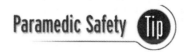

There are a number of risks in extubating emergency patients. The most obvious is overestimating the ability of the patient to protect his or her own airway.

With so much emphasis on endotracheal intubation, it is easy to forget the big picture: The optimal management of emergency patients requires outstanding ventilation and oxygenation. We frequently use an endotracheal tube to accomplish this goal, but you can still ventilate and oxygenate patients if intubation attempts fail. This chapter discusses some alternatives to maintaining oxygenation and ventilation when endotracheal intubation is impossible, impractical, not permitted, or has failed.

Everyone in emergency medicine eventually encounters a situation when a patient cannot be intubated. In the controlled setting of the operating room, 1% to 4% of surgical patients have "difficult" airways. Some studies estimate that about 1 in every 500 to 1,000 patients cannot be intubated, even by experienced anesthesiologists in the operating room.

It is reasonable to expect that the incidence of difficult airways is higher in prehospital emergency situations because of complications that are not typically encountered in anesthesia (full stomachs, environmental considerations, or trauma).

The incidence of repeated failure to secure an airway by intubation in prehospital emergency settings is hard to quantify. Clearly, there is variability based on the intubator's experience, amount of practice, and skill, but the inability to intubate is a reality. Although there is no universal quality indicator, an emergency system with a "failure to intubate" rate higher than 5% to 10% should take a critical look at their quality improvement process and take steps to improve individual and collective performance. Paramedics should be able to maintain a 90% to 95% successful intubation rate.

Although failure to intubate is a difficult problem, there are alternative actions that can be taken. First, do not forget the basics. Anytime you are having difficulty intubating, be sure to ventilate the patient with positive pressure ventilations and manage the airway with manual positioning and simple airway adjuncts (▶ Figure 12-1). Fortunately, only a small percentage of patients cannot be intubated *and* cannot be ventilated.

Endotracheal intubation is the established standard for definitive airway management. All the techniques described in this chapter are considered to be alternatives to intubation, typically used when endo-

tracheal intubation is impossible or otherwise contraindicated. None of these techniques provide the protection and therapeutic benefits of intubation. They should not be considered a substitution for intubation but rather an option when intubation is not possible.

Esophageal Airways

Esophageal airways were initially introduced in 1968 and became popular as a primary method of airway management for prehospital care providers in the early 1970s. The **esophageal obturator airway (EOA)** was endorsed by the American Heart Association in 1974 and has been used in prehospital settings. The effectiveness of esophageal airways is extremely controversial, and the issue is complicated by conflicting research findings. One of the main contributions of esophageal airways has been the continual refinement of design that has led to improved devices. Although they are not commonly used today, esophageal airways are available and have some advantages in specific situations.

The concept of an esophageal airway is simple. If you occlude the esophagus completely, all of the gas delivered under pressure to the patient will go into the lungs. Additionally, by placing an **obturator** in the esophagus, you effectively eliminate the risk of

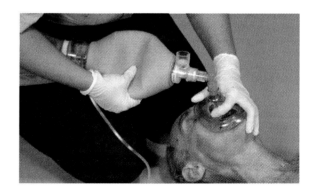

Figure 12-1 Anytime you are having difficulty intubating, be sure to ventilate the patient with positive pressure ventilations and manage the airway with manual positioning and simple airway adjuncts.

Paramedic Safety (Tip)

If you are unable to intubate the patient, *ventilate!*

regurgitation and subsequent aspiration. The common characteristic of esophageal airways is a long tube attached to a ventilation mask. The tube has a large inflatable balloon at its distal end, which serves as a cuff. The tube is inserted blindly into the esophagus, the mask is sealed to the patient's face, and the balloon is inflated. Ventilation is accomplished by positive pressure generated within the mask by a bag-valve device (▼ Figure 12-2).

Advantages and Disadvantages of Esophageal Airways

There are a number of advantages of esophageal airways over intubation. First, they require less technical skill than intubation. In theory, they can be properly used with less practice and continual skill maintenance. This may be particularly advantageous in rural settings where there is an infrequent need for airway management. Esophageal airways also provide excellent protection against vomiting.

Unfortunately, there are also numerous disadvantages of esophageal airways. The most significant is the fact that the device still requires a mask seal to ventilate the patient. Second, the esophageal airway does little to maintain a patent airway. Although the device prevents gastric insulation and regurgitation, the paramedic must still open the airway.

Poor mask seal and difficulty in manually opening the airway are two of the major reasons for hypoventilation when the airway is unprotected and are major technical problems associated with using esophageal airways.

Indications for Esophageal Airways

The esophageal airway can be used only in apneic patients without a gag reflex. In general, the indication for the use of an esophageal airway is an inability to intubate. The esophageal airways are considered a temporary airway device and must be removed after 2 hours.

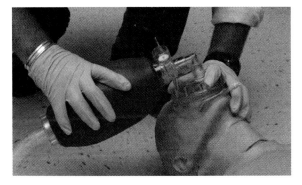

Figure 12-2 Esophageal airways prevent gastric inflation and regurgitation by obstruction of the esophagus.

Case Study

Case Study, Part 1

"They're late," your partner says to no one in particular. The two of you are standing outside of the ambulance garage, waiting for the day crew to come back from a cardiac arrest run. A few minutes later you can hear the sound of the ambulance's diesel motor coming toward you. As the crew pulls in, the call tones ring out from your pagers—dispatch is requesting your response to a report of an unconscious elderly woman. Quickly, the off-going crew provides a rapid-fire report of the rig's condition—"You have a couple of backboards, there should be oxygen in the jump bag, and we were able to restock the medication kit." En route, you can make out that two district cars are heading toward the same location.

As you walk onto the scene, you can see people congregated near the patio, where two police officers are performing CPR on a victim. An AED is attached to the victim's chest. Bystanders report that today is the patient's 65th birthday, and that about two hours into the party, the patient told her daughter that she felt very "warm" and stepped outside to get some air. Her husband found her a few minutes later, collapsed on the patio bench, gasping for air. Police officers arrived about 4 minutes after dispatch to find the patient unconscious and unresponsive, with agonal respirations and no pulse. The AED defibrillated once prior to your arrival. CPR was continued after the officers found no pulses or other signs of circulation after the delivered shock.

Your reassessment of the patient's initial presentation is as follows:

Initial Assessment

Recording time
0 minutes

Appearance
Cyanotic, supine on patio deck

Level of consciousness
Unconscious

Airway
Managed with head tilt-chin lift

Breathing
Apneic, assisted with BVM device (100% oxygen)

Circulation
Pulseless

Your partner hands you the airway kit. Unzipping the pack you reach for the laryngoscope handle—and to your surprise, you find it missing, along with several blades and endotracheal tubes! You realize that the off-going crew did not restock the airway kit after their last call. As if on cue, the patient vomits copiously. Quickly you and your team roll her onto her side, suctioning out her oral cavity.

Question 1: What are your concerns about managing this airway with only basic airway adjuncts?

Question 2: What are some noninvasive airway adjuncts that might be useful in a situation like this?

Contraindications to Use of Esophageal Airways

Esophageal airways should not be used in patients younger than 16 years. Because the cuff has to come to rest in the esophagus above the cardiac sphincter but below the carina, the airway can be used only in patients between 5 and 7 feet tall. In a shorter person, the cuff may come to rest in the sphincter itself, or the stomach. In a taller person, the cuff may come to rest in the esophagus above the level of the carina. When inflated, it may cause a partial obstruction in the trachea because the open end of the tracheal rings faces the esophagus.

No airway that is intended to be inserted into the esophagus should ever be used if the patient has any history of esophageal disease (such as esophageal varices, strictures, or diverticuli) or has ingested a caustic substance, because of the increased risk of esophageal rupture. The trachea must be protected before removal of an esophageal airway because vomiting then occurs in almost all patients. Intubation with an esophageal airway in place can be challenging.

Complications of Esophageal Airways

The most significant complication of esophageal airway insertion is inadvertent tracheal intubation. If tracheal placement goes unrecognized, the patient will receive no pulmonary ventilation. Confirmation of tube placement is just as important following esophageal airway placement as it is following endotracheal intubation, and the consequences of unrecognized misplacement are just as disastrous.

In addition to misplacement, the complication rate of esophageal airways is quite high. Hypoventilation due to poor mask seal and airway control is common. Esophageal rupture, while uncommon, is life threatening. Laryngospasm caused by excessive upper airway stimulation, as well as vomiting and aspiration, can occur during insertion or in failed attempts. If the cuff is left in place too long, or inflated with too much air, it can cause localized tissue necrosis.

Equipment for Esophageal Airways

The original esophageal airway was called the esophageal obturator airway (EOA) (▶ Figure 12-3). The EOA is no longer manufactured and very few are still in circulation. EOAs should not be used because of the inability to decompress the stomach prior to removal.

The **esophageal gastric tube airway (EGTA)** is a modification of the EOA. It consists of a mask attached to a plastic tube that is 34 cm long and 13 mm in diameter. The tube has a 35-mL balloon at its distal end. The EGTA has an opening at the distal tip of the esophageal tube, enabling a 16F gastric tube

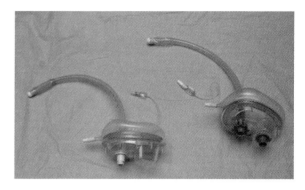

Figure 12-3 Esophageal obturator airway and esophageal gastric tube airway.

to be inserted for decompression of the stomach prior to removal of the esophageal airway. The mask has a 15/22-mm ventilation port enabling ventilation (▼ Figure 12-4).

Technique for Esophageal Airway Placement and Placement Confirmation

Remember that the goal of an EGTA is to occlude the esophagus. Therefore, the technique is intended to facilitate entry of the tube into the esophagus, *not* the trachea. If the procedure is followed correctly, esophageal placement occurs in most cases, but its position *must* be confirmed.

All of the alternative airway procedures before and after insertion are similar to the procedures discussed in the previous chapter. Therefore, only the differences from those procedures will be discussed here.

Procedures Before Insertion

As with every airway procedure, all equipment is checked and assembled before you start the technique. In particular, check the cuff of the esophageal airway and ensure that it holds 35 mL of air. The tube must be inserted into the mask before being inserted into the patient to prevent the tube from migrating too far into the airway. It should snap

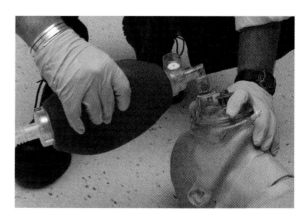

Figure 12-4 Ventilation with an EGTA in place.

firmly in place, with the curvature of the tube following the natural contour of the airway.

The patient should be preoxygenated before insertion. Ventilation should not be interrupted longer than 30 seconds to accomplish airway placement. This is rarely a problem because the procedure is blind and generally faster than endotracheal intubation

Finally, patient positioning is extremely important. In contrast to endotracheal intubation, where the goal of preintubation positioning is to align the axes of the airway, you *want* this tube to go into the esophagus. Therefore, the patient's head should be placed in the neutral or slightly flexed position.

Displace the Jaw Forward

With the head in the neutral or flexed position, insert the thumb of your gloved nondominant hand into the patient's mouth and lift the jaw. This action lifts the hyoid bone, pulling the base of the tongue off the posterior pharyngeal wall.

Insert the Esophageal Tube

Following the curvature of the tube, insert the device blindly into the posterior pharynx and (presumably) into the esophagus. Be gentle and stop advancing the tube if you meet resistance. Continue to advance it until you are able to seal the mask to the patient's face.

Inflate the Cuff

The device is inserted completely when the mask contacts the patient's face. Inflate the balloon with 35 mL of air. *Do not* inflate with additional air because this would significantly increase the risk of esophageal rupture and necrosis. Be sure to remove the syringe. If it remains attached, it will cause the balloon to deflate.

Procedures After Insertion

Following inflation of the balloon, obtain a mask seal, perform a head tilt-chin lift maneuver, and begin to ventilate the patient. Confirm the presence of breath sounds. Use other clinical indicators to continuously monitor the location of the tube. There are no specific requirements to secure the esophageal airway in place, but be careful with it. Inadvertent removal can be quite traumatic to the esophagus and can result in extensive vomiting.

Esophageal airways, although not frequently used anymore, can be very useful in prehospital emergency medicine. The EGTA is an excellent way to stop vomiting that may be making intubation impossible. Insert the EGTA and suction out any vomit in the mouth. Ventilate the patient through the EGTA for preintubation oxygenation. Remove the mask (but keep the tube in place) and intubate around the tube inserted in the esophagus.

Multi-lumen Airways

Esophageal airways are a misnomer because they do not provide a patent airway. Although the theoretical advantage of the esophageal obturator is clear, in practice it does not ensure a patent airway, and you cannot control ventilations well with an EGTA. Through the 1970s and 1980s, many people sought to develop an airway device that could be inserted blindly (obviating the need for laryngoscopy) and that would result in better airway management and ventilation. Two devices that have been developed are the __Pharyngotracheal Lumen Airway (PtL)__ and the __Combitube__ (▼ Figure 12-5).

Both the PtL and the Combitube have a number of improvements over their predecessors. These devices have a long tube that is blindly inserted into the airway. In contrast to esophageal airways, the tube can be used for esophageal obturation (if it is inserted into the esophagus, as is usually the case) or as an endotracheal tube (if it is inserted into the trachea). The other major improvement is the presence of an oropharyngeal balloon, which eliminates the need for a mask seal.

__Multi-lumen airways__ have a long tube that can be used for esophageal obturation or as an endotracheal tube, depending on where it goes following blind insertion into the airway. The device has two

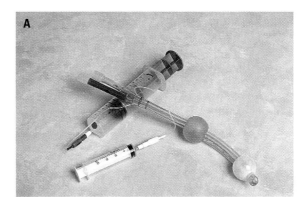

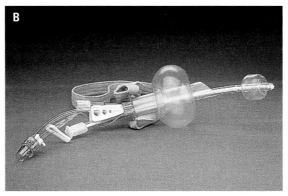

Figure 12-5 The Combitube (A) and Pharyngotracheal Lumen Airway (PtL) (B).

lumens, each with a 15/22-mm ventilation adapter. The proper port for ventilation depends on where the tube is located. Both multi-lumen airways have a proximal cuff, which is inflated in the oropharynx to eliminate the need for a face mask.

Advantages and Disadvantages of Multi-lumen Airways

Multi-lumen airways have many of the advantages of esophageal airways and have been engineered to decrease some of the disadvantages. The major advantage is that insertion is technically easier than endotracheal intubation and requires less experience and technical skill to perform. In effect, the airway cannot be improperly placed, because effective ventilation is possible if the tube goes into either the trachea or the esophagus. Because the procedure is performed with the patient in the neutral position, cervical spine movement is kept to a minimum. No mask seal is required to ventilate with either device.

Multi-lumen airways also provide some patency to the airway. If the tube is placed in the trachea, it functions exactly like an endotracheal tube, and no upper airway positioning is required. If the tube is placed into the esophagus (as most commonly occurs), the pharyngeal balloon creates an airtight seal in the oropharynx, making tongue position less of a factor in the maintenance of a patent airway. A jaw-thrust maneuver should easily alleviate any ventilatory difficulty that occurs if the epiglottis partially obstructs the airway.

Like esophageal airways, multi-lumen airways can be used only on deeply unconscious patients with no gag reflex. If the patient regains consciousness, the device must be removed. You must pay strict attention to the assessment of ventilation because ventilation in the wrong port results in no pulmonary ventilation. Multi-lumen airways are usually considered temporary airways. Although in some cases they have been used for prolonged ventilation, these devices are generally replaced as soon as possible. Intubating the trachea via direct laryngoscopy with a multi-lumen airway in place can be challenging.

Indications for Multi-lumen Airways

Multi-lumen airways are indicated for the airway management of deeply unconscious, apneic patients with no gag reflex, in whom endotracheal intubation is not possible, or has failed.

Contraindications for Multi-lumen Airways

Neither of the multi-lumen airways can be used in pediatric patients, and they should be used only for patients between 5 and 7 feet tall. (A smaller version of the Combitube, called the Combitube SA [small adult], can be used on adults more than 4 feet tall.) Because most of the time the tube is inserted into the esophagus, neither the PtL nor the Combitube should be used in patients who have a known pathologic condition of the esophagus or who have ingested caustic substances.

Complications of Multi-lumen Airways

Multi-lumen airways address many of the design limitations of esophageal airways. Experience with the devices is still somewhat limited, however. It is reasonable to assume that laryngospasm, vomiting, and possible hypoventilation may occur. Trauma may also result from improper insertion technique.

A few cases of difficult ventilation have occurred with multi-lumen airways. Ventilation may be difficult if the pharyngeal balloon pushes the epiglottis over the glottic opening. In all cases, the ventilation became easier when the device was withdrawn 2 to 4 cm.

Equipment for Multi-lumen Airways

The PtL consists of two tubes and two cuffs. The longer tube passes through the shorter, wider tube (▶ **Skill Drill 12-1**). The longer tube is 31 cm long and 8 mm in diameter and usually is inserted into the esophagus. This tube is open at its distal tip and has a balloon at its distal end. A semirigid stylet maintains the curvature and rigidity of the long tube and occludes the tip. The shorter tube is 21 cm long and is designed to come to rest with its tip deep in the oropharynx. A large low-pressure cuff is inflated proximal to the tip of the shorter tube. Both cuffs are inflated simultaneously with an in-series valve system that can be inflated with a bag-valve device. The short tube is made of hard plastic to resist damage from biting, and a strap goes around the head to secure the device (▼ **Figure 12-6**).

The Combitube consists of a single tube with two lumens, two balloons, and two ventilation attachments (▶ **Skill Drill 12-2**). One of the lumens is open at

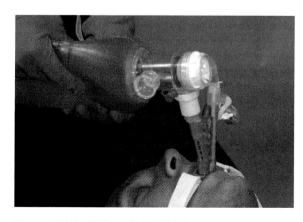

Figure 12-6 Ventilation with a PtL in place.

Skill Drill

12-1 Insertion of the PtL

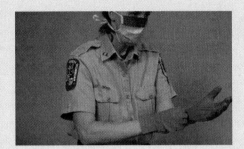

1 Take body substance isolation precautions (gloves and face shield).

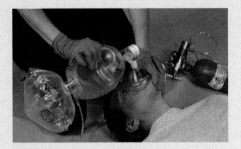

2 Preoxygenate the patient whenever possible with a bag-valve-mask device and 100% oxygen.

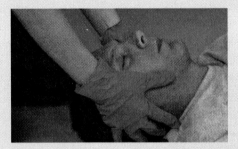

3 Place the patient's head in the neutral position.

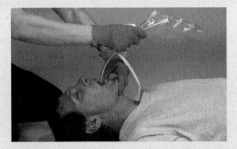

4 Open the patient's mouth with a tongue jaw-lift and insert the PtL in the midline of the patient's mouth.

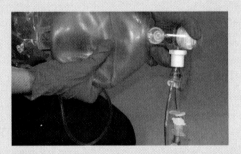

5 Inflate the proximal and distal cuffs.

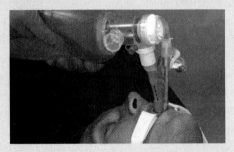

6 Ventilate the patient through the pharyngeal (green) tube first. If the chest rises, continue to ventilate through the green tube.

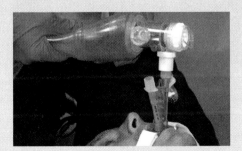

7 If the chest does not rise, remove the stylet from the clear tube and ventilate through the clear tube.

Skill Drill

12-2 Insertion of the Combitube

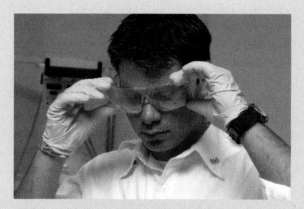

1 Take body substance isolation precautions (gloves and face shield).

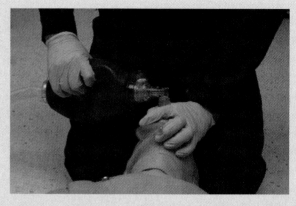

2 Preoxygenate the patient whenever possible with a bag-valve-mask device and 100% oxygen.

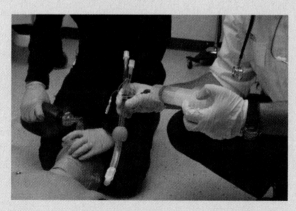

3 Gather your equipment.

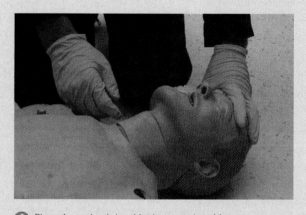

4 Place the patient's head in the neutral position.

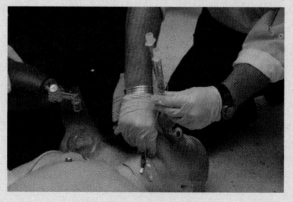

5 Open the patient's mouth with a tongue jaw-lift and insert the Combitube in the midline of the patient's mouth. Insert the tube until the incisors or alveolar ridge lie between the two reference marks.

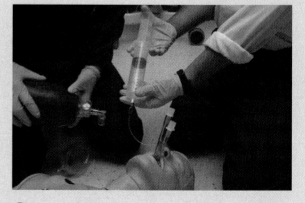

6 Inflate the pharyngeal cuff with 100 mL of air.

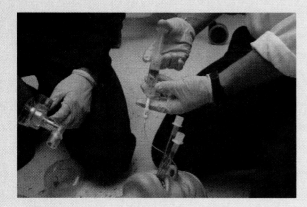

7 Inflate the distal cuff with 10 to 15 mL of air.

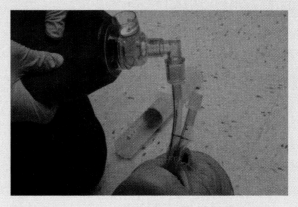

8 Ventilate the patient through the longest tube (pharyngeal) first. Chest rise indicates esophageal placement of distal tip (continue to ventilate).

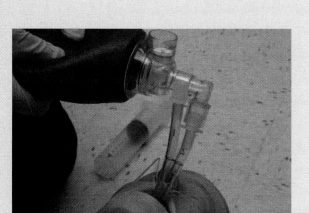

9 No chest rise indicates tracheal placement (switch ports and ventilate).

its distal end, and the other is closed. The closed lumen has side holes distal to the pharyngeal balloon. The proximal balloon is designed to be inflated with 100 to 140 mL of air and provide a pharyngeal seal. The distal balloon is inflated with 15 mL of air and either makes an airtight seal with the walls of the trachea (in the event of tracheal placement) or leads to esophageal obturation (in the event of esophageal placement) (▼ Figure 12-7).

Technique for Multi-lumen Airway Insertion

The advantage of multi-lumen airways is that you can use them to ventilate regardless of whether the tube goes into the esophagus or the trachea. While this is an advantage, it makes confirmation of ventilation *very* important. If you used the wrong port, the patient would receive *no pulmonary ventilation.* Confirmation of ventilation is a critical part of the procedure for using multi-lumen airways.

Procedures Before Insertion

Check and prepare all equipment. Check both cuffs and ensure that they hold air. The patient should be preoxygenated before insertion. Ventilation should not be interrupted for longer than 30 seconds to accomplish airway placement. This is rarely a problem because the procedure is blind and relatively fast. For both PtL and Combitube insertion, the patient's head should be placed in the neutral position.

Forwardly Displace the Jaw

With the patient's head in the neutral position, insert the thumb of your gloved nondominant hand into the patient's mouth and lift the jaw. This action lifts the hyoid bone and pulls the base of the tongue off the posterior pharyngeal wall.

Insert the Device

Following the curvature of the tube, insert the device blindly into the posterior pharynx. The Combitube

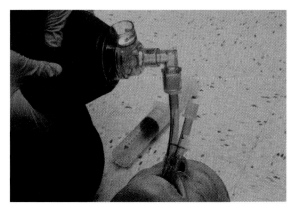

Figure 12-7 Ventilation with a Combitube in place.

is inserted until the incisors are between the two black lines printed on the tube. The PtL is inserted until the flange comes to rest on the teeth. Be gentle, and stop advancing the tube if you meet resistance.

Inflate the Cuffs

Both multi-lumen devices have two cuffs. In the PtL, the cuffs inflate together through an inline valve system. Attach a bag-valve device to the inflation adapter and inflate the cuffs until the pilot balloon is firm. Close the clamp to prevent air leakage. The Combitube has two independent inflation valves that must be inflated sequentially. The first inflation valve goes to the pharyngeal balloon and is inflated with 100 mL of air (this is printed on the pilot balloon). The second inflation valve inflates the distal balloon and is filled with 15 mL of air.

Procedures After Insertion

Following inflation of the balloons, begin to ventilate the patient. With the PtL, first ventilate the short tube (the one without the stylet); with the Combitube, ventilate the longer (blue) tube. Confirm the patient's chest rise and the presence of breath sounds. If there are no breath sounds and the chest does not rise and fall with ventilation, switch immediately to the other inflation port. Be sure to continuously monitor ventilations. Both multi-lumen airways are generally secure in the airway due to the large pharyngeal balloons. Nonetheless, the head strap of the PtL should be attached because inadvertent removal of a multi-lumen airway would be extremely traumatic.

▶ **Table 12-1** summarizes the indications, contraindications, advantages, disadvantages, complications, and special considerations of PtL airway insertion.

▶ **Table 12-2** summarizes the indications, contraindications, advantages, disadvantages, complications, and special considerations of Combitube insertion.

The Laryngeal Mask Airway

The laryngeal mask airway (LMA) is a relatively new airway management device that has become popular with anesthesiologists (▶ Figure 12-8). The LMA was invented by Dr. A. I. J. Brain at the London Hospital in 1981 and became commercially available in 1988. The device was originally developed as an alternative to facemask ventilation (as is commonly used during short surgical procedures) and endotracheal intubation (used for longer periods of anesthesia) in the operating room. Prior to the development of the LMA, no device provided a viable option for those cases of intermediate length that required more airway support than mask ventilation but did not require intubation.

Table 12-1
PtL Airway Insertion

Indications

- Alternative airway control when conventional intubation procedures have been unsuccessful or equipment is unavailable

Contraindications

- Children are too small for the tube
- Esophageal trauma or disease
- Caustic ingestion

Advantages

- Can ventilate with tracheal or esophageal placement
- No facemask needed to seal
- No special equipment is required
- Does not require the patient's head to be placed in the sniffing position

Disadvantages

- Cannot be used on patients who are awake
- Can only be used on adults
- Pharyngeal balloon mitigates but does not eliminate aspiration risk
- Can only be passed orally
- Extremely difficult to perform endotracheal intubation with the device in place

Complications

- Pharyngeal or esophageal trauma can occur due to poor technique
- Unrecognized displacement of tracheal tube into the esophagus
- Displacement of the pharyngeal balloon

Special Considerations

- Good assessment skills are essential to properly confirm placement
- Misidentification of placement has occurred
- Multiple confirmations of placement technique should be done

Table 12-2
Combitube Insertion

Indications

- Alternative airway control when conventional intubation procedures have been unsuccessful or equipment is unavailable

Contraindications

- Children are too small for the tube
- Esophageal trauma or disease
- Caustic ingestion

Advantages

- Rapid insertion
- No facemask needed to seal
- No special equipment is required
- Does not require the patient's head to be placed in the sniffing position

Disadvantages

- Impossible to suction the trachea when the tube is in the esophagus
- Cannot be used on patients who are awake
- Can only be used on adults
- Extremely difficult to perform endotracheal intubation with the device in place

Complications

- Pharyngeal or esophageal trauma can result from poor technique
- Unrecognized displacement of tracheal tube into the esophagus
- Displacement of the pharyngeal balloon

Special Considerations

- Good assessment skills are essential to properly confirm placement
- Misidentification of placement has occurred
- Multiple confirmations of placement technique should be done

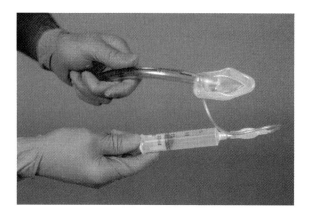

Figure 12-8 The laryngeal mask airway.

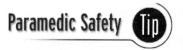

Paramedic Safety

The time to test the integrity of your cuff is before insertion, not after! Do not skip this critical step.

inflatable cuff conforms to the contours of the airway and makes a relatively airtight seal (▶ Figure 12-9).

Advantages and Disadvantages of the Laryngeal Mask Airway

The LMA has many advantages compared to ventilating the unprotected airway with a mask. The LMA has been shown to provide better oxygenation than mask ventilation with an oral airway, and ventilation with an LMA does not require the continual maintenance of a mask seal. Compared to an endotracheal tube, LMA insertion is easier and does not require laryngoscopy. There is significantly less risk of soft tissue, vocal cord, tracheal wall trauma, and dental trauma than with either endotracheal intubation or other forms of intubation that rely on esophageal obturation. The LMA provides protection from upper airway secretions and the tip of the LMA wedged into the proximal esophagus probably provides some obturation.

The main disadvantage of the LMA, especially in emergencies, is that it does not provide protection against aspiration. In fact, the LMA actually increases the risk of aspiration if the patient regurgitates because the patient's stomach contents would most likely be directed into the trachea. Experience in the operating room may not accurately predict the risk of aspiration for emergency patients because patients undergoing surgery have fasted prior to receiving anesthesia.

The LMA was not designed for emergency use. Although it is not a replacement for endotracheal intubation, the LMA may have a role in emergencies if intubation is not possible and the only option is mask ventilation. Because of the newness of the LMA, very few studies have been conducted on the use of the device in emergency situations. Emergency care practitioners are encouraged to be cautious about the use of the LMA until more studies have been conducted. Nonetheless, the positive experience of the LMA in the operating room suggests the LMA has some potential in emergency medicine. In emergency medicine the LMA should be considered better than mask ventilation, but inferior to endotracheal intubation.

The LMA is designed to provide a conduit from the glottic opening to the ventilation device. This is achieved by surrounding the opening of the larynx with an inflatable silicone cuff positioned in the hypopharynx. When properly inserted, the opening of the LMA is positioned right at the glottic opening. The tip of the device is inserted into the proximal esophagus, the lateral portions in the piriform fossa, and the upper border at the base of the tongue. The

Paramedic Safety

Like many other medical devices, equipment such as EOAs and multi-lumen airways have defined shelf-lives. Make sure to check expiration dates on a regular basis, especially if such devices are designed as back-up airways or otherwise are rarely used.

Documentation

If adverse events occur with the use of these airways, such as bleeding or trauma, be sure to document these occurrences on the patient's chart.

Did You Know ?

If you are having difficulty inserting a multi-lumen airway, you may be hanging up on the base of the tongue. Use a laryngoscope to lift the tongue out of the way.

During prolonged LMA ventilation, some air may be insufflated into the stomach because the seal made in the airway is not airtight. Because of the risk of aspiration, it is unlikely that the LMA will ever replace endotracheal intubation in prehospital emergency care. The LMA should not be considered a primary airway for emergency patients, but it may have a role. For a patient who cannot be intubated, the LMA should be considered superior to mask ventilation.

Indications for the Laryngeal Mask Airway

The LMA should be considered as one possible alternative to mask ventilation only in cases when the patient cannot be intubated.

Contraindications for the Laryngeal Mask Airway

The product literature for the LMA states that it should be used only in "fasting" patients. Unfortunately, this would eliminate all emergency patients. It could conceivably be considered a potential alternative to mask ventilation in the prehospital emergency setting but not as a replacement for intubation. You

Case Study

Case Study, Part 2

Fortunately, a multi-lumen airway is at the bottom of the airway kit, reserved for difficult intubations. It's been awhile since you last used one. And if the patient vomits again, you will have to stop ventilations and suction again. The multi-lumen device will at least help you control her airway better.

After examining the unit quickly, you begin to adjust the patient's head position for the insertion procedure. As you lift the head into an extended, "sniffing" position, your partner whispers urgently, "I don't think that's the right way to position her head!"

Question 3: Is your partner correct? If he is, what would be the correct position?

CASE STUDY

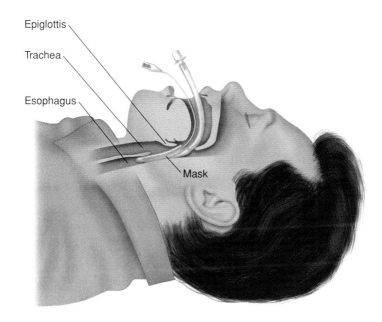

Epiglottis

Trachea

Esophagus

Mask

Figure 12-9 When properly positioned, the opening of the LMA is at the glottic opening, the tip is at the entrance of the esophagus, the lateral portions in the pyriform fossae, and the upper border at the base of the tongue.

must weigh the risk of aspiration against the risk of hypoventilation with mask ventilation in the context of a given clinical scenario.

The LMA is less effective in obese patients and should not be used in patients with morbid obesity. Patients who are pregnant or have hiatus hernias are at an increased risk for regurgitation and must be evaluated carefully if LMA use is considered. The LMA is ineffective for the ventilation of patients requiring high pulmonary pressures.

Complications of the Laryngeal Mask Airway

The biggest complications involve regurgitation and subsequent aspiration. The incidence of misplacement in the operating room is relatively low (1% to 5%) and appears to decrease with experience. Nonetheless, the paramedic should observe the patient for clinical indications of adequate ventilation (chest rise, breath sounds) during LMA ventilation. Hypoventilation of patients who require high ventilatory pressures can also occur. A few cases of upper airway swelling have been reported.

Equipment for the Laryngeal Mask Airway

The LMA comes in five sizes and is sized based on the patient's weight. The device consists of an inflatable cuff attached to an obliquely cut tube. The cuff provides a collar that is designed to position the opening of the tube at the glottic opening when inflated. Two vertical bars are present at the opening of the tube to prevent occlusion. The proximal end of the tube is fitted with a standard 15/22-mm adapter. The cuff has a one-way valve assembly and should be inflated with a predetermined volume of air (based on the size of the airway) (▶ Figure 12-10).

Technique for Laryngeal Mask Airway

Procedures Before Insertion

Check and prepare all equipment. Check the cuff of the LMA by inflating it with 50% more air than is required for that size airway. The cuff should then be completely deflated so that no folds appear near the tip. Deflation is best accomplished by pressing the device, cuff down, on a flat surface (▶ Figure 12-11). Lubricate the base of the device. The patient should be preoxygenated before it is inserted. Ventilation should not be interrupted for more than 30 seconds to accomplish airway placement. Place the patient in the sniffing position.

Insert Your Finger Between the Cuff and the Tube

Proper insertion of the LMA depends on holding the device properly. Place the index finger of your dom-

inant hand in the notch between the tube and the cuff. Open the patient's mouth.

Insert the Laryngeal Mask Airway Along the Roof of the Mouth

The key to proper insertion is to slide the convex surface of the airway along the roof of the mouth. Use your finger to push the airway against the hard palate. Once it slides past the tongue, the LMA will move easily into position.

Inflate the Cuff

Inflate the cuff of the LMA with the amount of air indicated for that size airway. If the LMA is properly positioned, it will move out of the airway slightly (1 to 2 cm) as it seats into position. This is a good indication that the LMA is in the correct position.

Procedures After Insertion

Following inflation of the cuff, begin to ventilate the patient. Confirm chest rise and the presence of breath sounds. Continuously and carefully monitor for aspiration in the tube. The LMA can be easily dislodged as

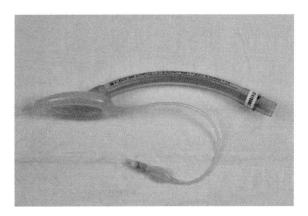

Figure 12-10 The LMA.

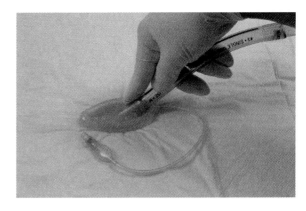

Figure 12-11 Press the LMA against a flat surface to remove all wrinkles from the cuff.

Paramedic Safety Tip

As an emerging device for prehospital use, the LMA may prove to be an effective alternative airway in cases where endotracheal intubation is not absolutely needed, but basic airway techniques may not be enough.

it was not designed for patients who are being transported. Carefully attend to the airway during any patient movement, and be prepared to mask ventilate if the LMA becomes dislodged.

One of the design features of the LMA is the fact that you can intubate *through* it. A 6.0 mm endotracheal tube can be passed through a size three or four LMA. The vertical bars are designed to allow a well-lubricated tube to pass straight through, and research in the operating room found a 90% success rate of endotracheal intubation following this technique. The Fasttrach LMA is actually designed to guide an endotracheal tube into the trachea, and may prove to be an alternative to direct laryngoscopy (▶ Figure 12-12).

▼ **Table 12-3** compares endotracheal intubation (ETI) to several nonsurgical alternative airway procedures.

Case Study

Case Study, Part 3

With your partner's assistance you reposition the head into a better, neutral position and grasp the jaw with one hand. With the other hand you insert the airway with surprising ease. After inflating the balloon, you check for tube placement by ventilating the correct tube. Seeing chest rise, you confirm tube placement by auscultating equal bilateral lung sounds.

Unfortunately, your efforts to resuscitate the patient fail to bring about spontaneous circulation; 45 minutes later you cease resuscitative efforts and turn your attention to comforting the family.

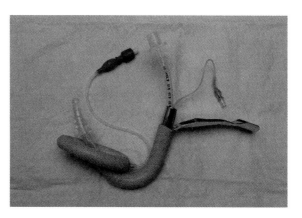

Figure 12-12 The Fasttrach LMA with a 6.0 endotracheal tube.

Table 12-3
Comparison of Endotracheal Intubation (ETI) to Nonsurgical Alternative Airway Procedures*

	Ease of Placement	Overcoming Obstruction	Prevention of Aspiration	Oxygenation	Ventilation	Complications	
Endotracheal intubation	Difficult	Excellent	Excellent	Excellent	Excellent	High	
Esophageal airways (EOA/EGTA)	Moderate	Poor	Good	Good	Good	High	Can only be done in deeply unconscious patients
PtL	Moderate	Poor	Good	Good	Very good	Low	
Combitube	Easy	Poor	Good	Good	Very good	Low	
LMA	Moderate	Poor	Poor	Very good	Excellent	Moderate	

*EOA indicates esophageal obturator airway; EGTA, esophageal gastric tube airway; PtL, pharyngeotracheal lumen airway; and LMA, laryngeal mask airway.

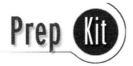

Chapter Summary

With practice and experience, you should be able to intubate 90% to 95% of emergency patients that you encounter. This means that 5% to 10% of your patients will be difficult or impossible to intubate in the emergency setting. It is important to remember that the goal of airway management is oxygenation and ventilation, not intubation. There are alternatives to intubation that can allow you to provide excellent oxygenation and ventilation, and you should be as skilled and comfortable with those alternatives as you are with techniques of endotracheal intubation.

Under certain conditions, devices that can block the esophagus can greatly improve the ability to manually open an airway and ventilate the patient. There are many limitations to these devices; as always, you must be familiar with indications and contraindications for their use and practice the techniques often.

Multi-lumen airways represent an improvement over esophageal airways in the ability to allow for ventilation to be performed. Like esophageal obturators, however, the insertion of the multi-lumen airway is a blind technique, requiring careful assessment to ensure adequate ventilation.

Vital Vocabulary

Combitube A dual-lumen airway device that is inserted blindly. You can ventilate the patient whether the tube is placed in the esophagus or the trachea.

esophageal gastric tube airway (EGTA) An esophageal airway device that is designed to occlude the esophagus, thus preventing regurgitation.

esophageal obturator airway (EOA) The original esophageal airway that is no longer manufactured or used because it does not allow for decompression of the stomach prior to removal.

laryngeal mask airway (LMA) An airway device that is inserted into the mouth blindly and comes to rest at the glottic opening. A flexible cuff is inflated, creating an almost airtight seal.

multi-lumen airways An airway device that has a single long tube that can be used for esophageal obturation or endotracheal tube ventilation, depending on where it comes to rest following blind positioning.

obturator A device that closes or blocks an opening.

pharyngotracheal lumen airway (PtL) A dual-lumen airway device that is inserted blindly into the mouth. The patient can be ventilated whether the tube is placed in the esophagus or into the trachea.

Case Study Answers

Question 1: What are your concerns about managing this airway with only basic airway adjuncts?

Answer: If the patient continues to vomit, the chances of aspiration will continue to increase. Additionally, even with careful monitoring the possibility of gastric distention exists with basic manual ventilation.

Question 2: What are some noninvasive airway adjuncts that might be useful in a situation like this?

Answer: There are several nonsurgical airway devices that might provide effective alternatives to endotracheal intubation. These include esophageal airways, such as the esophageal gastric tube airway, the multi-lumen airway, and the laryngeal mask airway.

Question 3: Is your partner correct? If he is, what would be the correct position?

Answer: Your partner is correct in this case. The patient's head position should be in a neutral position, with the jaw flexed forward for proper insertion position.

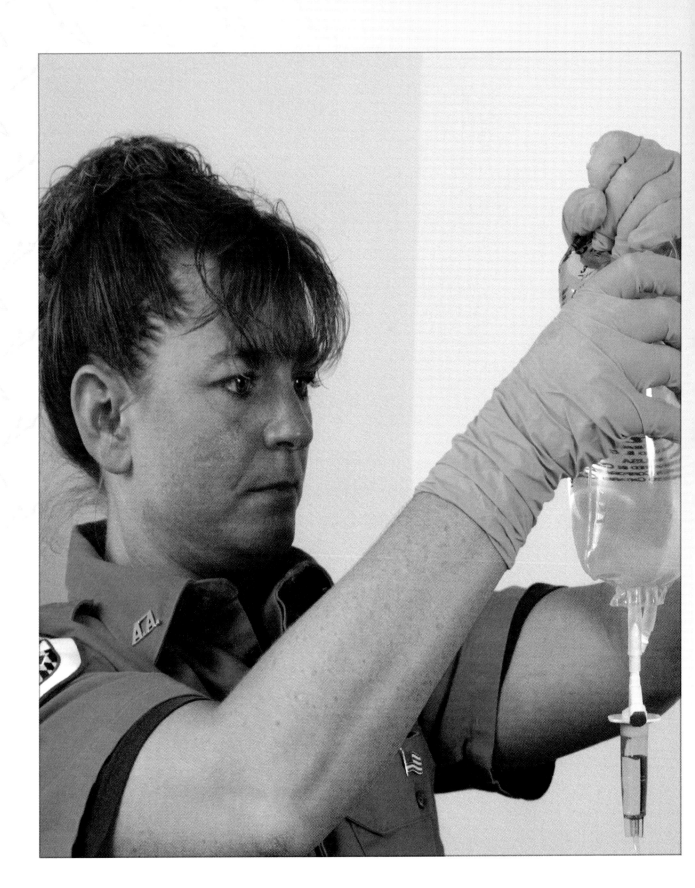

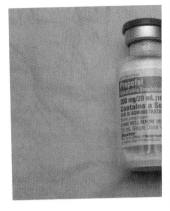

Figure 13-8 Propofol.

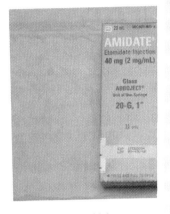

Figure 13-9 Etomidate.

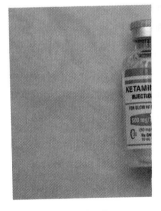

Figure 13-10 Ketamine.

Propofol

Propofol (Diprivan) is a
that has been developed a
diazepines and barbiturat
has a rapid onset, short
effect, powerful antegrad
little effect on the patien

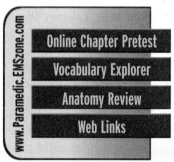

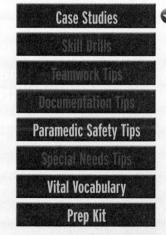

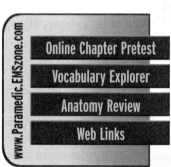

Objectives

Cognitive Objectives

2-1.65 Describe the indications, contraindications, advantages, disadvantages, complications, and equipment for rapid sequence intubation with neuromuscular blockade. (p 275)

2-1.66 Identify neuromuscular blocking drugs and other agents used in rapid sequence intubation. (p 275)

2-1.67 Describe the indications, contraindications, advantages, disadvantages, complications, and equipment for sedation during intubation. (p 268)

2-1.68 Identify sedative agents used in airway management. (p 268)

www.Paramedic.EMSzone.com

TECHNOLOGY

Online Chapter Pretest

Vocabulary Explorer

Anatomy Review

Web Links

FEATURES

Case Studies

Skill Drills

Teamwork Tips

Documentation Tips

Paramedic Safety Tips

Special Needs Tips

Vital Vocabulary

Prep Kit

Chapter

Ben

Ber
(Val
rela
as ε
pin
prc
wh
prc
as (
tioi
nec
be
prε
the
pli
ne
the
pr
be

ar
Fl
ni
m
ev

B

B
h
T
rε
(l
tl
c
r
c
r
r
ε

(
(
t
ε
i
(

lations are brief, uncoordinated twitch of small muscle groups in the face, neck, trunk, and extremities. These fasciculations are not harmful, but they tend to cause generalized muscle pain at the termination of paralysis.

The main advantage of depolarizing agents is the very rapid onset (60 to 90 seconds) of total paralysis and their relatively short duration of action (5 to 10 minutes). Succinylcholine is often used as an initial paralytic because its onset is fast and it wears off quickly. If you are unable to secure the patient's airway, you have to support the patient's ventilations only for a short period of time before the patient can breathe again on his or her own.

Succinylcholine should be used with caution in patients with hyperkalemia (patients with burns, crush injuries, and blunt trauma). Because its structure is similar to acetylcholine, succinylcholine can cause bradycardia, especially in children. Premedication with atropine prevents succinylcholine-induced bradycardia and should precede its administration in pediatric patients if at all possible.

Nondepolarizing Neuromuscular Agents

Nondepolarizing neuromuscular blocking agents also bind to the acetylcholine receptor sites, but unlike depolarizing neuromuscular blocking agents, they do not cause depolarization of the muscle fiber. When given in sufficient quantity, the amount of nondepolarizing medication exceeds the amount of acetylcholine in the synaptic cleft, and the critical threshold of depolarization cannot be achieved.

Curare is a nondepolarizing neuromuscular blocker that has been used for centuries as a poison on the tips of arrows and spears in Africa and South America. It was used medicinally from the 1940s to the 1960s, but much more effective agents have been developed. The most commonly used nondepolarizing neuromuscular blockers are vecuronium (Norcuron),

pancuronium (Pavulon), atricurium (Tracrium), and tubocurarine (Tubarine). Although there are minor differences among them, their general characteristics are similar (▼ Figures 13-12 and 13-13).

In general, nondepolarizing agents have a rapid onset of action (3 to 5 minutes) and a longer duration (30 to 90 minutes) than depolarizing agents. This fact makes nondepolarizing agents ideal when you want the patient to be paralyzed for a long period of time, such as after the airway has been secured and you need to manage the patient. If you administer only a depolarizing agent, you would have to give the medication either by infusion or re-bolus every 5 minutes, which significantly increases the risk of complications.

Nondepolarizing agents should not be given before the patient's airway is secured. If you are unable to intubate the patient, managing the airway of a paralyzed patient for a long time significantly increases the probability of vomiting and aspiration.

When nondepolarizing agents are administered in small quantities before a depolarizing agent, they prevent fasciculations. The mechanism for this is unknown, but reducing fasciculations significantly

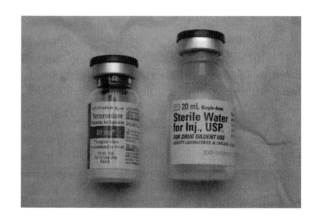

Figure 13-12 Vecuronium.

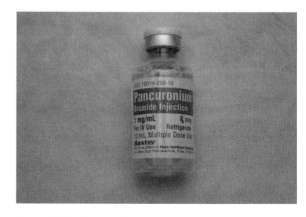

Figure 13-13 Pancuronium.

decreases the postparalysis muscle aches and should be done whenever time permits. The defasciculating dose is typically 10% of the normal dose and does not result in paralysis, but causes weakness.

Rapid-Sequence Intubation

Rapid-sequence intubation involves a specified set of procedures combined in rapid succession to induce general anesthesia and intubate a patient quickly. The sequence was originally developed in 1946 as a method of intubating obstetric patients who needed to be anesthetized but had full stomachs and therefore posed a high risk for aspiration. The procedure underwent a significant improvement in 1961, when Sellick first described the use of posterior cricoid pressure to reduce the risk of regurgitation further.

Although rapid-sequence intubation has been successfully performed for years in surgery, its use in the prehospital setting is relatively new. In fact, its use in hospital emergency departments has only become common in the last decade. *All* patients presenting to hospital emergency departments or encountered in prehospital situations are presumed to have, and usually do have, a full stomach. Intubation of these patients, therefore, must include decreasing the risk of aspiration. An adaptation of the steps for rapid-sequence intubation has great potential in emergency settings.

Rapid-sequence intubation represents a culmination and integration of all of your airway, problem-solving, and decision-making skills into one procedure. It includes the safe, smooth, and rapid induction of deep sedation and paralysis followed immediately by intubation. Many patients are candidates for rapid-sequence intubation, but it is generally used for conscious or combative patients who need to be intubated and who are unable or unwilling to cooperate.

The general steps for rapid-sequence intubation are the same for all patients, as discussed below. Different protocols are used, however, for hemodynamically stable patients and unstable patients.

Technique for Rapid-Sequence Intubation

Prepare the Patient and Equipment

The experience of being intubated is very scary for patients. Be sure to explain what you are going to do and that the patient will be asleep during the procedure. Reassure the patient that he or she will not feel or remember anything. Place the patient on a cardiac monitor and pulse oximeter.

Unlike most intubation procedures, rapid-sequence intubation gives you control. You often

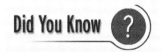

Before initiating rapid-sequence intubation, ask yourself whether you are going to be able to ventilate and intubate the patient. Rapid-sequence intubation should be attempted only if you have confidence that you will be able to intubate and ventilate the patient, or ventilate the patient without intubating, if necessary. Otherwise a patient who has been sedated and paralyzed will die. Above all else, *do no harm*.

have time to assemble your equipment and make sure that everything is in proper working order. In particular, be sure to have suction immediately available.

Preoxygenate

Adequately preoxygenate the patient to ensure that positive pressure ventilation is not necessary until rapid-sequence intubation has been successfully completed. Obviously, however, if the patient is not ventilating adequately on his or her own, you will need to assist with ventilations during the procedure itself. If the patient is breathing adequately, you should increase the FiO_2 to 1.0 (▼ Figure 13-14).

Premedicate

If time permits, consider administering any or all of the following medications:

1. A defasciculating dose of a nondepolarizing neuromuscular blocking agent (typically 10% of a normal dose)
2. Lidocaine to decrease the cardiovascular effects and increased intracranial pressure

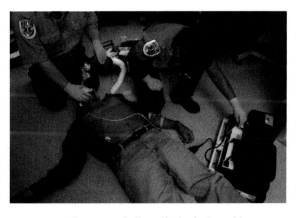

Figure 13-14 Preoxygenate the patient prior to rapid-sequence intubation.

associated with of upper airway stimulation (typically 1 mg/kg of body weight)

3. Atropine to decrease the incidence of bradycardia associated with the administration of succinylcholine (typically 0.5 mg)

Sedate

As long as the patient is hemodynamically capable of tolerating it (generally defined as having a systolic blood pressure over 90), administer a sedative agent to induce sedation and amnesia.

Paralyze

Immediately following administration of the sedative, administer succinylcholine. Paralysis will begin in 30 seconds and will be complete within 2 minutes.

Apply Posterior Cricoid Pressure

Immediately upon the loss of the eyelash reflex, have an assistant apply posterior cricoid pressure (▶ Figure 13-15). As long as the oxygen saturation is maintained, do not give positive pressure ventilation. Limiting positive pressure ventilation significantly decreases the risk of regurgitation.

Intubate

Intubate the trachea as carefully as possible (▶ Figure 13-16). Confirm tube placement and release cricoid pressure. Secure the tube as normal.

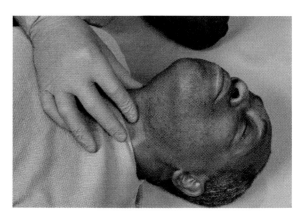

Figure 13-15 Cricoid pressure to limit the risk of regurgitation.

Maintain Paralysis and Sedation

When you are absolutely sure you have successfully intubated the patient, administer a nondepolarizing neuromuscular blocker for long-term paralysis. Continue to administer a sedative if the patient's blood pressure is adequate. Monitor the patient's heart rate and blood pressure to ensure that sedation is not wearing off or becoming inadequate.

While the general steps of rapid-sequence intubation are the same for all patients, some modification is necessary for unstable patients. If the patient's oxygen saturation drops at any point, however, you have

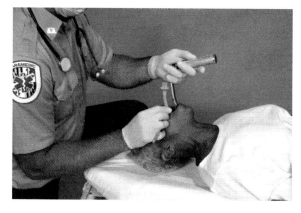

Figure 13-16 Intubate the trachea.

no choice but to ventilate. Do so carefully, with posterior cricoid pressure and slow (1.5- to 2-second) inspirations. If the patient is hemodynamically unstable, you have to judge whether sedation is appropriate or whether the risk of profound hypotension is too great to allow you to safely sedate the patient prior to inducing paralysis. ▶ **Box 13-2** lists sample protocols for rapid-sequence intubation in hemodynamically stable and unstable patients.

etomidate
agent.

intracrani
cranium tha
breathing ar

ketamine
qualities. It
(PCP). Ketan
because of
ated with it

nondepola
Also bind to
larizing neu
depolarizati

opioids/o
potent anal
emergency
induction, a

paralytics
blockade, tl
intubate cri
the procedu
intact gag r

propofol
oped as an

sedation
induce amn
benzodiaze

succinylc
blocking (pa
depolarizati
observed d

Box 13-2

Sample Protocols for Rapid-Sequence Intubation

For Hemodynamically Stable Patients

1. Prepare patient and equipment
2. Preoxygenate ($FiO_2 = 1.0$ for 3 to 5 minutes)
3. Consider defasciculating dose of nondepolarizing neuromuscular blocker, lidocaine, and/or atropine
4. Sedate
5. Administer succinylcholine
6. Cricoid pressure
7. Intubate, verify tube placement, release cricoid pressure
8. Administer nondepolarizing neuromuscular blocker and maintain adequate sedation

For Hemodynamically Unstable Patients

1. Prepare patient and equipment
2. Preoxygenate or ventilate as necessary
3. Consider sedation
4. Administer succinylcholine
5. Cricoid pressure
6. Intubate, verify tube placement, release cricoid pressure
7. Administer nondepolarizing neuromuscular blocker

important. To remove thick secretions, vomitus, or blood, a bulb syringe can be used for newborns and infants, and a soft suction catheter or a rigid-tip-catheter can be used for infants and children (▼ Figure 14-3 A-C) (▶ Skill Drill 14-1).

Head Tilt-Chin Lift Maneuver

When there is no suspicion of sustained trauma or cervical spine trauma, the head tilt-chin lift maneuver is appropriate for infants and children (▶ Skill Drill 14-2).

Jaw-Thrust Without Head-Tilt Maneuver

The jaw-thrust (without head tilt) maneuver is used when there is suspected trauma or cervical spine

injury or if the child is found to be unconscious and the mechanism of injury is not clear (▶ Skill Drill 14-4). The jaw-thrust maneuver is also beneficial when a child is having a seizure. The jaw thrust maneuver can be used simultaneously while providing BVM ventilation. Hold the mask to the patient's face, while still grasping the angles of the jaw (jaw thrust).

Modified Jaw-Thrust Maneuver

The modified jaw-thrust maneuver is also used for opening the airway when cervical spine trauma is suspected. This maneuver also provides some degree of spinal immobilization (▶ Skill Drill 14-3).

Airway Adjuncts

Airway adjuncts such as an oropharyngeal airway or a nasopharyngeal airway are often useful to help keep the airway open. Even with the proper use of airway maneuvers as described previously, the large tongue of a child can obstruct the airway. These adjuncts can be used alone or with BVM ventilation. The key to their use in children is proper size, proper insertion technique, and observing the indications and contraindications to their use.

Oropharyngeal Airway

The indications for use of an oropharyngeal airway (▶ Skill Drill 14-5) include respiratory insufficiency, airway obstruction, and seizures. Contraindications include the presence of a gag reflex and a history of possible ingestion of caustic or petroleum-based substances.

To determine the appropriate airway size, use a length-based resuscitation tape or confirm the correct size visually by placing the airway next to the patient's face, with the flange at the level of the front teeth (central incisors) and the bite block parallel to the hard palate. The tip of the oropharyngeal airway should be the angle of the jaw (▼ Figure 14-4).

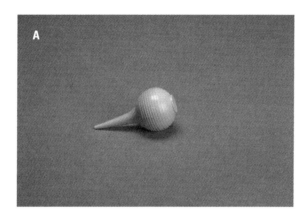
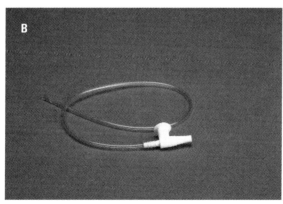
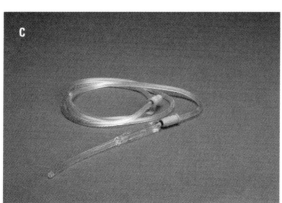

Figure 14-3 A. Bulb syringe. B. Suction catheter. C. Rigid tip catheter.

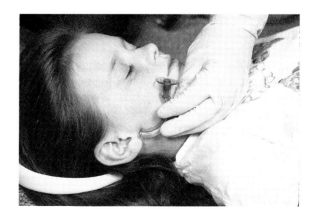

Figure 14-4 Place an OP airway next to the face, with the flange at the level of the central incisors and the bit block segment parallel to the hard palate.

Skill Drill

14-1 Suctioning with a Bulb Syringe

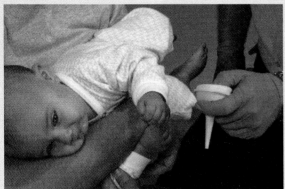

1 Squeeze the bulb away from the infant to remove air.

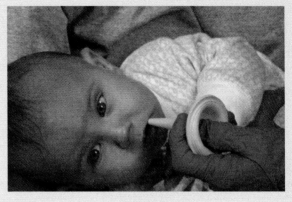

2 Open the infant's mouth and insert the tip of the syringe at the side of the mouth. Advance the syringe tip into the mouth to suction thin secretions. Do not insert the syringe tip into the soft tissues at the back of the mouth.

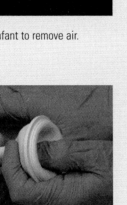

3 Open the infant's nostril slightly and suction the nose. Insert the tip of the syringe straight back into the nostril.

Several complications can occur with the use of oropharyngeal airways in children. If the oropharyngeal airway is too small, it can push the tongue back and actually cause obstruction of the airway. If it is too large, it can directly obstruct the airway. In addition, pharyngeal bleeding can result, especially if the oropharyngeal airway needs to be rotated into position (▶ Figure 14-5).

Nasopharyngeal Airway

The indications for use of a nasopharyngeal airway are the same as those for the use of an oral airway: respiratory insufficiency, airway obstruction, and seizures. The contraindications are different and include: nasal

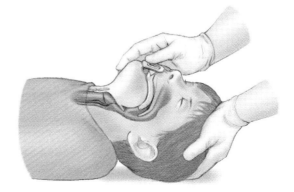

Figure 14-5 If the OP airway is too small, the tongue may be pushed into the pharynx, obstructing the airway.

Skill Drill

14-2 Head Tilt-Chin Lift Maneuver

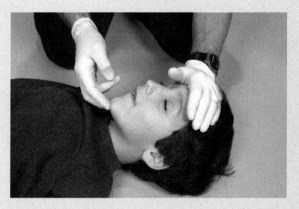

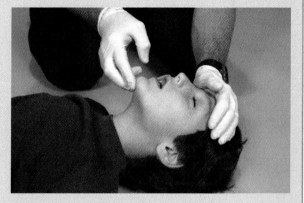

1 With the patient supine, place one hand on the forehead and several fingers on the chin.

2 Tilt the head back and lift the chin.

Skill Drill

14-3 Modified Jaw-Thrust Maneuver

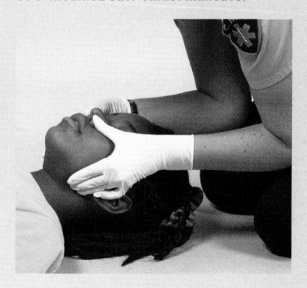

1 With the patient supine, position yourself above the child's head.

2 Place your fingers behind the angle of the lower jaw/ mandible and push the jaw upward.

Skill Drill

14-4 Jaw-Thrust Maneuver without Head-Tilt

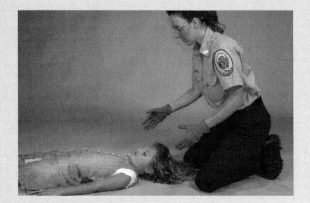

1 With the patient supine, position yourself above the child's head.

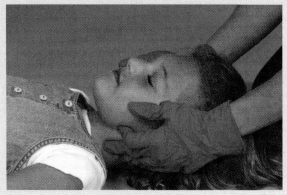

2 Position your third, fourth, and fifth fingers along the child's neck to maintain spinal immobilization.

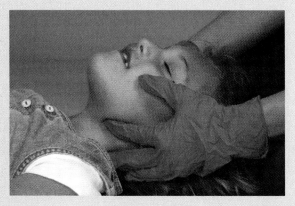

3 Position your second finger and thumb on the angle of the lower jaw/mandible, and push the child's jaw upward.

obstruction, possible basilar skull fracture, major nasofacial or maxillofacial trauma, and age younger than 1 year. In contrast to the oropharyngeal airway, the nasopharyngeal airway is sometimes tolerated in patients with an intact gag reflex (▶ Skill Drill 14-6).

To determine the appropriate airway size, use a length-based resuscitation tape, or compare the nasopharyngeal airway to the patient's face. The outside diameter of the nasopharyngeal airway should be less than the diameter of the child's nasal passage. Place the airway next to the face and measure from the tip of the nose to the tragus of the ear. If there is an adjustable flange, move it up or down the tube to obtain the correct length (▶ Figure 14-6).

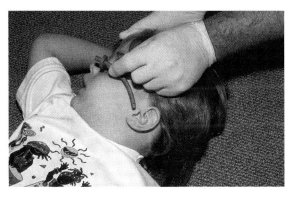

Figure 14-6 Place the NP airway next to the face and measure from the tip of the nose to the tragus of the ear.

Skill Drill

14-5 Inserting an Oropharyngeal Airway

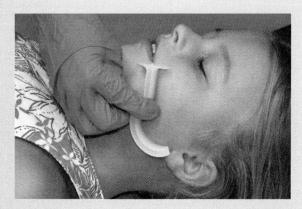

① Measure the oropharyngeal airway.

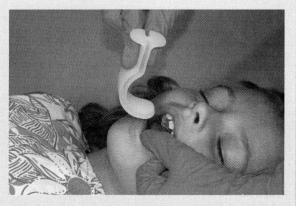

② Point the tip of the airway toward the roof of the patient's mouth (the hard palate), and depress the tongue with the curved portion of the airway.

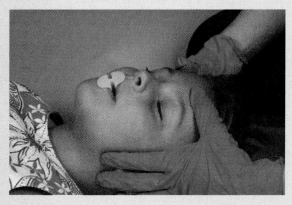

③ Place the oropharyngeal airway into the patient's mouth until the flange rests against the lips. When the flange is at the lips, gently rotate the airway 180°.

Complications of nasopharyngeal airway insertion include pharyngeal bleeding, adenoid tissue laceration, obstruction of the tube with secretions or blood, laryngospasm, and vomiting. If the nasopharyngeal airway is too long, vagal stimulation or esophageal entry can occur.

Artificial Ventilation of Pediatric Patients

The ventilation of pediatric patients has special implications. Although it is not more difficult, most paramedics have more experience treating adults and therefore are often anxious when treating children.

The use of a BVM device to assist with ventilations is indicated for infants and children in the following situations:

- Apnea

- Respiratory failure

- Respirations that are too fast or too slow to provide adequate oxygenation

- Unresponsive children

- When the addition of oxygen alone fails to improve the child's color

- Oxygen saturation via pulse oximetry remains less than 90% despite 100% oxygen administration

Skill Drill

14-6 Inserting a Nasopharyngeal Airway

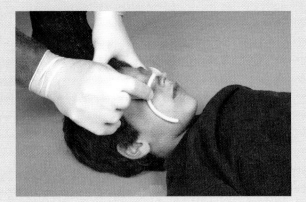

1 Measure the airway.

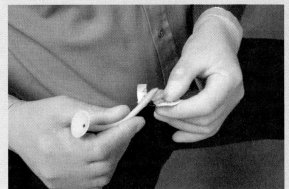

2 Lubricate the airway tip.

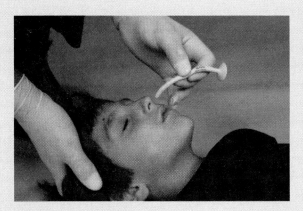

3 Advance the airway along the floor of the nares.

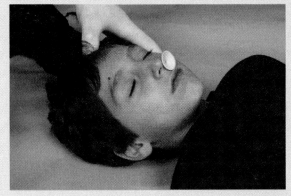

4 Advance the airway until the flange is against the outside of the nostril.

While BVM ventilation or other means of assisted ventilation do not provide a definitive airway by themselves, they are often all that is necessary during EMS resuscitation and transport. Furthermore, specific contraindications to intubation, including facial trauma, that would make successful intubation unlikely, and partial airway obstruction with good air exchange constitute indications for ventilation with a BVM device.

Although the indications and contraindications for providing BVM artificial ventilation are no different between children and adults, there are several differences in artificial ventilation techniques. First, it is critical to have available and to use the correct equipment size for the child being treated. Second, it

is important to use the correct ventilatory rate for the child's age group: 30 breaths/min for infants, 20 breaths/min for children, and 12 breaths/min for adults. Third, it is important to understand the proper use of pop-off valves that are present on several ventilation bags. In children, a higher inspiratory pressure may be required, so the pop-off valve should be blocked or disabled (▶ Figure 14-7). Ventilation is also more likely to cause gastric distention in a child, so cricoid pressure is often useful.

Selecting the Correct Mask Size

The mask should extend from the bridge of the nose to the cleft of the chin. A clear/transparent mask is beneficial, as any secretions from the mouth can be

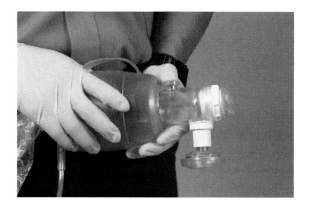

Figure 14-7 If a pop-off valve is present, occlude it to permit delivery of higher inspiratory pressures.

Table 14-1	
BVM Sizes Based on Age	
Age	**Bag size**
Birth to 1 year of age	at least 450 mL
1-8 years of age	pediatric BVM (at least 450 mL) preferred; however, an adult BVM (1,500 mL) can be used if the bag is not fully inflated
Greater than 8 years	adult size (1,500 mL)

visualized. Another important feature of a properly sized mask is that it serves to minimize the amount of dead space, thereby limiting the rebreathing of exhaled carbon dioxide.

Pediatric ventilation masks are not simply smaller versions of adult masks because there are important anatomic differences that affect mask design. The heads of infants and children are more ball-shaped than an adult's, which is more oblong. Infants also have a flat nasal bridge. Pediatric masks, therefore, are more rounded than triangular (▼ Figure 14-8). It is critical to choose the proper mask size to extend from the bridge of the nose to the cleft of the chin. It is important to avoid compressing the child's eyes because ocular trauma and/or vagal stimulation can occur.

Selecting the Appropriate Bag Size

The chest wall of a child is compliant and does not need much pressure or volume to obtain a rise. A large ventilation bag that is used on adults therefore is too big for a small child. If a large ventilation bag needs to be used, however, it is not necessary to empty it to deliver adequate breathing to a child. On the other hand, a pediatric bag may not have enough tidal volume for a 10-year-old child.

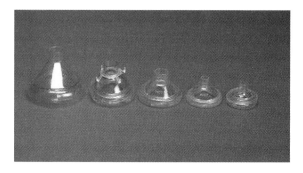

Figure 14-8 Pediatric masks are more rounded than adult masks.

To determine the correct ventilation bag size, three factors must be known—the patient's age, weight, and appropriate tidal volume (volume of air exchanged with each breath). The tidal volume is approximately 8 mL/kg in children and 8 to 10 mL/kg in infants. Another method for calculating tidal volume is to estimate the child's weight using a length-based resuscitation tape. This tape is likely to tell you the correct mask and ventilation bag size as well. ▲ Table 14-1 provides general guidelines for the selection of the most appropriate-sized BVM based on the child's age.

Bag-Valve-Mask Technique Tips

When you place the mask over the child's mouth and nose, avoid the temptation to push on the apex of the mask to obtain a better seal. This pressure can result in compression on the eyes, which can cause vagal stimulation and bradycardia.

The EC Clamp

To perform an EC clamp, place your thumb on the child's mask at the apex and your index finger on the mask at the chin (C grip). With gentle pressure, push down on the mask to establish an adequate seal. Position your third, fourth, and fifth fingers (the E) along the bony ridge of the jaw/mandible, as you would using the jaw-thrust technique. Avoid placing these fingers on the soft tissue under the chin. Pull the jaw into the mask (▶ Figure 14-9). Ventilation using the EC clamp can be done by either the one- or the two-rescuer technique for providing BVM ventilation. (▶ Skill Drills 14-7 and 14-8).

To ensure that you ventilate the patient at an age-appropriate rate, use the "squeeze, release, release" method. Begin ventilation by saying "squeeze," providing just enough ventilation to result in chest rise. To avoid gastric distention, do not overventilate the

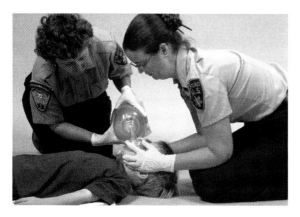

Figure 14-9 The EC clamp technique will facilitate proper hand placement for good mask-to-face seal.

patient. Allow adequate time for exhalation. After each ventilation, begin releasing the bag and say "release, release." Continue to ventilate using the "squeeze, release, release" method. Ventilation rates based on the child's age are as follows:

- Infants, 30 breaths/min
- Children, 20 breaths/min
- Adolescents, 12 breaths/min

Assess adequacy of BVM ventilation by looking for chest rise and fall, auscultating for breath sounds at the third intercostal space in the midaxillary line bilaterally, and looking for improvement in the child's color, pulse rate, and/or pulse oximetry.

Cricoid Pressure

Cricoid pressure (the Sellick maneuver) can and should also be used with pediatric patients. Locating the cricoid ring may be more challenging because the laryngeal prominence is less obvious. Only minimal pressure is needed, and excessive pressure can actually cause tracheal compression and airway obstruction. In some cases, paramedics with significant practice and large hands can open the child's airway, obtain a mask seal, and perform posterior cricoid pressure all with one hand (▶ Figure 14-10) (▶ Skill Drill 14-9).

Flow-Restricted, Oxygen-Powered Ventilation Devices

The flow-restricted, oxygen-powered ventilation device (FROPVD) should not be used in infants and children. The flow is too high for children and is therefore likely to cause gastric distention. It could also result in a pneumothorax. When used in adolescents (or adults), cricoid pressure should be maintained in order to limit gastric distention.

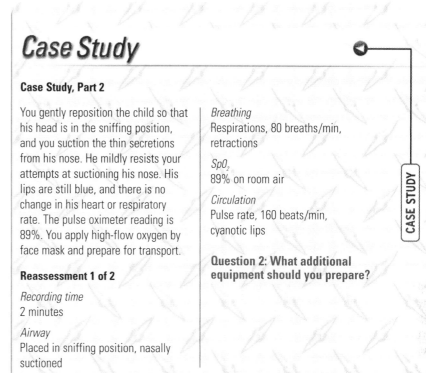

Case Study

Case Study, Part 2

You gently reposition the child so that his head is in the sniffing position, and you suction the thin secretions from his nose. He mildly resists your attempts at suctioning his nose. His lips are still blue, and there is no change in his heart or respiratory rate. The pulse oximeter reading is 89%. You apply high-flow oxygen by face mask and prepare for transport.

Reassessment 1 of 2

Recording time
2 minutes

Airway
Placed in sniffing position, nasally suctioned

Breathing
Respirations, 80 breaths/min, retractions

SpO₂
89% on room air

Circulation
Pulse rate, 160 beats/min, cyanotic lips

Question 2: What additional equipment should you prepare?

Pediatric Endotracheal Intubation

Although endotracheal intubation has been considered the gold standard for out-of-hospital airway management, recent studies have suggested that effective BVM ventilation can be as effective for EMS

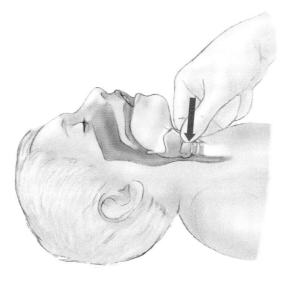

Figure 14-10 Performing posterior cricoid pressure with one hand.

Skill Drill

14-7 Pediatric BVM Ventilation Using One-Rescuer Technique

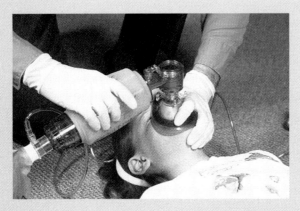

1 Choose the proper mask and seal it to the child's face.

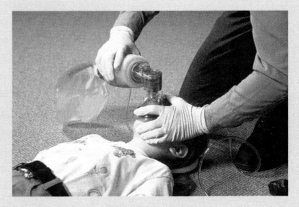

2 Squeeze the bag smoothly and allow adequate time for exhalation.

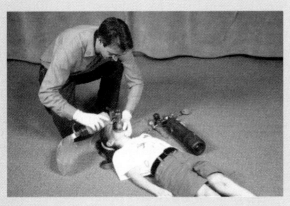

3 Assess effectiveness by watching bilateral rise and fall of the chest, and do not overinflate.

systems with short transport times (▶ Skill Drill 14-10). Indications for pediatric endotracheal intubation are as follows:

- cardiopulmonary arrest
- respiratory arrest
- respiratory failure
- traumatic brain injury
- unresponsiveness
- inability to maintain a patent airway
- need for prolonged hyperventilation
- need for endotracheal administration of resuscitative medications

While some of these indications are similar to those for BVM ventilation, endotracheal intubation is indicated when BVM ventilation is ineffective. Once again, the most important part of pediatric endotracheal intubation is preparation and equipment selection. Some of the anatomic differences (listed previously) between children and adults play a role in performing a successful intubation, as proper airway position is critical.

Laryngoscope Handle and Blades

Any size laryngoscope handle can be utilized, although some prefer the thinner pediatric handles. Straight (Miller, or Wis-Hipple) blades are preferred as they make it easy to lift the floppy epiglottis. If a

Skill Drill

14-8 Pediatric BVM Ventilation Using Two-Rescuer Technique

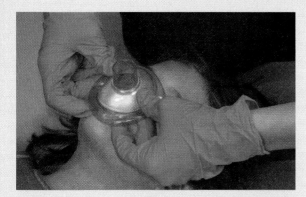

1 Rescuer 1 chooses the proper size mask and seals it to the patient's face using the spread/mold/seal technique.

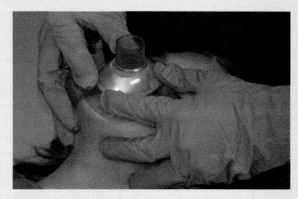

2 Seal the mask to the patient's face. With gentle pressure, push down on mask to establish an adequate seal.

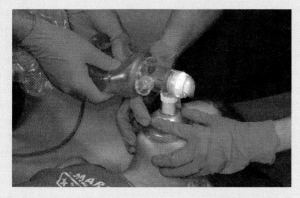

3 Rescuer 2 ventilates the patient while rescuer 1 maintains the mask seal and an adequate airway.

curved (Macintosh) blade is used, the tip of the blade is positioned in the vallecula to lift the jaw and epiglottis to visualize the vocal cords.

The appropriately sized blade extends from the patient's mouth to the tragus of the ear. Acceptable means of measuring include using a length-based resuscitation tape or employing the following general guidelines:

- Premature newborn, size 0 straight blade
- Full-term newborn to 1 year, size 1 straight blade
- 2 years to adolescent, size 2 straight blade
- Adolescent and above, size 3 straight or curved blade

Teamwork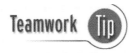

While responding to a pediatric call, if the age of the patient is known, some of the necessary equipment can be prepared en route and placed at the top of the pediatric bag (if one exists). If the patient's age is not known, one provider should quickly assess the patient and provide initial care while the other provider obtains the appropriate-sized equipment. If intubation is required, one provider should provide assisted ventilation while the other provider prepares and hands the equipment, applies cricoid pressure, and monitors the patient.

Skill Drill

14-9 Performing Cricoid Pressure on Children

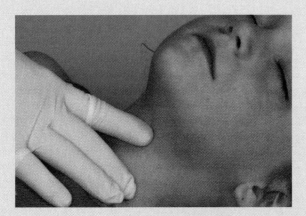

1 Locate the cricoid ring by palpating the trachea for a prominent horizontal band below the thyroid cartilage and cricothyroid membrane.

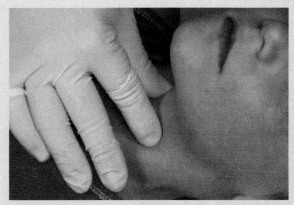

2 Apply gentle downward pressure using one fingertip in infants and the thumb and index finger in children. Avoid excessive pressure as this can cause tracheal compression and airway obstruction.

Endotracheal tube size can be selected utilizing a length-based resuscitation tape; for children older than 1 year, use this formula: age (in years) ÷ 4 + 4 (for example, a 4-year-old would need a 5.0 tube: [4 ÷ 4] + 4 = 5.0); anatomic clues, such as the size of the child's fifth digit or nares; or general guidelines (▶ **Table 14-2**).

One key point is to use uncuffed tubes until 8 to 10 years of age. A cuff at the cricoid ring is unnecessary to obtain a seal in young children. Furthermore, a cuff can cause ischemia and damage the mucosa of the trachea at this location. It is important to have a tube one size smaller as well as one size larger than expected always available for situations in which there is variability in upper airway diameter.

The appropriate depth for insertion is 2 to 3 cm beyond the vocal cords. The tube should then be inserted an additional 2 to 3 cm. The depth should be recorded as the mark at the corner of the child's mouth. For uncuffed tubes, there is often a black glottic marker to use as a guide. When you see this line go through the vocal cords, stop. For cuffed tubes, when the cuff is just below the cords, stop. Another guideline is to insert the tube to a depth three times the inside diameter of the endotracheal tube minus 1. (For example a 3.5-mm tube should be inserted to 10.5 − 1 = 9.5 cm).

The use of a stylet is based on personal preference. If you use a stylet, insert it into the endotracheal tube stopping at least 1 cm from the end of the tube. Pediatric stylets will fit into tubes sized 3.0 to 6.0 mm, whereas the adult stylets are used for tubes sized 6.0 mm and above. With the stylet in place, bend the endotracheal tube into a gentle upward curve. In some cases, bending the tube into the shape of a hockey stick is beneficial.

Preoxygenation

The child should be preoxygenated with a BVM device and 100% oxygen for at least 30 seconds prior to attempting intubation using the "squeeze, release, release" technique previously described. Adequate preoxygenation cannot be overemphasized because respiratory failure or arrest is the most common cause of cardiac arrest in the pediatric population. During this time, you must also ensure that the child's head is in the proper position—the neutral position for those with suspected spinal trauma or the sniffing position for those without trauma. An airway adjunct can be inserted if needed to ensure adequate ventilation.

Additional Preparation

Stimulation of the parasympathetic nervous system and bradycardia can occur during intubation; therefore, a cardiac monitor should be applied if available. A pulse oximeter should be utilized prior to, during, and after the intubation attempt in order to monitor the patient's pulse rate and oxygen saturation.

In addition, suction apparatus should be readily available to clear oral secretions from the child's airway before, during, or after intubation.

Intubation Technique

Open the patient's mouth by applying thumb pressure on the chin. Some patients may require use of the cross-finger technique: Use your thumb and index finger or thumb and third finger to push the upper and lower teeth apart. If an oral airway has been inserted, remove it. If needed, suction the child's mouth and pharynx to clear any secretions.

Hold the laryngoscope handle in your left hand, using your thumb and second (index) and third (middle) finger to hold the handle (the "trigger finger" position). Insert the laryngoscope blade in the right side of the patient's mouth sweeping the tongue to the left side and keeping the tongue under the blade. Advance the blade straight along the tongue, while applying gentle traction upward along the axis of the laryngoscope handle at a 45° angle. Never press the blade against the teeth or gums of a child. A child's teeth do not have the strong root system of an adult, so they could be loosened or cracked more easily during a traumatic intubation attempt.

When the blade passes the epiglottis, gently lift the epiglottis if you are using a straight blade. If you are using a curved blade, the tip of the blade should be placed in the vallecula, and the jaw, tongue, and blade lifted gently at a 45° angle.

Identify the vocal cords and other normal anatomic landmarks. If they are not visible, have your partner apply gentle cricoid pressure. Additional gentle suctioning may be needed to clearly view the vocal cords.

Case Study

Case Study, Part 3

Once the infant is moved to the ambulance, you begin BVM ventilation with an infant-sized mask and pediatric ventilation bag at a rate of 30 breaths/min using the one-rescuer technique. The infant does not fight your ventilation attempts, and in fact his pulse oximeter reading climbs to 95%. His pulse rate is 140 beats/min, his blood pressure is 90/60 mm Hg, and his lips are pink. His capillary refill drops to 2 seconds; his hands and feet are pink and warm. Upon auscultation with bagging, you still hear bilateral expiratory wheezing, but breath sounds are heard in all lung fields.

Reassessment 2 of 2

Recording time
5 minutes

Airway
Open, clear of obstructions

Breathing
BVM ventilation, 30 breaths/min, bilateral expiratory wheezing

SpO$_2$
95% (ventilated with 100% oxygen)

Circulation
Pulse rate, 140 beats/min; capillary refill, 2 seconds; skin is pink and warm

Question 3: Is BVM ventilation adequate for the remainder of this transport?

Question 4: What transport factors would change your opinion?

Question 5: What patient factors would change your opinion?

CASE STUDY

Table 14-2
General Guidelines for Selecting Pediatric Endotracheal Tubes

Age	Endotracheal tube, mm	Insertion depth, cm
Premature infant	2.0–2.5 uncuffed	5.0–8.0
Newborn	3.0–3.5 uncuffed	8.0–9.5
Infant to 1 year	3.5–4.0 uncuffed	9.5–11.0
Toddler (2–4 years)	4.0–5.0 uncuffed	11.0–14.0
Preschool (5–6 years)	5.0–5.5 uncuffed	14.0–15.5
School age (6–10 years)	5.5–6.5 uncuffed	15.5–18.5
School age (10–12 years)	6.5 cuffed	18.5
Adolescent	7.0–8.0 cuffed	20.0–23.0

Skill Drill

Skill Drill 14-10 Performing Pediatric Endotracheal Intubation

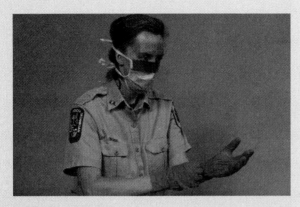

1 Take body substance isolation precautions (gloves and face shield).

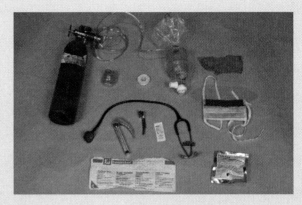

2 Check, prepare, and assemble your equipment.

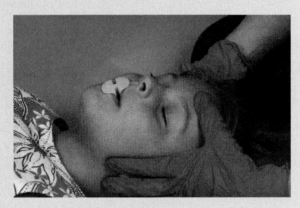

3 Manually open the patient's airway and insert an adjunct if needed.

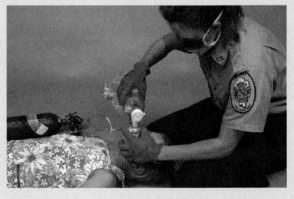

4 Preoxygenate the child with a BVM device and 100% oxygen for at least 30 seconds.

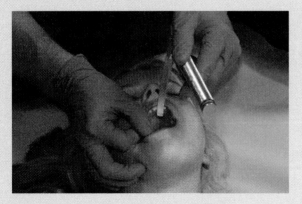

5 Insert the laryngoscope blade in the right side of the mouth and sweep the tongue to the left. Lift the tongue with firm, gentle pressure. Avoid using the teeth or gums as a fulcrum.

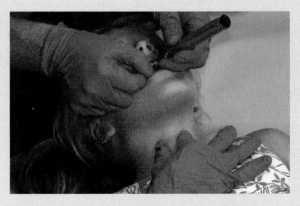

6 Identify the vocal cords. If the cords are not visible, instruct your partner to apply cricoid pressure.

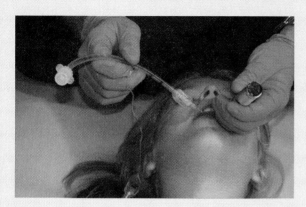

7 Introduce the endotracheal tube in the right corner of the patient's mouth.

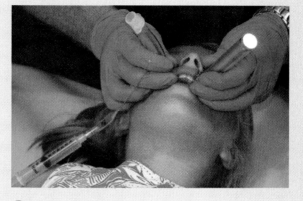

8 Pass the endotracheal tube through the vocal cords to approximately 2 to 3 cm below the vocal cords. Inflate the cuff if a cuffed tube is used.

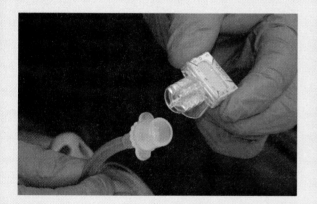

9 Attach an end-tidal carbon dioxide detector.

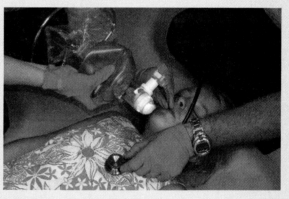

10 Attach the BVM device, ventilate, and auscultate for equal breath sounds over each lateral chest wall high in the axillae. Ensure absence of breath sounds over the abdomen.

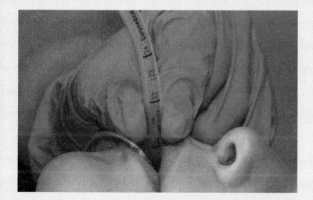

11 Secure the endotracheal tube, noting the placement of the distance marker at the patient's teeth or gums and reconfirm tube placement.

Paramedic Safety Tip

Although paramedics should wear appropriate body substance isolation attire for all EMS calls, it is important to remember to wear a visor or protective eyewear, a disposable mask, and gloves while performing endotracheal intubation.

Hold the tube in your right hand, and insert the tube from the right-hand corner of the patient's mouth. Do not pass the tube through the channel of the laryngoscope blade, as you will lose site of the vocal cords. Guide the tube through the vocal cords, and advance the tube until the glottic/vocal cord mark is positioned just beyond the vocal cords (approximately 2 to 3 cm). Record the depth of the tube as measured at the right-hand corner of the patient's mouth, and remove the laryngoscope blade. Remove the stylet from the tube if one was used. Be sure to hold the tube securely at the level of the mouth while removing the stylet to avoid inadvertent extubation. Next, recheck the tube depth to be certain it did not displace during stylet removal. If you are using a cuffed tube, inflate the cuff until the pilot balloon is full. Suction the tracheal tube if there is fluid present. Attach the tube to a ventilation bag and 100% oxygen. Release cricoid pressure.

Confirm proper endotracheal tube placement using one or more of several techniques. Look for bilateral chest rise during ventilation. Listen to the lungs bilaterally at the midaxillary line at the third intercostal space. You should listen for two breaths in each location. If breath sounds are decreased on the left side, the tracheal tube may be positioned too deep and aimed toward or in the right mainstem bronchi. To correct this, listen to the left side of the chest while ventilating and slowly withdrawing the tube, until breath sounds are equal on both sides. Re-record the depth of the tube.

Breath sounds travel easily in a child because of a child's small chest size. It is important to listen over the patient's stomach to ensure that there are no bubbling or gurgling sounds in the epigastric region. These sounds indicate esophageal intubation. If noted, the tube should be removed, and the intubation procedure reattempted. Additional methods to confirm appropriate tracheal tube position include improvement in the child's skin color, pulse rate, pulse oximetry/oxygen saturation, exhaled CO_2 detectors, and esophageal intubation detection

devices. If the tube is properly positioned, hold the tracheal tube firmly in place and secure the tube with tape or a commercially available device.

Reconfirm tube placement by listening for bilateral breath sounds as well as sounds in the epigastric region. It is important to reconfirm tube placement not only after securing the tube but after any patient movement (for example, onto the stretcher or into the ambulance), because tubes can easily become dislodged. Remember to record and frequently monitor the depth of the tube. Once tube position has been confirmed, resume assisted ventilation and oxygenation.

If during the intubation attempt you realize the tube is too large or the vocal cords and glottic landmarks cannot be identified, stop the intubation attempt and ventilate the patient with the BVM device and 100% oxygen. Modify your equipment selection appropriately, and start the procedure from the beginning. If intubation cannot be accomplished after two attempts, discontinue attempts, and resume BVM ventilation for the remainder of the transport.

Securing the Endotracheal Tube

While there are several methods of using tape to secure endotracheal tubes (▶ **Skill Drill 14-11**), no single method is fail-safe. One person should always hold the tube in place while another secures the device.

Confirmation of Endotracheal Tube Position

Three methods to confirm endotracheal tube position include clinical assessment, use of end-tidal carbon dioxide devices, and use of esophageal aspiration bulbs or syringes. Most of the process of confirmation of endotracheal tube placement is identical to that used in adults. However, there are several important factors that must be remembered when using some of these devices in children.

- The adult colorimetric end-tidal carbon dioxide detector cannot be used in children weighing less than 15 kg. (The pediatric one can be used in any infant or child).

- The esophageal bulb or syringe cannot be used in children younger than 5 years weighing less than 20 kg.

- The carbon dioxide detector must be removed from the ET tube prior to endotracheal drug administration.

Indications for Immediate Tracheal Tube Removal

- No chest rise with ventilation

- Presence of epigastric gurgling sounds or vomitus in tracheal tube

Skill Drill

14-11 Securing an Endotracheal Tube

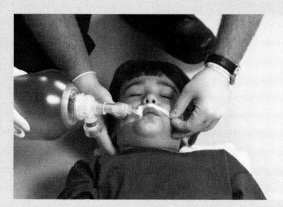

1 With the tube positioned at the corner of the mouth, tear a strip of tape and anchor one end to the side of the face. Wrap it around the tube several times and anchor the other end over the maxilla.

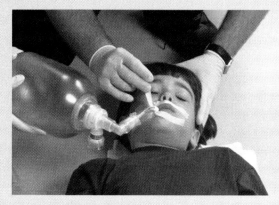

2 Wrap another piece of tape around the tube and anchor it over the mandible.

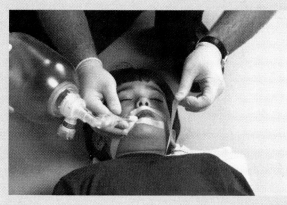

3 Reinforce the tape around the child's neck.

• Failure to confirm proper tube position with detection devices

Complications of Endotracheal Intubation

• Unrecognized esophageal intubation

• Induction of emesis and aspiration

• Hypoxia resulting from prolonged intubation attempts

• Damage to teeth, soft tissues, and intraoral structures

Documentation Tip

Pulse rate and oxygen saturation should be documented before, during, and after an intubation attempt. Once the tube has been positioned, document the depth of the tube as measured at the right-hand corner of the patient's mouth.

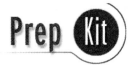

Chapter Summary

To ensure proper airway positioning, it is important to understand the anatomic differences between a child and adult airway.

The use of manual airway maneuvers is often easier in children than in adults.

Airway adjuncts can be beneficial in children, but it is imperative to use the correct size.

Selecting the proper equipment size is critical to being able to adequately ventilate infants and children. Utilizing a length-based resuscitation tape can simplify this task.

The "squeeze, release, release" technique allows for adequate ventilation (and exhalation) rates for infants, children, and adolescents.

Either one- or two-rescuer BVM ventilation techniques can be used in children. The two-rescuer technique is preferable for a trauma patient, or when one rescuer cannot achieve a good seal and provide adequate ventilation.

Although endotracheal intubation constitutes definitive airway management, in many cases BVM ventilation and oxygenation are sufficient to manage a pediatric airway problem.

Availability and use of appropriately sized equipment are critical to successful ventilation and intubation of an infant or child.

Intubation is a multi-step procedure often requiring two people. Use your partner, and work together!

Once an endotracheal tube is in place, reconfirm position after any patient movement.

Continue to reassess the patient during transport.

Vital Vocabulary

cricoid pressure The application of pressure to the cricoid cartilage in order to compress the esophagus.

EC clamp A technique of positioning the fingers for bag-valve-mask ventilation in order to maintain an effective mask-to-face seal.

flow-restricted, oxygen-powered ventilation device (FROPVD) A manually-triggered ventilatory device used for assisting ventilations in both conscious and unconscious patients.

nasopharyngeal airway A flexible rubber tube that is inserted into the nostril and into the nasopharynx in order to lift the tongue off of the airway.

neutral position A position of the head in which the head is neither extended nor flexed. This position is maintained in patients with potential spinal injury as well as when maintaining the airway of an infant or child.

occiput The rounded posterior aspect of the skull.

oropharyngeal airway A firm plastic device that is inserted into the oropharynx and maintains airway patency by lifting the tongue off of the airway.

resuscitation tape A length-based measuring tape used in the emergency care of pediatric patients that provides general guidelines such as endotracheal tube sizes and medication doses.

sniffing position Upright position in which the child's head and chin are positioned slightly forward to keep their airway open, such as if the child were sniffing or smelling a flower.

tidal volume The volume of air (in milliliters) that is moved in and out of the respiratory system in a single breath.

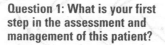

Case Study Answers

Question 1: What is your first step in the assessment and management of this patient?

Answer: You must first ensure a patent airway in this child, which will involve properly positioning the head and suctioning secretions from the mouth and nose as needed.

Question 2: What additional equipment should you prepare?

Answer: It is clear that this child is not improving despite proper positioning of the head, suctioning, and 100% supplemental oxygen. You must be prepared to initiate BVM ventilations with 100% oxygen and prepare the necessary equipment in order to accomplish this.

Question 3: Is BVM ventilation adequate for the remainder of this transport?

Answer: Yes. Because BVM ventilation was effective, intubation was not required for this patient at this time.

Question 4: What transport factors would change your opinion?

Answer: If there is a prolonged transport time, endotracheal intubation may be beneficial as it provides a definitive airway and results in less gastric distention. A patient that is awake, even an infant, may prove to be difficult to intubate for several reasons. It may be difficult to adequately open the airway to visualize the vocal cords, and the vocal cords may open and close, making tube placement difficult.

Question 5: What patient factors would change your opinion?

Answer: If the patient begins to deteriorate en route (less activity, lower oxygen saturation, lower heart rate), despite adequate BVM ventilation, endotracheal intubation is indicated even for short transports.

CASE STUDY ANSWERS

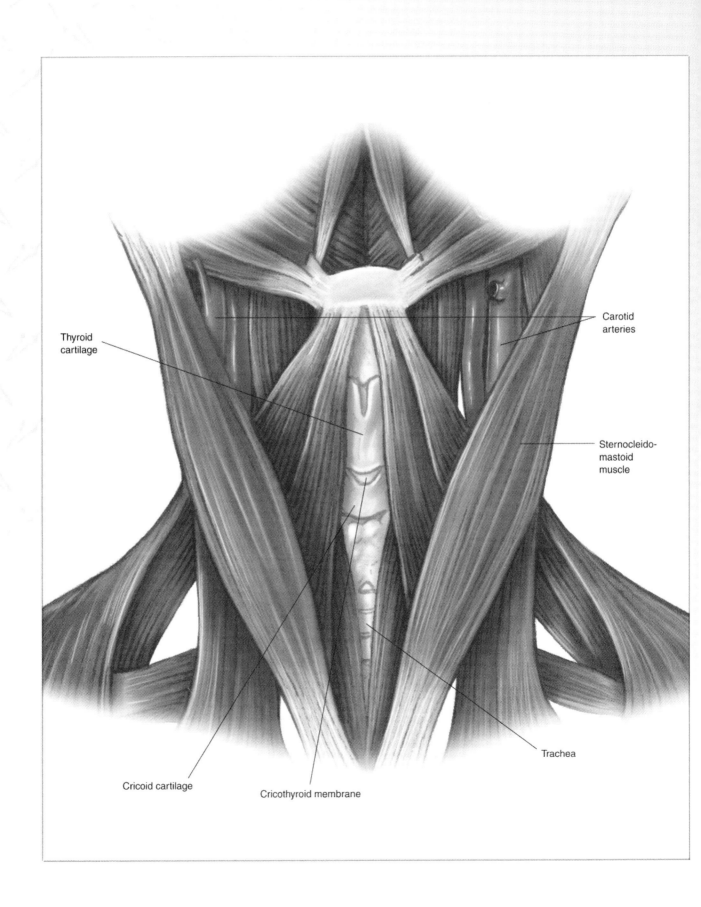

Thyroid cartilage

Carotid arteries

Sternocleido-mastoid muscle

Cricoid cartilage

Cricothyroid membrane

Trachea

Objectives

Cognitive Objectives

2-1.70 Describe the indications, contraindications, advantages, disadvantages, and complications for performing an open cricothyrotomy. (p 310)

2-1.71 Describe the equipment and technique for performing an open cricothyrotomy. (p 310)

2-1.72 Describe the indications, contraindications, advantages, disadvantages, complications, and technique for transtracheal catheter ventilation (needle cricothyrotomy). (p 315)

Psychomotor Objectives

2-1.104 Intubate the trachea by the following method:
- Open cricothyrotomy (p 306) (Skill Drill 15-1)

2-1.107 Perform transtracheal catheter ventilation (needle cricothyrotomy). (p 312) (Skill Drill 15-2)

www.Paramedic.EMSzone.com

TECHNOLOGY

- Online Chapter Pretest
- Vocabulary Explorer
- Anatomy Review
- Web Links

Chapter FEATURES

- Case Studies
- Skill Drills
- Teamwork Tips
- Documentation Tips
- Paramedic Safety Tips
- Special Needs Tips
- Vital Vocabulary
- Prep Kit

Preceding chapters of this book have provided you with many tools that will enable you to secure and maintain a patent airway in a variety of patients. Fortunately, in most cases, the paramedic is able to secure a patent airway with relative ease using conventional methods that are either basic (BVM device and oral airway) or advanced (endotracheal intubation). There are, however, situations in which the patient's condition or other uncontrollable factors preclude the use of these conventional airway techniques. At this point a more aggressive and invasive approach must be taken to secure the airway and maximize the chances of your patient's survival.

Two methods of securing an airway can be used when conventional means fail—the open (surgical) cricothyrotomy and transtracheal catheter ventilation (nonsurgical or needle cricothyrotomy).

Anatomy Review

When palpating the anterior midline of the neck, you must be familiar with several key landmarks (▼ Figure 15-1). The most obvious prominence is the upper aspect of the <u>thyroid cartilage</u> (Adam's apple), which is easier to palpate in men than in women. Inferior to the thyroid cartilage is the <u>cricoid cartilage</u>, a less prominent feature, which is somewhat more difficult to palpate. The vocal cords lie approximately 1 cm above the cricoid cartilage. Collectively, the thyroid and cricoid cartilages form the <u>larynx</u>, or voice box.

Inferior to the larynx, several additional firm prominences are palpable in the anterior midline of the neck, most notably the cartilaginous rings of the trachea. The trachea bifurcates into the left and right mainstem bronchus (carina). Bilateral to the inferior larynx and upper trachea lies the thyroid gland, which unless enlarged, is usually not palpable.

Between the thyroid cartilage and cricoid cartilage is a soft depression, the <u>cricothyroid membrane</u>, which is a thin sheet of connective tissue (fascia) that joins the thyroid and cricoid cartilages. The cricothyroid membrane is covered only by skin,

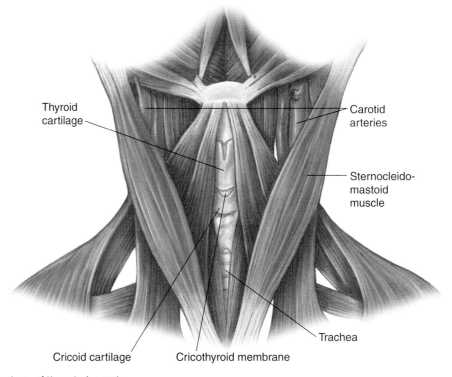

Figure 15-1 Anatomy of the anterior neck.

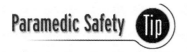

Paramedic Safety Tip

Incising the cricothyroid membrane vertically will minimize the risk of inadvertent laceration of the external jugular veins.

which makes it an ideal entry point should rapid access to the airway be required.

You will encounter a few important blood vessels in the immediate region of the cricothyroid membrane. The superior cricothyroid vessels run at a transverse angle across the upper third of the cricothyroid membrane. If cricothyrotomy is performed across the lower third of the membrane, these vessels should not be encountered. The external jugular veins run vertically and are located lateral to the cricothyroid membrane. If the cricothyroid membrane is incised vertically when performing a cricothyrotomy, the jugular veins can be avoided altogether.

When performing cricothyrotomy, you should expect to encounter minor bleeding from the subcutaneous and small skin vessels as you incise the cricothyroid membrane. This bleeding, however, should be easy to control with light pressure after the tube has been inserted into the trachea.

Cricothyrotomy

Cricothyrotomy is an emergent surgical procedure that involves incising the cricothyroid membrane with a scalpel and inserting an endotracheal or tracheostomy tube (▼ Figure 15-2) directly into the subglottic area (below the vocal cords) of the trachea. When

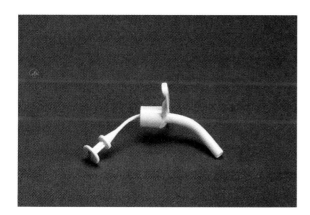

Figure 15-2 Tracheostomy tube.

Case Study

Case Study, Part 1

You and your partner, who volunteer for a rural EMS system, are watching TV when you are dispatched to the intersection of 5th Street and Elm Avenue for a major motor vehicle crash. You arrive at the scene a short time later. Local law enforcement is already at the scene and is directing traffic. You see your patient, a young male, who was removed from his car prior to your arrival. He is lying motionless on the sidewalk with obvious trauma to the facial area. There are no other victims. Your partner immediately assumes manual control of the patient's head to stabilize his cervical spine as you conduct an initial assessment.

You make the following determinations on your initial assessment:

Initial Assessment

Recording time
0 minutes

Appearance
Motionless, massive maxillofacial trauma

Level of consciousness
Unresponsive

Airway
Blood gurgling from his mouth with each breath.

Breathing
Slow and shallow

SpO₂
80% (room air)

Circulation
A weak and rapid radial pulse is detected.

Skin signs
Cool, clammy, pale

Question 1: What is your most immediate concern with this patient?

Question 2: What management must you provide during the initial assessment?

performed via this method, the technique is referred to as an "open" cricothyrotomy (▶ Skill Drill 15-1).

The advantages of open cricothyrotomy are that it can be performed quickly, it is technically easier than performing a tracheostomy, and it can be performed without manipulating the cervical spine, which is especially advantageous since many cricothyrotomies are indicated in patients with severe trauma, specifically massive facial trauma. Relative to its advantages, there are few disadvantages of cricothyrotomy, which include difficulty in performing the procedure in children (younger than 8 years), or in patients with short, muscular, or fat necks.

In contrast to needle cricothyrotomy, an open cricothyrotomy is more difficult to perform; however, inserting a larger bore tube (such as an endotracheal

Skill Drill

15-1 Performing an Open Cricothyrotomy

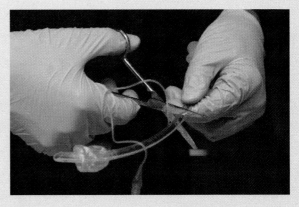

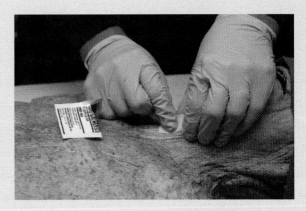

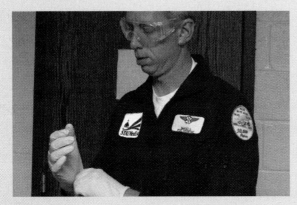

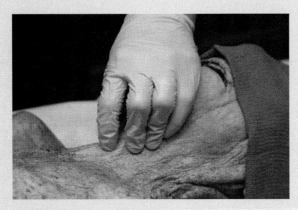

1 Take body substance isolation precautions (gloves and face shield).

2 Check, assemble, and prepare the equipment.

3 With the patient's head in a neutral position, palpate for and locate the cricothyroid membrane.

4 Cleanse the area with an iodine-containing solution.

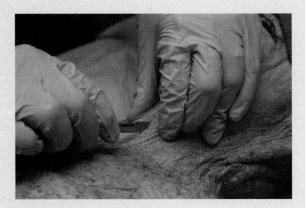

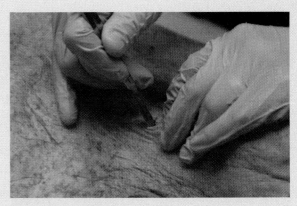

5 Stabilize the larynx and make a 1- to 2-cm vertical incision over the cricothyroid membrane.

6 Puncture the cricothyroid membrane and make a horizontal cut 1 cm in each direction from the midline.

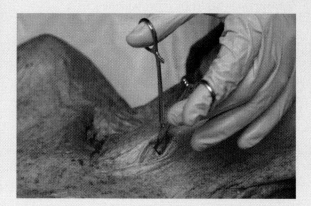

7 Spread the incision apart with curved hemostats.

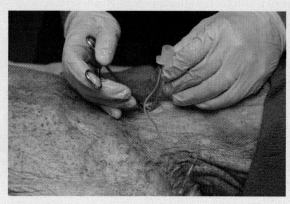

8 Insert the tube into the trachea.

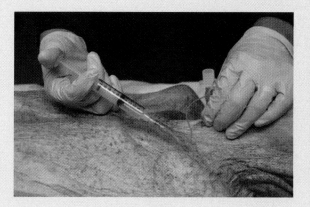

9 Inflate the distal cuff of the tube.

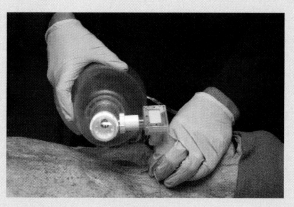

10 Attach an end-tidal carbon dioxide detector in-between the tube and the bag-valve-mask device.

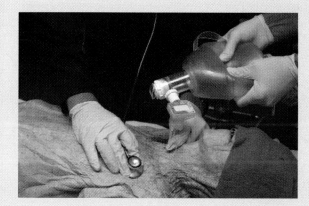

11 Ventilate the patient and confirm correct tube placement by auscultating the apices and bases of both lungs and over the epigastrium.

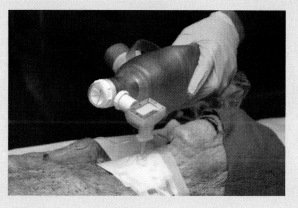

12 Secure the tube with a commercial device or tape. Reconfirm correct tube placement and resume ventilations at the appropriate rate.

tube or tracheostomy tube) enables you to achieve greater tidal volumes, which facilitates more effective oxygenation and ventilation. Needle cricothyrotomy will be covered later in this chapter.

Indications

Cricothyrotomy is indicated when you are unable to secure a patent airway with more conventional means (BVM ventilation or intubation). Cricothyrotomy is not the preferred means of initially securing a patient's airway. Even if you are unable to intubate a patient but can provide an effective mask-to-face seal and adequate tidal volume with a BVM device, cricothyrotomy would not be appropriate.

Situations that may preclude you from securing the airway by other means include severe maxillofacial trauma, complete upper airway obstruction, and the inability to open the patient's mouth.

Patients with severe maxillofacial trauma (▼ Figure 15-3) can present a challenge to even the most experienced paramedic. Such patients frequently have associated mandibular fractures, which would make it extremely difficult to maintain an effective mask-to-face seal with a BVM device. Posterior lacerations of the tongue with severe oropharyngeal bleeding are also commonly associated with maxillofacial trauma. Visualization of the upper airway anatomy would be extremely difficult without performing frequent airway suctioning to prevent aspiration, which would delay intubation and increase patient hypoxia.

Patients with a complete upper airway obstruction would also prevent successful endotracheal intubation or BVM ventilation. A foreign body that is completely obstructing the glottic opening would obviously preclude you from passing an endotracheal

tube through the vocal cords. Patients who have severe upper airway swelling secondary to epiglottitis, acute anaphylaxis, or airway burns would also be difficult to intubate because the view of the airway anatomy would be significantly obscured. In addition, BVM ventilation in these patients would likely only produce negligible tidal volume.

Patients with head injuries and whose teeth are clenched (**trismus**) may require cricothyrotomy, especially if you do not have the resources or protocols to perform rapid sequence intubation. Secondarily, head injury, which is frequently accompanied by facial trauma, contraindicates nasal intubation or the placement of a nasopharyngeal airway, especially if fluid is draining from the patient's ears or nose (▼ Figure 15-4). This fluid may be cerebrospinal fluid, which would indicate either a basilar skull fracture or a fracture of the cribriform plate. If nasal intubation is attempted in these patients, inadvertent placement of the endotracheal tube or nasopharyngeal airway into the cranial vault may occur.

Contraindications

As mentioned previously, if you are able to secure the airway by less invasive techniques, cricothyrotomy would be contraindicated. Other contraindications include the inability to identify the anatomic landmarks (cricothyroid membrane), crushing injuries to the larynx and tracheal transaction, which would likely result in placement of the tube outside of the trachea if cricothyrotomy were attempted, underlying anatomic abnormalities (such as trauma, tumors, subglottic stenosis), and in small children who are younger than 8 years. The larynx of a small child is generally unable to support a tube large enough to produce effective ventilation without causing damage

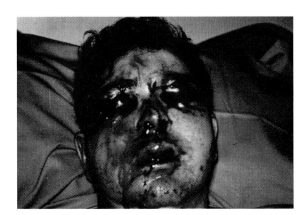

Figure 15-3 Patients with maxillofacial trauma pose a challenge to even the most experienced intubator.

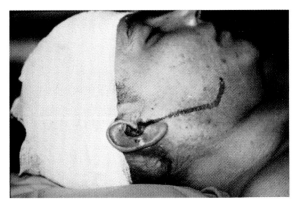

Figure 15-4 Endotracheal intubation may not be possible in patients with head injury and trismus. Nasotracheal intubation is contraindicated in patients with head injury and drainage from the ears or nose.

to the larynx. In children, you would be safer performing a needle cricothyrotomy, which will be described later in this chapter. In cases where cricothyrotomy is contraindicated, the paramedic must transport rapidly to the closest appropriate facility, where an emergency tracheostomy can be performed. Tracheostomy is not a skill typically performed in the field by paramedics.

Complications

The potential complications associated with open cricothyrotomy can be minimized by using proper technique. Although this is a rapid airway securing technique, you must approach the situation both with care and the intent of performing the technique correctly the first time.

You should expect minor bleeding while performing a cricothyrotomy. More severe hemorrhage is usually secondary to the inadvertent laceration of a major vessel, the external jugular vein, which lies lateral to the larynx. Incising the cricothyroid membrane vertically will minimize this potential complication as well as the risk of damaging the thyroid gland. Gently inserting the tube once the incision has been made will minimize the risk of perforating the esophagus or damaging the laryngeal nerves.

The goal in performing a cricothyrotomy is to perform the procedure rapidly. Taking too long to perform a cricothyrotomy would result in unnecessary hypoxia to the patient, which may cause additional complications, including cardiac dysrhythmias, permanent brain injury, or cardiac arrest. Frequent practice on a cadaver (if available) or a special cricothyrotomy manikin will maximize your ability to perform this procedure quickly if it is needed.

If you are able to correctly identify the anatomic landmarks and ensure proper tube placement after cricothyrotomy has been performed, inadvertent placement of the tube outside the trachea will be

---

Case Study

Case Study, Part 2

You immediately suction the patient's oropharynx. Visual inspection of the patient's mouth reveals a lacerated tongue with oropharyngeal bleeding. You also note deformity and instability of his mandible. You direct your partner to stabilize the patient's head with his knees and begin assisting ventilations with a BVM device. You complete a rapid trauma assessment, which reveals the following findings:

Rapid Trauma Assessment

Recording time
2 minutes after patient contact

Head
Depression to the frontal region of the skull, massive maxillofacial trauma with oropharyngeal bleeding

Neck
No jugular venous distention, trachea midline, no cervical spine deformity

Chest
Multiple abrasions, breath sounds weak, but equal bilaterally

Abdomen
Unremarkable

Pelvis
Stable

Lower extremities
Unremarkable

Upper extremities
Unremarkable

Posterior
Unremarkable

Your partner reports that the oropharyngeal bleeding is continuing despite frequent suctioning. In addition, he is having difficulty maintaining a mask-to-face seal because of the patient's mandibular fracture.

Question 3: How will you remedy this patient's airway problem?

CASE STUDY

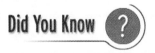

Frequent practice of this technique on a cadaver or specialized manikin will maximize your ability to perform cricothyrotomy rapidly.

minimized. Tube misplacement should be suspected when **subcutaneous emphysema** is encountered after performing a cricothyrotomy. Subcutaneous emphysema occurs when air infiltrates the subcutaneous layers of the skin, and is characterized by a "crackling" sensation when palpated.

As with any procedure performed under the less than desirable environment of the prehospital setting, there is always a risk of infection to the patient. Open cricothyrotomy would clearly pose a greater risk of patient infection in comparison to other, less invasive emergency interventions such as endotracheal intubation or intravenous therapy. Even though you will be performing cricothyrotomy in an emergent attempt to secure the patient's airway, care should be taken to maintain aseptic technique as much as possible.

▶ **Table 15-1** summarizes the indications, contraindications, advantages, disadvantages, and complications of performing an open cricothyrotomy.

Equipment

Commercially manufactured cricothyrotomy kits are available (▼ Figure 15-5). If such a kit is not available, at a minimum you must prepare the following equipment:

- Scalpel
- Endotracheal tube or a tracheostomy tube (6.0-mm minimum)
- Commercial device (or tape) for securing the tube
- Curved hemostats
- Suction apparatus
- Sterile gauze pads for minor bleeding control
- BVM device attached to 100% oxygen

Technique

Once you determine that an open cricothyrotomy is needed, you must proceed rapidly, yet cautiously. You will obviously encounter some bleeding during the procedure. Proper body substance isolation precautions, including use of gloves and a face shield, must be followed.

First, you must identify the proper landmark, which is relatively easily accomplished by placing the patient's head in a neutral position, palpating the thyroid and cricoid cartilages, and then locating the cricothyroid membrane in-between the two cartilages.

Again, attempting to maintain maximum aseptic technique, cleanse the area with iodine and avoid touching the area once cleansed. While you are

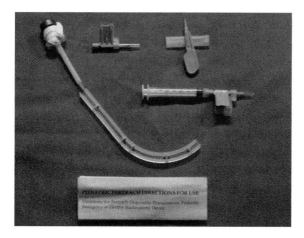

Figure 15-5 Cricothyrotomy kit.

Table 15-1
Open Cricothyrotomy

Indications
- Delayed or inability to intubate or ventilate by other means
- Severe maxillofacial trauma
- Complete upper airway obstruction
- Posterior laceration of the tongue
- Inability to open the patient's mouth

Contraindications
- Inability to identify the anatomic landmarks
- Crush injury to the trachea
- Tracheal transaction
- Underlying anatomic abnormality (such as trauma, tumor, subglottic stenosis)

Advantages
- Rapidly performed
- Technically easier than performing a tracheostomy
- Does not manipulate the cervical spine

Disadvantages
- Difficult to perform in children younger than 8 years
- Difficult to perform in patients with short, muscular, or fat necks

Complications
- Incorrect tube placement/false passage
- Prolonged execution time
- Thyroid gland or laryngeal nerve damage
- Perforation of the esophagus
- Severe bleeding
- Subcutaneous emphysema
- Infection

locating and preparing the site, your partner should be preparing your equipment as well as ensuring that the cardiac monitor and pulse oximeter are attached to the patient.

While stabilizing the larynx with one hand, make a 1- to 2-cm vertical incision over the cricothyroid membrane. Some advocate making an additional 1-cm incision horizontally across the membrane to facilitate easier placement of the tube. If you choose to do this, remember that the thyroid gland and external jugular veins are lateral to the area and can be unnecessarily damaged if the horizontal incision it too long. Once the incision has been made, insert the curved hemostats into the opening and spread it apart. Your partner should be available to control any bleeding that might occur.

With the trachea exposed, gently insert a 6.0-mm cuffed endotracheal tube or a 6.0 tracheostomy

(Shiley) tube and direct it into the trachea. Once in place, inflate the distal cuff with the appropriate volume of air, which is typically 5 to 10 mL. Attach the BVM device to the standard 15/22-mm adapter on the proximal end of the tube and ventilate while your partner auscultates to ensure the presence of clear breath sounds bilaterally as well as the absence of epigastric sounds. If epigastric sounds are heard, you have likely perforated and inadvertently inserted the tube into the esophagus.

Additional confirmation can be accomplished by attaching an end-tidal carbon dioxide detector in-line between the tube and the BVM device. After confirming proper tube placement, secure the tube with either a commercial device or tape, ensure that any minor bleeding has been controlled, and continue to ventilate at the appropriate rate.

Needle Cricothyrotomy

Needle cricothyrotomy also uses the cricothyroid membrane as an entry to the airway; however, instead of incising the cricothyroid membrane and inserting a tube, a 14- to 16-gauge over-the-needle catheter (angiocath) is inserted through the membrane and into the trachea. Adequate oxygenation and ventilation are then achieved by attaching a high-pressure jet ventilator (▼ Figure 15-6) to the

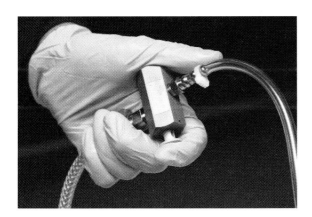

Figure 15-6 High-pressure jet ventilator.

Case Study

Case Study, Part 3

Recognizing that your partner is not able to secure a patent airway because of the patient's continued oropharyngeal bleeding and mandibular fracture, you determine that endotracheal intubation is indicated. Anticipating a potentially difficult intubation, you decide to perform the procedure while en route to the hospital. As you continue to perform oropharyngeal suctioning for 15 seconds and BVM ventilation for 2 minutes, the patient is loaded into the ambulance and transport is initiated. A law enforcement officer, who is a certified EMT-B, accompanies you in the back of the ambulance for assistance.

After preparing the necessary equipment, you attempt endotracheal intubation, but are unable to perform effective direct laryngoscopy because the patient has a mandibular fracture. You are briefly able to visualize the upper airway but you cannot see the vocal cords beyond the blood in the patient's airway.

Question 4: What are your options for airway management at this point?

Question 5: Would a dual-lumen airway be a viable alternative? Why or why not?

CASE STUDY

hub of the catheter. Needle cricothyrotomy is frequently used as a temporizing measure until a more definitive airway can be obtained (such as open cricothyrotomy or tracheostomy).

Needle cricothyrotomy with transtracheal catheter ventilation (▶ Skill Drill 15-2) is faster and technically easier to perform than an open cricothyrotomy. Additionally, like the open cricothyrotomy, it can be performed without manipulating the cervical spine. In contrast to the open cricothyrotomy, there are fewer complications, specifically a lower risk of causing damage to adjacent structures because you are not using a scalpel to perform the procedure. Needle cricothyrotomy also allows for subsequent endotracheal intubation attempts because it uses a smaller bore catheter, thus allowing an endotracheal

2

Skill Drill

15-2 Performing Needle Cricothyrotomy and Transtracheal Catheter Ventilation

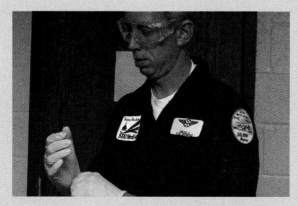

1 Take body substance isolation precautions (gloves and face shield).

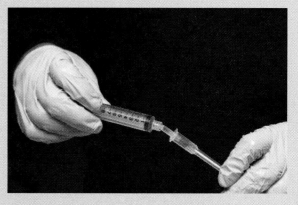

2 Attach a 14- to 16-gauge intravenous catheter to a 10-mL syringe containing approximately 3 mL of sterile saline or water.

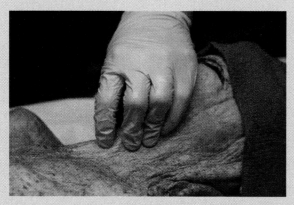

3 With the patient's head in a neutral position, palpate for and locate the cricothyroid membrane.

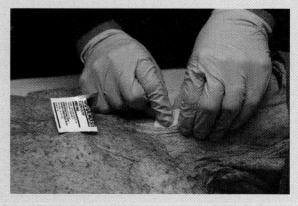

4 Cleanse the area with an iodine-containing solution.

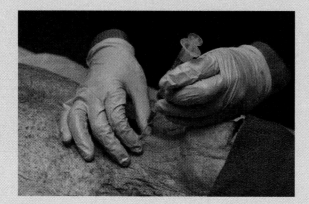

5 Stabilize the larynx and insert the needle into the cricothyroid membrane at a 45° angle towards the feet.

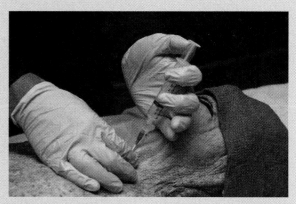

6 Aspirate with the syringe to determine correct catheter placement.

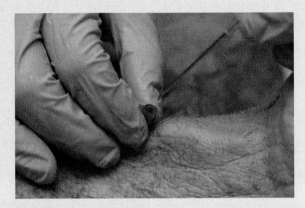

7 Slide the catheter off of the needle until the hub of the catheter is flush with the patient's skin.

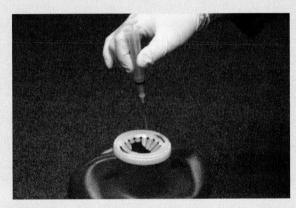

8 Place the syringe and needle in a puncture-proof container.

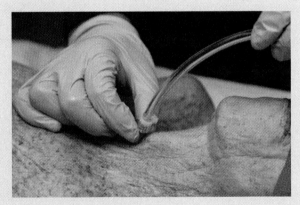

9 Connect one end of the oxygen tubing to the catheter and the other end to the jet ventilator.

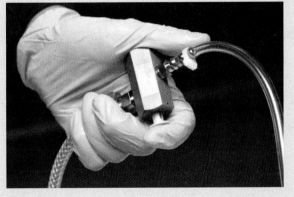

10 Open the release valve on the jet ventilator and adjust the pressure accordingly to provide adequate chest rise.

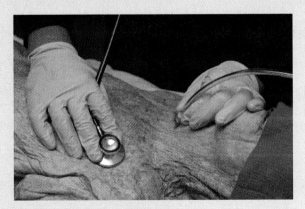

11 Auscultate the apices and bases of both lungs and over the epigastrium to confirm correct catheter placement.

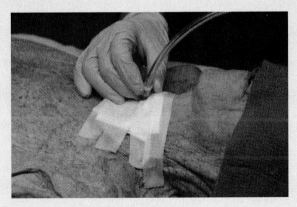

12 Secure the catheter with a 4" × 4" gauze pad and tape. Continue ventilations while frequently assessing for adequate ventilations and any potential complications.

tube to easily pass beside it. This could be particularly beneficial if you do not have the equipment or protocols to perform an open cricothyrotomy.

There are, however, some disadvantages to performing a needle cricothyrotomy. Using a smaller bore tube (the angiocath) to ventilate the patient does not provide protection from aspiration as an endotracheal or tracheostomy tube would if you performed an open cricothyrotomy. A larger bore tube would clearly fill the diameter of the trachea, thus protecting it from esophageal regurgitation. Another disadvantage is that it requires a specialized, high-pressure jet ventilator in order to deliver adequate tidal volume. Additionally, the jet ventilator will expend high volumes of oxygen very rapidly.

Indications

The indications for needle cricothyrotomy and transtracheal catheter ventilation are essentially the same as for the open cricothyrotomy—the inability to ventilate the patient by other, less invasive techniques, severe maxillofacial trauma, inability to open the patient's mouth, and uncontrolled oropharyngeal bleeding. Again, it must be emphasized that this procedure is not the preferred initial means of obtaining a patent airway. Other, less invasive techniques should be attempted prior to performing a needle cricothyrotomy.

Contraindications

If the patient has a complete airway obstruction above the site of catheter insertion, needle cricothyrotomy should not be performed. Exhalation is not as effective using a small-bore catheter when compared with a large-bore tube (such as an endotracheal tube or tracheostomy tube). Also, expiration via the glottic opening is not possible because the airway is completely obstructed superior to the catheter insertion site. As the result of minimal and ineffective exhalation, the high-pressure ventilator used with needle cricothyrotomy would cause an increase in intrathoracic pressure, thus resulting in **barotrauma** and a potential pneumothorax. Barotrauma can also be caused by overinflation of the lungs with the jet ventilator, so care must be taken to open the release valve only until the chest adequately rises.

If the equipment necessary to perform transtracheal catheter ventilation is not readily available, you should opt to perform an open cricothyrotomy. If you do not have protocols to perform an open cricothyrotomy and/or you do not have a jet ventilator on your ambulance, there is an alternative, although less effective, method of ventilating the patient via needle cricothyrotomy.

Attach a 7- to 7.5-mm endotracheal tube adapter into the barrel of a 10-mL syringe. Next, connect the syringe to the intravenous catheter that has been placed through the cricothyroid membrane. Connect the bag-valve device to the endotracheal tube adaptor and begin ventilations. Although you will not be able to deliver near the tidal volume that you would be able to if you were using a jet ventilator, this may be your only alternative to at least provide some oxygenation and ventilation until a more definitive airway can be obtained at the emergency department.

Complications

With proper technique, complications associated with needle cricothyrotomy can be significantly reduced. Improper catheter placement can result in severe bleeding secondary to damage of adjacent structures. Even if the catheter is correctly placed, excessive air leakage around the insertion site can cause subcutaneous emphysema. If too much air infiltrates into the subcutaneous space, compression of the trachea and subsequent obstruction could occur.

Extreme care must be exercised when ventilating the patient with a jet ventilator. The release valve should only be opened long enough for adequate chest rise. Overinflation of the lungs can result in barotrauma, which carries the risk of pneumothorax.

▶ **Table 15-2** summarizes the indications, contraindications, advantages, disadvantages, and complications of performing a needle cricothyrotomy.

Equipment

The following pieces of equipment are needed in order to perform needle cricothyrotomy and transtracheal catheter ventilation:

- Large-bore IV catheter (14 to 16 gauge)
- 10-mL syringe
- 3 mL of water or saline
- Oxygen source (50 psi)
- High-pressure jet ventilation device and oxygen tubing

Technique

As with any procedure or contact with the patient, you must adhere to body substance isolation precautions. Blood may splatter, especially if the patient is combative. A face shield should be worn as well.

In preparing your equipment, draw up approximately 3 mL of sterile water or saline into a 10-mL syringe and attach the syringe to the IV catheter.

Table 15-2
Needle Cricothyrotomy

Indications

- Delayed or inability to intubate or ventilate by other means
- Severe maxillofacial trauma
- Posterior laceration of the tongue
- Inability to open the patient's mouth

Contraindications

- Total airway obstruction (inspiratory and expiratory)
- Equipment not immediately available

Advantages

- Rapidly performed
- Provides adequate ventilation when performed properly
- Does not interfere with subsequent endotracheal intubation attempts
- Does not manipulate the cervical spine

Disadvantages

- Requires a high-pressure jet ventilator
- Rapidly expends high volumes of oxygen
- May not afford adequate protection from aspiration

Complications

- Bleeding from improper catheter placement
- Subcutaneous emphysema from air leakage around the catheter site or undetected laryngeal trauma
- Airway obstruction caused by excessive bleeding or subcutaneous air that compresses the trachea
- Barotrauma as the result of overinflation of the lungs

Case Study

Case Study, Part 4

Because you are unable to effectively manage this patient's airway, you determine that an open cricothyrotomy is warranted. You perform the technique successfully, confirm correct placement, and secure the tube. You immediately begin ventilating the patient and within a matter of a few minutes, noting that his oxygen saturation has increased to 94%, which is up from the initial reading of 80%. After attaching a cardiac monitor, you reassess the patient and note the following findings:

Vital Signs

Recording time
12 minutes after patient contact

Skin signs
Pale, cool

Pulse rate/quality
110 beats/min, stronger at the radial

Blood pressure
98/58 mm Hg

Respiratory rate/depth
Assisted at 20 breaths/min

Pupils
Dilated, equal, reactive

SpO$_2$
94% (transtracheally ventilated)

Electrocardiogram
Sinus tachycardia

Upon arrival at the emergency department, you give your verbal report to the attending physician, who commends you and the law enforcement officer. The patient is placed on a mechanical ventilator and taken to radiology for a CT scan.

CASE STUDY

Next, place the patient's head in a neutral position and locate the cricothyroid membrane. If time permits, cleanse the area with an iodine-containing solution.

While stabilizing the patient's larynx, carefully insert the needle into the midline of the cricothyroid membrane at a 45° angle towards the feet (caudally). You should feel a pop as the needle penetrates the membrane. After the pop is felt, insert the needle approximately 1 cm further, and then aspirate with the syringe. If the catheter has been correctly placed, you should be able to easily aspirate air and see the saline or water bubbling within the syringe. If blood is aspirated or if you meet resistance, you should reevaluate the placement of the catheter because it is likely that the catheter is outside the trachea.

After confirming correct placement of the catheter, advance the catheter over the needle until the catheter hub is flush with the skin, then withdraw the needle and place it in a puncture-proof container. Next, attach one end of the oxygen tubing to the catheter and the other end to the jet ventilator.

Begin ventilations by opening the release valve on the jet ventilator and observing for adequate chest rise. Auscultation of breath and epigastric sounds will further confirm correct catheter placement. In order to prevent overexpansion of the lungs and subsequent barotrauma, it is important that you turn the release valve off as soon as you see the chest rise. Exhalation will occur passively via the glottis. To achieve adequate oxygenation and ventilation, you should ventilate the patient at least 20 times per minute.

Secure the catheter in place by placing a folded 4" × 4" gauze pad under the catheter and secure it in place with tape. After securing the catheter, you continue ventilations while frequently assessing the patient for adequacy of ventilations as well as for potential complications (such as subcutaneous emphysema from incorrect placement).

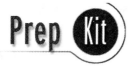

Prep Kit

Chapter Summary

In most cases, the paramedic is able to secure a patent airway with relative ease using conventional methods such as BVM ventilation or endotracheal intubation.

Situations such as massive maxillofacial trauma, oropharyngeal bleeding, or the inability to ventilate the patient by conventional means requires a more aggressive and invasive approach to managing the airway.

When performed correctly, both the open cricothyrotomy and needle cricothyrotomy can provide rapid access to the patient's airway and effective oxygenation and ventilation.

Your resources, protocols, and the patient's condition will guide you as to which technique is most appropriate.

Frequent practice will allow you to maintain proficiency should you need to perform these invasive airway procedures in a real emergency.

Vital Vocabulary

<u>barotrauma</u> Trauma caused by excessive pressure, specifically increased intrathoracic pressure secondary to overinflation of the lungs.

<u>cricoid cartilage</u> The cartilaginous prominence inferior to the thyroid cartilage. The cricoid cartilage is less prominent and more difficult to palpate than the thyroid cartilage.

<u>cricothyroid membrane</u> The narrow indentation in between the thyroid and cricoid cartilages. The cricothyroid membrane is the site used to gain rapid access to the airway during an open or needle cricothyrotomy.

<u>cricothyrotomy</u> Rapid access to the airway by incising the cricothyroid membrane, inserting an endotracheal tube or tracheostomy tube into the trachea, and ventilating the patient.

<u>high-pressure jet ventilator</u> A ventilatory device used in conjunction with a large-bore IV catheter to perform transtracheal catheter ventilation.

<u>larynx</u> Collectively, the thyroid and cricoid cartilages.

<u>needle cricothyrotomy</u> Inserting a large-bore IV catheter through the cricothyroid membrane and into the trachea.

<u>Shiley</u> A type of tracheostomy tube inserted through the cricothyroid membrane and into the trachea during an open cricothyrotomy.

<u>subcutaneous emphysema</u> The infiltration of air into the subcutaneous (fatty) layer of the skin.

<u>thyroid cartilage</u> The cartilaginous prominence superior to the cricoid cartilage; also known as the Adam's apple.

<u>transtracheal catheter ventilation</u> Ventilating a patient with a high-pressure jet ventilator attached to a large-bore IV catheter that was inserted through the cricothyroid membrane and into the trachea.

<u>trismus</u> Tetanic muscle spasms resulting in clenching of the teeth.

Case Study Answers

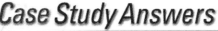

Question 1: What is your most immediate concern with this patient?

Answer: Clearly, this patient's airway is not patent. He is unconscious, which prevents him from maintaining his airway spontaneously. In addition, the massive maxillofacial trauma and oropharyngeal bleeding are putting his airway and respiratory system in immediate jeopardy from aspiration. You must act quickly to secure his airway and manage his inadequate breathing.

Question 2: What management must you provide during the initial assessment?

Answer: There are two major problems that you must address simultaneously. The oropharyngeal bleeding must be suctioned in order to prevent aspiration. Secondly, his slow, shallow breathing must be managed with assisted ventilations in order to increase his respiratory rate and tidal volume, both of which will improve oxygenation. To manage both problems, you must perform oropharyngeal suction for 15 seconds, and then provide assisted ventilations with a BVM device for 2 minutes. You should continue this alternating pattern of suctioning and ventilations until the airway is clear of blood. Remember, the airway must be kept clear at all times. With an unconscious patient, an oropharyngeal airway should be inserted to assist in maintaining airway patency. A nasopharyngeal airway would not be indicated because of his head injury.

Question 3: How will you remedy this patient's airway problem?

Answer: Continued oropharyngeal bleeding will result in aspiration unless corrective action is taken immediately. This bleeding is not easily controlled, and you must protect the trachea and lungs. Additionally, the mandible, which is relied on in maintaining an adequate mask-to-face seal, is fractured, making BVM ventilations ineffective. Endotracheal intubation will remedy these problems; however, you must realize that the mandibular fracture may make intubation extremely difficult or impossible and that oropharyngeal bleeding may obstruct your view of the vocal cords.

Question 4: What are your options for airway management at this point?

Answer: At this point, you have exhausted other means of airway control, to include bag-valve mask ventilations, and endotracheal intubation attempts. At this point, your only viable options are to secure this patient's airway surgically with an open cricothyrotomy, or, if locally established protocols will not allow this, a needle cricothyrotomy. Whichever technique you choose, you must perform it now, or the patient will die. Continue to keep the patient's airway clear of blood with suction during the technique.

Question 5: Would a dual-lumen airway be a viable alternative? Why or why not?

Answer: The dual-lumen airway would not be considered a viable option in this patient. Because the dual-lumen airway (such as a Combitube or PtL) is blindly inserted into the airway, it typically comes to rest in the esophagus. Although this would protect the airway from esophageal regurgitation, it still leaves the trachea vulnerable to aspiration secondary to the oropharyngeal bleeding that this patient is experiencing. Frequent suctioning therefore would still be required.

CASE STUDY ANSWERS

www.Paramedic.EMSzone.com

Special Airway Situations
Dental Appliances

Dental appliances can take on many different forms and are commonly encountered in the older population, a population that needs emergent intubations most commonly secondary to medical conditions. The most common dental appliances are dentures, upper or lower or both, bridges, and individual teeth.

Often, it is not the dental appliance itself that hinders your ability to perform a safe and effective intubation, but identifying dentures and bridges early on and removing them will be critical in performing the endotracheal intubation efficiently. Not identifying the dental appliance correctly will make the intubation more difficult to obtain. The less experienced paramedic may become overly concerned with the presence of prominent teeth and thus not concentrate effectively on the task at hand. Furthermore, the oropharyngeal anatomy may be somewhat distorted by the presence of the dental appliance. These factors will decrease the likelihood of successful intubation and thus endanger the airway.

The dental appliance can always become loose and enter the posterior oropharynx. During the insertion of large airway appliances such as an LMA, the airway may become obstructed and ventilations may not be possible. As Blaschke and Chen[1] described in their case report, even a complete set of dentures may lead to a nearly complete obstruction of the airway, almost causing death of the patient.

Prior to intubation it is critical to look at the oropharynx. If the patient is conscious, ask the patient if he or she wears dentures or has bridges. In any patient with an airway obstruction, consider a dental appliance as the possible obstruction. Evidence that the patient may be wearing dentures includes a smooth gum line, a perfectly aligned full set of teeth in an older person, or the hard palate area that is covered by the roof of the denture. Secondary clues might be denture cleaning material present in the household. Bridges are more difficult to recognize. Metal hooks onto adjacent natural teeth may provide confirmation. Again, smooth, perfectly aligned teeth in an older person with otherwise flawed dentition may be another clue. You will also be likely to notice dentures when proceeding to intubate and finding very prominent teeth or a loose appliance.

Airway management, once the dental appliance has been removed, is the same as for all patients, although possibly a bit easier, as teeth may be lacking. Dental appliances should be removed before intubation is attempted. If the patient is awake and alert, he or she may remove the dental appliance. Dentures are very expensive so it is important to store them in a clean, safe environment. If possible, place them in a cup and a labeled brown bag to be transported with the patient. If a cup and bag are not available, even placing them into the patient's pocket for safekeeping until arrival at the hospital may be acceptable. If the patient has an airway obstruction caused by a dental appliance, performing the usual steps in clearing an obstruction, such as abdominal thrusts, direct laryngoscopy, and use of the Magill forceps may be indicated. Great care will need to be taken in cases of bridges, as these often contain sharp metal ends that may lacerate the posterior pharynx or larynx.

Once the intubation has been successful and the tube secured, removal of dental appliances at that time is technically difficult and dangerous as it may cause tube dislodgement in the process. The risk of oropharyngeal infections also increases when the dental appliances are not removed and cleaned over time in an intubated patient.

Mandibular Wiring

Another dental appliance which necessitates a special approach is mandibular wiring. The use of mandibular wiring to manage mandibular fracture can provide a challenge in an emergent situation. With a wired mandible, it is very difficult to adequately control the tongue, thus decreasing your ability to ventilate the patient effectively. The presence of mandibular wiring is usually obvious, with metal wiring attached to the jaw and teeth. The mouth will be in a slightly open position and will not be able to fully open or close. If you cannot open or close a patient's jaw, search for wires.

The presence of mandibular wiring will make oral intubation impossible. If not contraindicated, naso-tracheal intubation may be necessary to ensure an open airway. If you cannot perform nasal intubation, you may need to use bolt cutters to cut the metal wiring and gently open the airway to gain access to the oropharynx. The wire ends may protrude and represent a danger to the patient and providers. You can tape needle caps or pen caps over them to protect soft tissue. The mandible will need to be supported. Major jaw instability may represent a relative contraindication to orotracheal intubation, possibly requiring the need for an emergent cricothyrotomy.

Epiglottitis

Epiglottitis, or acute swelling of the epiglottis and supraglottic tissues, is caused by the bacterium *Haemophilus influenzae*. Although epiglottitis can strike adults, it occurs more commonly in children between the ages of 6 months and 7 years. Epiglottitis is especially frightening for paramedics because of the relatively rapid appearance of life-threatening signs of airway occlusion, often within 24 hours of the complaint of a sore throat. Rapid identification and careful, judicious use of appropriate airway management are crucial to good patient outcome.

Initial presentation of epiglottitis includes complaints of sore throat and fever. As the illness progresses and tissue swelling increases, the patient will attempt to compensate for the resulting airway constriction by sitting upright and avoiding efforts that could aggravate the condition, such as coughing, swallowing, and speaking. The child will likely drool and refuse to take anything by mouth, especially in later stages. In-hospital diagnostics include lateral neck radiographs and blood values. However, prehospital suspicion of epiglottitis will be made primarily on clinical presentation. A child who presents with tachypnea, accessory muscle use, and appears septic and listless must be evaluated quickly but carefully!

Ideally, the definitive airway treatment of the supra-acute epiglottic patient will occur in the operating room, where direct visualization and control of the airway may be attempted under optimal conditions and in the hands of the most experienced medical personnel. Manipulation and visualization of the epiglottic airway should be avoided until this point.

Rapid transport should be initiated as soon as epiglottitis is suspected. Avoid direct visualization of the airway as much as possible. Complete an initial assessment and gather information on the history of the illness, administering oxygen as soon as possible. Above all, comfort the patient! Your calm, reassuring approach will go a long way in minimizing

the chances of the patient experiencing a completely occluded airway.

As with other patients with severe airway problems, it is important to balance the administration of oxygen without having the patient experience the undue stress of feeling suffocated by a nonrebreathing mask. Blow-by oxygen may be sufficient for the patient who is ventilating adequately. Reassess the patient's condition frequently, carefully noting the patient's mental status and respiratory tidal volume. If the patient becomes increasingly obtunded, assist ventilations using a bag-valve-mask (BVM) device, and high-flow oxygen may become necessary.

A child with epiglottitis who is unresponsive because of hypoxia needs to be ventilated. The airway may be managed with basic airway maneuvers and an appropriately sized BVM device. The expert use of a BVM device requires both adequate equipment and careful, real-time adjustment of the pediatric airway in order to be effective. In terms of equipment, a well-sized mask is critical for ensuring a face-mask seal. As you are ventilating the patient, you may make subtle adjustments of the patient's neck and jaw in order to establish the most patent airway. If possible, two rescuers should work together to manage the ventilatory effort, one to manage the mask-face seal and airway adjustments, and the other to compress the bag.

If basic airway maneuvers fail, you will have to consider advanced airway techniques. An oral intubation may be attempted, although the normal structures for visualization will be absent. A chest thrust may cause some air trapped in the lungs to escape, causing a bubble to appear where the glottic opening should be. An uncuffed endotracheal tube one or two sizes smaller than normal may be inserted, and ventilation resumed as normal, followed by auscultation of lung sounds to confirm tube placement and/or electronic carbon dioxide monitoring. If oral intubation appears unlikely or unsuccessful, an emergency cricothyrotomy may be necessary.

Chest Trauma

The patient with chest trauma is at risk for problems with ventilation and, therefore, oxygenation, resulting from decreased lung volume. Many injuries to the chest result in air or blood occupying space in the pleural cavity, which disrupts contact between the parietal and visceral pleura. This, in turn, prevents the generation of negative intrapulmonary pressure so that the flow of air into the affected lung is limited. As the pleural space fills with air or blood, the lung is further compressed. In the patient with pulmonary contusion, gas exchange across the respiratory membrane is impaired because of an increased diffusion distance across the capillary-alveolar interface. These are critical problems resulting in ventilation-perfusion mismatch that must be detected and managed in the initial assessment of the patient.

Specific injuries that interfere with ventilation because of chest trauma include simple pneumothorax, tension pneumothorax, open pneumothorax, hemothorax, bronchial laceration, ruptured diaphragm, rib fractures, flail chest, and pulmonary contusion. Although these injuries are often discussed as discrete problems, they may, and often do, coexist in patients. Mechanisms of injury that may result in chest trauma include motor vehicle collisions, falls, assaults, industrial accidents, and penetrating trauma.

In order to detect chest trauma and its effect on breathing, the chest of the patient with a significant mechanism of injury must be exposed in the initial assessment. The assessment requires careful inspection, auscultation, and palpation of the chest.

- Inspection must include examination for:
  - Signs of respiratory distress, such as tachypnea, retractions of intercostal and supraclavicular areas, and flaring of the nares.
  - Deviation of the trachea, although keep in mind that this is a late sign and its absence does not rule out tension pneumothorax.
  - Asymmetry of the chest or paradoxical movements of the chest wall.
  - Bruises or open wounds.
- Auscultation includes listening without a stethoscope for noisy breathing and for air entering the chest through any open wounds. The stethoscope should be quickly used in the initial assessment to determine the presence or absence of breath sounds and the equality of breath sounds if present bilaterally.
- Palpation of the chest includes examination for subcutaneous emphysema, instability of the ribs and sternum, symmetry, and tracheal deviation.
- Percussion of the chest, if conditions permit, may help distinguish between a pneumothorax and a hemothorax.

The management of the patient with chest trauma always includes the administration of 100% oxygen. The patient's ventilation must be monitored and assisted if the rate or tidal volume is inadequate to maintain pulmonary ventilation. In addition to specific measures for chest trauma, the patient often requires endotracheal intubation for adequate airway management and ventilation.

Open Pneumothorax

An open pneumothorax occurs when an opening in the chest wall is large enough to become the preferential pathway for air to enter the thoracic cavity. Smaller open chest wounds tend to be self-sealing. With each expansion of the chest cavity more air enters the pleural space on the affected side. The increasing amount of air progressively collapses the lung on the affected side so that it cannot be ventilated. The immediate treatment of an open pneumothorax is to seal the opening in the chest wall to prevent additional air from entering the pleural space. If need be, this can be done with a gloved hand until appropriate materials are available.

Materials used for an occlusive dressing must be three to four times the size of the opening in the chest to prevent them from being drawn into the chest cavity with inspiration. Petrolatum gauze, sturdy foil, or plastic wrap may be used because air cannot pass through them. Asking the patient, if he or she is able, to cough just as the dressing is being placed over the wound may help minimize the amount of air trapped in the pleural space. The dressing should be secured on three sides so that it is pulled against the opening on inspiration, preventing air from entering, but allowing for air to exit the chest through the untaped side on exhalation to prevent conversion to a tension pneumothorax. If signs of tension pneumothorax develop, the dressing should be removed on exhalation to allow air to exit the pleural space, and then be replaced.

Tension Pneumothorax

Tension pneumothorax occurs when a defect in the lung, usually from blunt trauma, is significant enough that it cannot seal itself. Air enters the pleural space on each inspiration, but cannot exit. Pressure continues to build in the thoracic cavity with each inspiration. Initially the lung on the affected side will be compressed by increasing intrathoracic pressure. If uncorrected, increasing pressure will continue to compress the vena cava, the mediastinum, and the contralateral lung.

Tension pneumothorax is rapidly fatal and must be treated immediately by releasing the air trapped under pressure in the thoracic cavity by creating an opening in the chest wall through which the air can escape, thus decompressing the structures of the thorax. This is performed in the prehospital setting through needle thoracostomy. Needle thoracostomy is accomplished by inserting a large-bore (14-gauge) over-the-needle catheter of sufficient length to penetrate the patient's chest wall into the pleural space on the affected side. The preferred site is the second intercostal space anteriorly in the midclavicular line, although the fourth intercostal space laterally in the midaxillary line may also be used. With a successfully performed needle thoracostomy, a rush of air under pressure will exit through the catheter. The catheter is then secured in place. Creation of a flutter valve is not necessary, because the diameter of the catheter is much smaller than that of the trachea, through which air will enter preferentially. As with open pneumothorax, high-pressure ventilation is contraindicated.

Simple Pneumothorax

Simple pneumothorax occurs when air is trapped in the pleural space but the defect in the lung does not continue to allow additional air into the pleural space. Depending on the percentage of pleural space volume filled with air, there can be a significant ventilation-perfusion mismatch. Prehospital treatment of a simple pneumothorax is supportive. The patient needs 100% oxygen as well as airway management and assistance with ventilation if indicated. The patient must be continually monitored to detect signs of a developing tension pneumothorax.

Hemothorax

Although hemothorax leads to a reduction in ventilatory capacity, the major concern in the patient with a hemothorax is hypovolemia caused by the volume of blood that can be contained in each hemithorax. The prehospital treatment of the patient with a suspected hemothorax includes administration of 100% oxygen and support of the airway and ventilation. If signs of hypovolemia are present, the judicious administration of intravenous crystalloids is indicated.

Bronchial Laceration

Laceration of a bronchus occurs primarily from penetrating trauma of the chest. Even with prompt management, this is often a lethal injury. The lung on the affected side cannot be ventilated and large amounts of inspired air enter the affected pleural cavity. There may be massive subcutaneous emphysema. Attempts to ventilate the unaffected lung lead to increased air in the affected pleural space. In the prehospital setting, treatment for a lacerated bronchus is not specific, but supportive. Again, high-pressure ventilation is contraindicated.

Flail Chest

Flail chest, the fracture of three or more adjacent ribs in two or more places each, interferes with the normal expansion of the chest wall and the ability to generate sufficient negative intrathoracic pressure. As the intercostal muscles contract to elevate the ribs, the detached segment collapses. In addition, the patient will experience significant pain with breathing and

will minimize inspiratory depth in an attempt to decrease the pain. The patient needs 100% oxygen, and if ventilation is inadequate, the patient will require positive pressure ventilation via an endotracheal tube. If the patient has an intact gag reflex and spontaneous respirations, nasotracheal intubation, once accomplished, may be more comfortable for the patient. In some cases, the patient with a flail chest may also be a candidate for rapid sequence induction or medication-assisted intubation.

Rib Fractures

The pain associated with rib fractures in the conscious patient causes the patient to attempt to control the pain by minimizing inspiration, resulting in hypoventilation. Assisting the patient in splinting the injured ribs may allow for adequate inspiratory effort. In selected patients, analgesia will allow for deeper breathing. In addition to administering 100% oxygen, the patient may require ventilatory support.

Pulmonary Contusion

Pulmonary contusion is common in blunt trauma, but can also complicate penetrating trauma to the lung. Disruption of the capillary-alveolar interface with the accumulation of blood or fluid in the alveoli interferes with pulmonary ventilation, resulting in ventilation-perfusion mismatch. Often, the onset of ventilatory difficulty caused by pulmonary contusion is delayed beyond the prehospital period. Suspected pulmonary contusion is treated with 100% oxygen, positive pressure ventilation if indicated, and avoidance of fluid overload to avert aggravation of pulmonary edema.

Ruptured Diaphragm

Rupture of the diaphragm or significant penetrating trauma involving the diaphragm may disrupt the function of the diaphragm and allow the abdominal contents to enter the thoracic cavity. Expansion of the lungs is impeded by the introduction of abdominal organs into the thorax. Depending on the degree of restriction of lung expansion, this may cause considerable hypoventilation and dyspnea. Occasionally, the presence of bowel sounds upon auscultation of the thorax indicates rupture of the diaphragm; however, the presence of bowel sounds is not reliably present. Therefore, the absence of bowel sounds in the thorax does not rule out a ruptured diaphragm in the presence of a suspicious mechanism. Rupture of the diaphragm should be suspected with any mechanism that creates a sudden and dramatic increase in intra-abdominal pressure. In addition to supporting oxygenation and ventilation, if the presence of hypovolemia creates a contraindication, the head of the backboard can be elevated slightly to allow gravitation of the organs inferiorly to relieve compression of the lungs. The use of the abdominal section of a pneumatic antishock garment in the patient with a ruptured diaphragm will lead to increased difficulty breathing resulting from further herniation of the abdominal contents into the thorax and is therefore contraindicated.

Chest trauma presents considerable risk of problems related to ventilation of the lungs. Immediate recognition of life-threatening chest trauma and intervention to maximize ventilatory capacity and oxygenation are critical in the prehospital setting. Although the patient with chest trauma requires aggressive prehospital management, the use of manually triggered oxygen-powered ventilation devices is contraindicated in the presence of disrupted pulmonary integrity.

The key to the prehospital management of chest trauma is an immediate but thorough assessment to detect injuries and inadequate ventilation. In addition to oxygenation and isolation of the airway for ventilation, the staples of airway management, some specific life-threatening chest injuries require additional intervention to improve or to prevent further compromise of lung volume. The prehospital care provider must recognize the indications for these procedures and perform them adeptly and without hesitation.

Reference

[1]Blaschke U, Chen EY. Foreign body in upper airway. Unsuspected cause of obstruction. *Postgrad Med.* 1989;86(3):235–237.

Page numbers in *italics* designate captions, tables, and skill drills.

Chapter 1

Opener © Eddie M. Sperling; **1-1** © Mark C. Ide.

Chapter 3

Opener © Eddie M. Sperling; **3-5** © Custom Medical Stock Photo.

Chapter 4

4-4 © Photodisc/Getty Images; **4-10** © Logical Images/Custom Medical Stock Photo; **4-11** © Photodisc/Creatas.

Chapter 5

5-12 Venturi mask provided courtesy of Salter Labs, www.salterlabs.com; **5-15** © Mediscan/Visuals Unlimited, Inc.; **5-17** © Use of the text, images, drawings, and materials is made with the permission of ResMed Limited. ResMed Limited owns the copyright in the text, images, drawings and materials and ResMed Limited reserves all rights; **Skill Drill 5-6** Venturi mask provided courtesy of Salter Labs, www.salterlabs.com.

Chapter 8

Opener © Bruce Ayers/The Bridgeman Art Library/Getty Images, Inc.

Unless otherwise indicated, photographs were supplied by the Maryland Institute of Emergency Medical Services System, the American Academy of Orthopaedic Surgeons, or Jones and Bartlett Publishers. Illustrations are by Imagineering, JB Woolsey, Rolin Graphics, and Studio Montage.

Additional Photo Research:
Kimberly Potvin

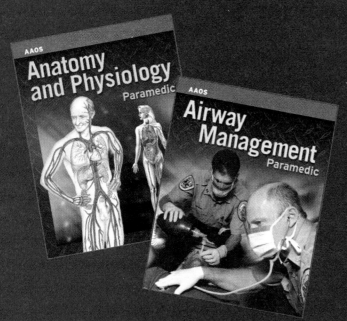
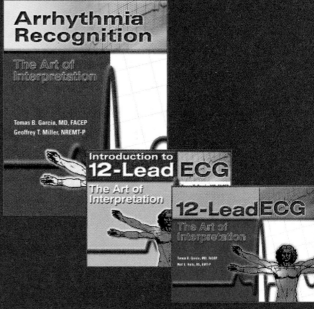
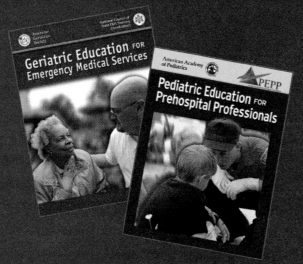
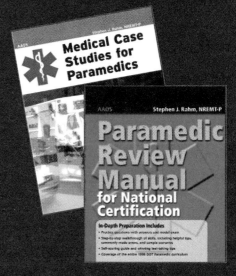
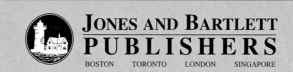